A Clinical Guide to Chinese Herbs and Formulae

For Churchill Livingstone

Publisher: Mary Law
Project Editor: Dinah Thom
Copy Editor: Susan Hunter
Production Controller: Nancy Arnott
Sales Promotion Executive: Hilary Brown

A Clinical Guide to Chinese Herbs and Formulae

Foreword by Giovanni Maciocia
GM CAc (Nanjing)
Acupuncturist and Chinese Herbalist; Lecturer,
Norsk Akupuncktur Skole, Oslo, Norway; Lecturer,
Acupuncture Foundation of Ireland, Dublin,
Republic of Ireland; Honorary Lecturer, Nanjing
College of Traditional Chinese Medicine, Nanjing,
People's Republic of China

Translated by Jin Hui De
Doctor of Chinese Medicine; Associate Professor,
International Acupuncture Training Centre and Head
of Interpreter Group, Nanjing College of Traditional
Chinese Medicine, Nanjing, People's Republic of
China

Subject Editor: Francesca Diebschlag
BAc MIROM MRCHM
Lecturer, The London School of Acupuncture and
Traditional Chinese Medicine, London, UK

Chen Song Yu

Director of the Teaching and Research Section of Chinese
Materia Medica,
Nanjing College of Traditional Medicine,
Nanjing, People's Republic of China

Li Fei

Director of the Teaching and Research Section of Prescription,
Nanjing College of Traditional Chinese Medicine, Nanjing,
People's Republic of China

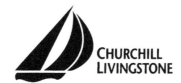

CHURCHILL
LIVINGSTONE

EDINBURGH LONDON MADRID MELBOURNE NEW YORK
AND TOKYO 1993

CHURCHILL LIVINGSTONE
An imprint of Harcourt Publishers Limited

© Longman Group Limited 1993
© Harcourt Brace and Company Limited 1998
© Harcourt Publishers Limited 2000

 is a registered trademark of Harcourt Publishers Limited

First edition 1993
  Reprinted 1994
  Reprinted 1996
  Reprinted 1998
  Reprinted 2000 (twice)

ISBN 0 443 04680 8

British Library of Cataloguing in Publication Data
A catalogue record for this book is available from the
British Library.

Library of Congress Cataloguing in Publication Data
Chen, Songyu.
    A clinical guide to Chinese herbs and
  formulae/Chen Songyu, Li Fei; translated by Jin
  Hui De; subject editor, Francesca, Diebschlag;
  foreward by Giovanni Maciocia.
        p.   cm.
    Includes index.
    ISBN 0-443-04680-8
    1. Herbs – Therapeutic use.   2. Medicine,
  Chinese.   I. Li, Fei.   II. Diebschlag, Francesca.
  III. Title.
    [DNLM: 1. Formularies, Homeopathic.   2.
  Medicine, Chinese Traditional   3. Plants,
  Medicinal – China.   WB50 JC6 C4645c]
  RM666.H33C52   1992
  615'.321'0951 – dc20
  DNLM/DLC
  for Library of Congress   92-22810
                                CIP

The
publisher's
policy is to use
paper manufactured
from sustainable forests

Printed and bound by Antony Rowe Ltd, Eastbourne

Contents

Foreword

The essence of Chinese herbal medicine is in the art of adapting a formula to a particular patient's disharmony. An adapted formula is like a mirror reflection of a particular imbalance of Qi. The harmonization of herbs within a formula is comparable to the balancing of acupuncture points within a treatment. However, balancing the herbs within a prescription is all the more intricate as careful account should be taken of the tastes of the herbs.

After diagnosing the patient's disharmony and deciding on a strategy of treatment with an appropriate formula, adapting it must take into account many different factors: the constitution of the patient, the state of his or her digestive system, his or her mental-emotional state, the combination of tastes and energies within the formula, and the harmonization of herbs with different movements (floating or sinking, ascending or descending). Taking all these factors into account, to adapt the chosen formula to the unique patient's disharmony is a very delicate and intricate task.

Such a task can be carried out if one masters not only the action of herbs and formulae, but also the differentiation between herbs and formulae with similar functions. The main emphasis of this book is exactly to illustrate how to combine herbs and how to differentiate between single herbs and formulae in relation to one's chosen treatment strategy. The book does this admirably and fills a gap in the existing literature on Chinese herbal medicine. The case histories are an invaluable part of the book illustrating how formulae are adapted in practice.

The authors of this book, Professors Chen Song Yu and Professor Li Fei are eminent teachers from the Nanjing College of Traditional Chinese Medicine which is one of the foremost institutions for the teaching of Chinese medicine. Between them, they have accumulated over 60 years of clinical practice and teaching, and they are the authors of many important textbooks of Chinese herbal medicine.

The translator of the book, Associate-Professor Jin Hui De is head of the interpreters' group of the Nanjing College of Traditional Chinese Medicine. He was co-translator of the now famous 'Essentials of Chinese Acupuncture' as well as many other Chinese medicine textbooks in English. He is uniquely qualified to translate medical texts as he is also a doctor of Chinese medicine.

This book is therefore a welcome addition to the scanty literature on Chinese herbal medicine and one that deserves to be in every practitioner's clinic.

1993   *Giovanni Maciocia*

Subject Editor's Preface

This book has five parts:

Part 1 points out similarities and differences between herbs of a similar nature or action.

Part 2 describes combinations of two or more herbs that commonly appear as a group within larger formulae.

Part 3 analyzes individual herbs according to their actions on the Zang Fu.

Part 4 sets forth guiding principles in formulating prescriptions according to the various treatment methods, and compares formulae within each such category.

Part 5 deals with specific pathological patterns or diseases, demonstrating the clinical use of formulae with case histories.

Throughout the text, words having a specific meaning within the context of TCM are capitalized (e.g. Qi, Blood, Wind-Cold), while words used according to their usual English meaning appear in lower case (e.g. blood, cold).

Each herb is identified by both its Pin Yin name and its Latin name the first time it is mentioned; thereafter, only the Latin name is used. Each formula is identified by its Pin Yin name and its English translation the first time it is mentioned; thereafter, only the English name is used. Appendices cross-index the Pin Yin and Latin names of herbs, and the Pin Yin and English names of formulae, for easy reference.

Formulae given within the text and case histories are generally variations of classic formulae, modified as they would be in clinical practice. For the classic formulae themselves, please refer to any standard reference work on Chinese herbal formulae, such as *Formulas and Strategies* by Bensky and Barolet.

1993   *F.D.*

Part 1:
A comparison of the actions and indications of some common Chinese herbs

Comparing the actions and indications of Chinese herbs facilitates both familiarization with the herbs and their correct selection in clinical work. Herbs with similar actions and indications can be substituted for each other.

Herbs that Release the Exterior   **1**

A. Herbs that disperse Wind-Cold

■ HERBA EPHEDRAE and RAMULUS CINNAMOMI

- *Ma Huang and Gui Zhi*

Similarities
— Both strongly disperse Wind-Cold due to their pungent and warm nature. They are indicated for severe Exterior Cold syndromes in Winter. When used in combination these two herbs effectively induce diaphoresis.

Differences
— Herba Ephedrae is pungent, bitter and warm in nature. It promotes the dispersing function of the Lungs, stops cough, soothes wheeze and promotes diuresis. It is thus indicated for cough and wheeze in Excess patterns due to impairment of the dispersing function of the Lung and for oedema due to invasion of Wind.
— Ramulus Cinnamomi is pungent, sweet and warm in nature. In combination with Herba Ephedrae it treats Exterior patterns of the Excess type; in combination with Radix Paeoniae Alba it treats Exterior patterns of the Deficient type (see Fig. 1.1). It warms and invigorates Yang and removes obstructions from the channels and collaterals. It is thus also indicated for oedema and dysuria due to blockage of Yang Qi by Phlegm and retained fluids, Chest Bi syndrome, abdominal pain due to Interior Cold complicated with deficiency of the Middle Burner, Cold Bi syndrome, irregular menstruation, dysmenorrhoea and amenorrhoea.

In combination with
HERBA EPHEDRA

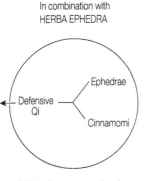

Both herbs are pungent and disperse the Defensive level, thus "Releasing the Exterior" in Excess patterns of exterior invasion.

In combination with
RADIX PAEONIAE ALBA

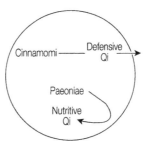

Cinnamomi disperses the Defensive level, while Paeoniae astringes Nutritive Qi, thus "Harmonizing Ying and Wei Qi" in Deficiency patterns of exterior invasion.

Fig. 1.1 Actions of Ramulus Cinnamomi.

■ FOLIUM PERILLAE, HERBA SCHIZONEPETAE and RADIX LEDEBOURIELLAE

- *Zi Su Ye, Jing Jie and Fang Feng*

Similarities
— All three disperse Wind-Cold. All are mild in nature and are commonly used in the treatment of Exterior Wind-Cold patterns. They can be used in combination, or may be substituted for each other.

Differences
— Folium Perillae is more effective in dispersing Cold than Wind. It also circulates Qi, harmonizes the Middle Burner, stops vomiting and prevents miscarriage. It is thus indicated in Exterior patterns of Wind-Cold complicated with stagnation of Qi, presenting with symptoms of distension and fullness in the epigastrium and abdomen.
— Herba Schizonepetae is more effective in eliminating Wind than Cold. It expresses skin eruptions and stops bleeding. As it is only mildly warm in nature, it can be used in combination with other herbs in the treatment of Exterior Wind-Heat syndromes.
— Radix Ledebouriellae is an important herb to eliminate Wind. It Releases the Exterior, eliminates Dampness, relieves pain, stops convulsion and relieves itching by eliminating Wind. It is thus indicated for headache, Bi syndromes, tetanus and rubella, all of which are caused by invasion of External Wind.

■ RHIZOMA SEU RADIX NOTOPTERYGII, RADIX ANGELICAE DAHURICAE and HERBA ASARI

- *Qiang Huo, Bai Zhi and Xi Xin*

Similarities
— All disperse Wind-Cold and relieve pain, and are thus indicated for Exterior symptoms such as headache and general aching, headache due to Wind and Bi syndromes due to Wind, Cold and Dampness.

Differences
— Rhizoma seu Radix Notopterygii is warm and dry in nature. It effectively disperses Wind-Damp, and is thus indicated for Exterior syndromes complicated with Dampness, headache involving the Tai Yang channel and Wind-Damp Bi syndromes affecting the upper body.
— Radix Angelicae Dahuricae eases the nose, relieves carbuncles and clears vaginal discharge by drying up Dampness. It is an important herb for headache involving the Yang Ming channel and for various disorders on the head and face.
— Herba Asari is pungent, warm and aromatic in nature. It disperses Cold, relieves pain, resolves fluid retained in the Lungs and eases the nose. When taken in large doses, this herb consumes Qi and Yin, thus producing stuffiness of the chest and respiratory paralysis; it is therefore not advisable to administer doses of more than 3 g, especially as a powder.

■ HERBA ELSHOLTZIAE and HERBA AGASTACHIS

- *Xiang Ru and Huo Xiang*

Similarities
— Both are pungent, warm and aromatic in nature. Both clear Summer Heat and Release the Exterior and are thus indicated for the common cold due to Summer Heat or Dampness during the Summer.

Differences
— Herba Elsholtziae is a strong diaphoretic. There is a saying: 'Xiang Ru in Summer is like *Ma Huang* in Winter'. It also promotes diuresis and is thus indicated for oedema. Herba Agastachis fragrantly resolves Dampness and thus also harmonizes the Middle Burner to relieve vomiting.

■ FRUCTUS XANTHII AND FLOS MAGNOLIAE

- *Cang Er Zi and Xin Yi Hua*

Similarities
— Both disperse Wind-Cold and ease the nose and are thus important herbs for rhinitis (Fig. 1.2).
— Fructus Xanthii not only expels Wind-Damp and relieves pain in Bi syndromes and headache, but also expels Wind and relieves itching in rubella and eczema.

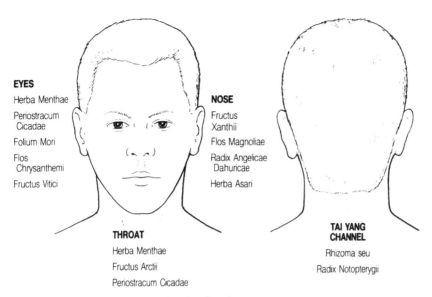

Fig. 1.2 Herbs that eliminate Wind from the head and neck.

B. Herbs that disperse Wind-Heat

■ **HERBA MENTHAE, FRUCTUS ARCTII and PERIOSTRACUM CICADAE**

● *Bo He, Niu Bang Zi and Chan Tui*

Similarities
— All three disperse Wind-Heat, ease the throat and express skin rashes. They are thus indicated for Exterior Wind-Heat patterns, sore throat, rubella and measles when the rash has not fully erupted.

Differences
— Herba Menthae is pungent and cool in nature and strongly Releases the Exterior by promoting diaphoresis. It also clears heat in the head and eyes and promotes the smooth circulation of Liver Qi. This herb is usually added to a decoction in the last few minutes of cooking.
— Fructus Arctii clears heat and toxins, relieves swelling, stops cough, moistens the Large Intestine and relieves constipation. It is thus indicated for the Fire Poison of carbuncles and mumps, for cough due to Lung Heat and for Exterior Wind-Heat patterns complicated with constipation.
— Periostracum Cicadae expels Wind and treats convulsions. It is thus indicated for

redness of the eyes, infantile convulsions and tetanus due to Wind-Heat in the Liver channel. It is used in large doses for the treatment of convulsion, but in small doses otherwise.

■ **FOLIUM MORI and FLOS CHRYSANTHEMI**

● *Sang Ye and Ju Hua*

Similarities
— Both expel Wind-Heat and clear Heat from the head and eyes. They also clear Heat from the Liver and improve vision. They are thus indicated for Exterior Wind-Heat patterns with headache and red eyes and for red eyes and dizziness due to Heat in the Liver.

Differences
— Folium Mori clears Heat from the Lung, moistens dryness and stops cough and is thus indicated for cough due to Dry Heat.
— Flos Chrysanthemi clears Heat from the Liver, improves vision and expels Fire Poison. Yellow Flos Chrysanthemi is more effective in dispersing Wind-Heat and expelling Fire Poison and is thus often used in the treatment of Exterior patterns. White Flos Chrysanthemi is more effective in clearing Liver Heat and improving vision and is thus often used to treat Interior patterns.

■ FRUCTUS VITICIS, RADIX ANGELICAE DAHURICAE and FLOS CHRYSANTHEMI

- *Man Jing Zi, Bai Zhi and Ju Hua*

Similarities
— All are commonly used in the treatment of headache due to invasion of External Wind (Fig. 1.3).

Differences
— Fructus Viticis acts similarly to Flos Chrysanthemi in expelling Wind Heat and clearing Heat from the head and eyes. However, Fructus Viticis strongly relieves pain and is only slightly cold in nature. It can thus be used to treat Wind-Cold headache when combined with Radix Angelicae Dahuricae, Rhizoma seu Radix Notopterygii and Radix Ledebouriellae.
— Radix Angelicae Dahuricae expels Wind-Cold and is thus indicated for Wind-Cold headache on the Yang Ming channel.

■ RADIX BUPLEURI, RADIX PUERARIAE AND RHIZOMA CIMICIFUGAE

- *Chai Hu, Ge Gen and Sheng Ma*

Similarities
— All Release the Exterior, reduce fever and raise the Qi of the Middle Burner. They are thus indicated for fever due to External Invasion and for sinking of Central Qi.

Differences
— Radix Bupleuri and Radix Puerariae are often combined to Release the Exterior and reduce fever. Radix Bupleuri enters the Shao Yang channel and treats alternating fever and chills due to Shao Yang disharmony. Radix Puerariae enters the Yang Ming channel and treats a feverish sensation of the body, with thirst and stiffness of the neck and back.
— Radix Bupleuri and Rhizoma Cimicifugae both raise Central Qi and are thus often used in the treatment of prolapse due to sinking of Central Qi.
— Radix Puerariae and Rhizoma Cimicifugae both express skin eruptions and are thus used in the early stage of measles or for any skin rash which has not fully erupted.
— Radix Bupleuri also promotes the smooth circulation of Liver Qi and is thus an important herb for Stagnant Liver Qi. Radix Puerariae promotes Body Fluids and relieves thirst, and is thus indicated for thirst during febrile diseases as well as for Thirsting and Wasting syndromes. Rhizoma Cimicifugae clears Heat and Poison, and is thus indicated for swelling, pain and erosion of the gums, mouth ulcers and erysipelas on the face.

Questions

1. Compare and contrast the actions of Herba Ephedrae and Ramulus Cinnamomi in Releasing the Exterior. What other

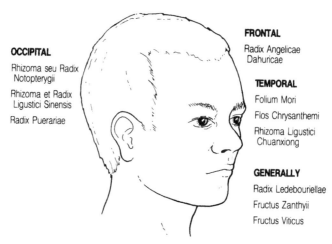

Fig. 1.3 Herbs that treat headache due to Wind.

actions do they have? What diseases do they treat?

2. Differentiate the actions of Radix Ledebouriellae, Rhizoma seu Radix Notopterygii, Radix Angelicae Dahuricae, Folium Mori, Flos Chrysanthemi and Fructus Viticis in the treatment of headache.

3. Compare and contrast the actions and indications of Radix Bupleuri, Radix Puerariae and Rhizoma Cimicifugae.

2   *Herbs that clear Heat*

A. Herbs that clear Heat and quell Fire

■ **GYPSUM FIBROSUM AND RHIZOMA ANEMARRHENAE**

● *Shi Gao and Zhi Mu*

Similarities
— Both clear Full Heat at the Nutritive (Ying) level, and Lung and Stomach Fire. They are thus indicated for febrile disease at the Nutritive (Ying) level, for cough and wheeze due to Lung Heat and for headache, toothache and Wasting and Thirsting syndromes due to Stomach Heat.

Differences
— Gypsum Fibrosum is extremely cold in nature and has a strong action in clearing Full Heat. Calcined Gypsum Fibrosum is used externally to astringe skin ulcers and promote tissue regeneration. It is thus indicated for boils, ulcers, burns and eczema.
— Rhizoma Anemarrhenae clears both Full and Empty Heat. It nourishes Yin, quells Fire, promotes Body Fluids and moistens dryness. It is thus indicated for dry cough, tidal fever, night sweats and nocturnal emissions due to Lung and Kidney Yin deficiency.
— Raw Gypsum Fibrosum is prescribed in large doses for oral administration. It should be broken into pieces and decocted prior to the addition of other ingredients of the prescription. Due to its extremely cold nature, it is contraindicated where there is Spleen Yang deficiency. Rhizoma Anemarrhenae is also cold in nature, and moistens the intestines. For this reason it is contraindicated where there is Spleen deficiency giving rise to loose stools.

■ **RHIZOMA PHRAGMITIS, RADIX TRICHOSANTHIS, FOLIUM PHYLLOSTACHYOS, and HERBA LOPHATHERI**

● *Lu Gen, Tian Hua Fen, Zhu Ye, and Dan Zhu Ye*

Similarities
— All are sweet and cold in nature and clear Lung and Stomach Heat. They treat External Heat at the Qi level, and Internal Heat patterns of the Lung and Stomach with symptoms of fever and thirst.

Differences
— Rhizoma Phragmitis is more effective in clearing Lung Heat with symptoms of cough and lung abscess. It also clears Stomach Heat, stops vomiting, promotes Body Fluids and alleviates thirst.
— Radix Trichosanthis clears Heat and promotes Body Fluids. It is often used where fluids have been consumed by febrile disease, and for Thirsting and Wasting syndromes. It moistens the Lung and resolves Phlegm and is thus used to treat productive cough due to Lung Dryness. It also relieves swelling and drains pus in cases of boils and carbuncles caused by Fire Poison.
— Folium Phyllostachyos clears Heat, particularly Heart Heat. It relieves restlessness and promotes diuresis. It is thus indicated for pathogenic Heat at the Qi and Nutritive (Ying) levels, urinary disorders due to Heat and mouth and tongue ulcers.
— Herba Lophatheri is similar to Folium Phyllostachyos in action, but is less effective in clearing Heart Heat and relieving restlessness. However, it is more effective in clearing Heat generally and in promoting diuresis.

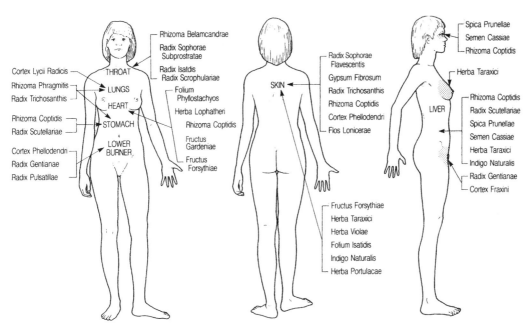

Fig. 2.1 Differentiation of Herbs that clear Heat according to area of action.

■ RHIZOMA COPTIDIS, RADIX SCUTELLARIAE and CORTEX PHELLODENDRI

● *Huang Lian, Huang Qin, and Huang Bai*

Similarities

— All are bitter and cold in nature and clear Heat, quell Fire, dry Dampness and clear Poison. They are often combined in cases of Heat and Fire in all three Burners (Fig. 2.1). They all treat Damp-Heat, including Damp-Heat in the intestines presenting with signs of dysentery, as well as Fire Poison patterns. Due to their cold and bitter nature, all three can damage the Yang and digestive Qi; due to their bitter and dry nature, they can consume Yin. They should be used carefully in cases of Spleen Yang deficiency or Yin deficiency.

Differences

— Rhizoma Coptidis strongly clears Heart, Stomach and Liver Heat and Poison. It is thus indicated for Heart Fire Blazing with symptoms of restlessness, mouth and tongue ulcers or coma, for retention of Damp-Heat with discomfort in the epigastrium, for Liver Fire giving rise to eye disorders and for carbuncles and ulcers due to Fire Poison.

— Radix Scutellariae clears Lung Heat, reduces Gall Bladder Fire, clears Heat to prevent miscarriage, cools the Blood and stops bleeding. It is thus indicated for cough and wheeze due to Lung Heat or Fire, Shao Yang syndrome with hypochondriac pain and jaundice, threatened abortion due to Heat and spitting of blood and epistaxis due to Blood Heat.

— Cortex Phellodendri reduces Empty Heat, clears Damp-Heat from the Lower Burner and relieves jaundice. It is thus indicated for nocturnal emissions and hypersexuality due to Empty Fire in the Lower Burner, as well as for Damp-Heat giving rise to symptoms such as festering ulcers, eczema, paralysis of the lower limbs, painful joints, turbid urine, leucorrhoea and jaundice.

■ RADIX SOPHORAE FLAVESCENTIS

● *Ku Shen*

— Radix Sophorae Flavescentis is similar to Cortex Phellodendri in its action of clearing Heat and drying Dampness. It also kills parasites and relieves itching in the treatment of eczema, scabies, leucorrhoea, generalized pruritus and pruritus vulvae. It promotes diuresis and is thus used for oedema and urinary disturbance due to Damp-Heat. It is reported that this herb also treats cardiac arrhythmia. Due to its very bitter and cold nature, it may damage the digestion if taken in large doses or over a long time. It is often used as an ingredient of patent remedies in the form of a pill or powder, or is applied externally.

■ **RADIX GENTIANAE, FRUCTUS GARDENIAE, SPICA PRUNELLAE and SEMEN CASSIAE**

● *Long Dan Cao, Zhi Zi, Xia Ku Cao and Jue Ming Zi*

Similarities
— All four clear Liver Heat and improve vision and are thus indicated for headache and eye disorders due to Liver Fire.

Differences
— Radix Gentianae has a strong action in reducing Liver Fire and clearing Damp-Heat in the Liver Channel. It is thus indicated for high fever, convulsions and headache due to Heat or Fire in the Liver Channel, and for Damp-Heat in the Lower Burner giving rise to symptoms such as swelling in the pubic region, swelling and pain of the scrotum, pruritus vulvae and a thick yellow vaginal discharge.
— Fructus Gardeniae clears Heart Heat, relieves restlessness, clears Damp-Heat and Poison, cools Blood and stops bleeding. It is thus indicated for stuffiness of the chest and restlessness due to Heart Heat, jaundice and urinary disturbance due to Damp-Heat, spitting of blood, epistaxis and haematuria due to Heat in the Blood, and for carbuncles and ulcers due to Fire Poison.
— Spica Prunellae clears Liver Heat and Stagnation and is thus indicated for headache, dizziness, and redness of the eyes due to Liver Fire and Liver Yang Rising, as well as for tuberculosis of the lymph nodes and simple goitre.
— Semen Cassiae is more effective in clearing Liver Heat and improving vision and is thus indicated for eye disorders due to Liver Heat and Fire. It also moistens the intestines and relieves constipation with dry stool.

B. Herbs that clear Heat and Fire Poison

■ **FLOS LONICERAE AND FRUCTUS FORSYTHIAE**

● *Jin Yin Hua and Lian Qiao*

Similarities
— Both herbs clear Heat and Poison and are thus indicated for all Fire Poison patterns including febrile disease, boils, carbuncles and ulcers.

Differences
— Flos Lonicerae also clears Summer Heat and treats dysentery with bleeding due to Fire Poison. Caulis Lonicerae is similar to Flos Lonicerae in clearing Heat and removing obstructions in the channels. Both treat Febrile Bi syndrome.
— Fructus Forsythiae clears Heart Fire and disperses masses. It is thus indicated for febrile disease at the Nutritive (Ying) level and Heat in the Heart, as well as for carbuncles, boils and ulcers due to Fire Poison, and tuberculosis of the lymph nodes. It is especially useful for skin disease.

■ **HERBA TARAXACI AND HERBA VIOLAE**

● *Pu Gong Ying and Zi Hua Di Ding*

Similarities
— Both clear Heat and Poison, and are thus indicated for carbuncles, boils and ulcers due to Fire Poison.

Differences
— Herba Taraxaci is especially effective in treating mastitis. It also clears Heat in the Liver and Gall Bladder and Damp-Heat. It is thus indicated for hypochondriac pain and jaundice due to Damp-Heat in the Liver and Gall Bladder, epigastric pain due to Stomach Heat and urinary disease due to Heat.
— Herba Violae is especially effective in treating carbuncles, boils and ulcers due to its strong action in eliminating Fire Poison. It also cools Blood and stops bleeding.

■ FOLIUM ISATIDIS, RADIX ISATIDIS AND INDIGO NATURALIS

● *Da Qing Ye, Ban Lan Gen and Qing Dai*

Similarities
— All these medicines come from the same plant and are thus similar in their action. All three clear Heat and Poison and cool Blood. They are indicated for febrile disease with Fire Poison, as well as for carbuncles, boils and ulcers due to Fire Poison.
— Folium Isatidis is often used in the treatment of febrile disease. It has a strong action in cooling Blood and eliminating Poison and it promotes the healing of skin eruptions.
— Radix Isatidis is also commonly used in the treatment of febrile disease and is especially effective for viral infections. It is more effective than Folium Isatidis in eliminating Fire Poison, relieving swelling and easing the throat.
— Indigo Naturalis cools Blood, stops bleeding and clears Liver Fire. It is thus indicated for bleeding due to Blood Heat, headache due to Liver Fire and convulsions due to Liver Heat. It is often applied to Fire Poison lesions externally in the form of a powder.

■ HERBA ANDROGRAPHITIS AND RHIZOMA PARIDIS

● *Chuan Xin Lian and Zao Xiu*

Similarities
— Both herbs clear Heat and Poison and are thus indicated for all Fire Poison patterns.

Differences
— Herba Andrographitis is widely used in the treatment of various infections, particularly of the intestinal tract and respiratory system. It is similar to Rhizoma Coptidis in nature and action. Rhizoma Paridis is indicated for poisonous snake bites and cancer. It clears Heat and stops convulsions, and is thus indicated for infantile convulsions or any convulsion due to high fever.

■ HERBA HOUTTUYNIAE, RHIZOMA BELAMCANDAE AND RADIX SOPHORAE SUBPROSTRATAE

● *Yu Xing Cao, She Gan and Shan Dou Gen*

Similarities
— All three herbs clear Lung Heat and are thus indicated for cough and sore throat.

Differences
— Herba Houttuyniae is primarily used to treat cough and lung abscess due to Heat in the Lung.
— Rhizoma Belamcandae and Radix Sophorae Subprostratae are primarily used to treat sore throat. Rhizoma Belamcandae also resolves Phlegm and regulates Qi, and is thus indicated for cough with profuse sputum and wheeze. Radix Sophorae Subprostratae has a strong action in clearing Heat and relieving swelling and is thus indicated for inflammation of the throat, and for cancer.

■ HERBA PORTULACAE, RADIX PULSATILLAE AND CORTEX FRAXINI

● *Ma Chi Xian, Bai Tou Weng and Qin Pi*

Similarities
— All three herbs clear Heat in the intestines and are thus indicated for diarrhoea and dysentery.

Differences
— Herba Portulacae also treats eczema, carbuncles, swelling and uterine bleeding.
— Radix Pulsatillae treats dysentery with bleeding due to Fire Poison. It is effective against both bacillary dysentery and amoebic dysentery.
— Cortex Fraxini clears Damp-Heat and is thus indicated for Damp-Heat leucorrhoea. It also clears Liver Heat and improves vision and is thus indicated for eye disorders due to Liver Fire.

■ CAULIS SARGENTODOXAE AND HERBA PATRINIAE

● *Hong Teng and Bai Jiang Cao*

Similarities
— Both clear Heat and Poison and move Blood

and are thus indicated for appendicitis, as well as abdominal pain in women due to stagnation of Qi and Blood.

Differences
— Caulis Sargentodoxae is more effective in moving Blood and is thus indicated for contusions and sprains, irregular menstruation and Wind-Damp Bi syndrome.
— Herba Patriniae is more effective in clearing Heat and draining pus and is thus indicated for carbuncles, boils and ulcers due to Fire Poison.

■ HERBA HEDYOTIS DIFFUSAE, HERBA SCUTELLARIAE BARBATAE AND RHIZOMA SMILACIS GLABRAE

● *Bai Hua She She Cao, Ban Zhi Lian and Tu Fu Ling*

Similarities
— All three clear Heat and Poison and eliminate Dampness and are thus indicated for cancer and syphilis.

Differences
— Herba Hedyotis Diffusae and Herba Scutellariae Barbatae are often used in the treatment of cancer and poisonous snake bite. Rhizoma Smilacis Glabrae is often used in the treatment of venereal diseases such as syphilis.

C. Herbs that clear Full Heat and Empty Heat and cool Blood

■ CORNU RHINOCERI ASIATICI AND CALCULUS BOVIS

● *Xi Jiao and Niu Huang*

Similarities
— Both clear Heart and Liver Heat, cool Blood and clear Fire Poison and are thus indicated for coma and convulsion due to pathogenic Heat at the Nutritive (Ying) and Blood levels.

Differences
— Cornu Rhinoceri Asiatici cools Blood, stops

bleeding, relieves skin eruptions, clears Heat and expels Wind, and is thus indicated for bleeding and skin eruptions due to Blood Heat, as well as for Liver Wind due to Heat. Cornu Bubali can be substituted, but must be prescribed in larger doses (15–30 g).
— Calculus Bovis is more effective in clearing Heart Heat and opening the orifices, as well as in clearing Heat and Fire Poison, and is thus indicated for coma in febrile diseases, and Fire Poison patterns. Calculus Bovis Factitius can be substituted.

■ RADIX REHMANNIAE, RADIX SCROPHULARIAE, CORTEX MOUTAN RADICIS AND RADIX PAEONIAE RUBRA

● *Sheng Di Huang, Xuan Shen, Mu Dan Pi, and Chi Shao*

Similarities
— All clear Heat and cool Blood and are thus indicated for pathogenic Heat at the Nutritive (Ying) and Blood levels, and for haemorrhagic patterns due to Heat.

Differences
— Radix Rehmanniae and Radix Scrophulariae are both sweet and cold in nature. They nourish Yin and promote Body Fluids and are thus indicated for Yin Deficiency. Radix Rehmanniae is more effective in cooling Blood and stopping bleeding (Fig. 2.2). Radix Scrophulariae is more effective in nourishing Yin and clearing Fire and Fire Poison, and is thus indicated for sore throat, tuberculosis of the lymph nodes and carbuncles, boils and ulcers due to Fire Poison.
— Cortex Moutan Radicis and Radix Paeoniae Rubra also invigorate Blood circulation and treat Blood Stasis, and are thus indicated for Blood Heat complicated by Stasis. They also clear Liver Fire. Cortex Moutan Radicis clears Empty Heat and is thus indicated for tidal fever. Radix Paeoniae Rubra is more effective in moving Blood and treating Stasis, but does not stop bleeding.

Radix Rehmanniae	Radix Rehmanniae Praeparata
Cold	Warm
Cools Blood (and stops bleeding)	Tonifies Blood
Clears Heat	
Tonifies Yin (and promotes Body Fluids)	Tonifies Yin

Fig. 2.2 Actions of Radix Rehmanniae.

■ HERBA ARTEMISIAE CHINGHAO, CORTEX LYCII RADICIS, RADIX AMPELOPSIS AND RADIX STELLARIAE

● *Qing Hao, Di Gu Pi, Bai Wei and Yin Chai Hu*

Similarities
— All clear Empty Heat and are thus indicated for fever and tidal fever due to Yin Deficiency and for persistent low-grade fever in the late stage of febrile disease.

Differences
— Herba Artemisiae Chinghao clears both Full and Empty Heat, as well as Summer Heat. It is indicated in the treatment of malaria.
— Cortex Lycii Radicis clears Lung Heat and is thus indicated in haemoptysis due to Lung Heat. It also treats hypertension and diabetes.
— Radix Ampelopsis cools Blood and is thus indicated in the treatment of Blood Heat in women.
— Radix Stellariae is more effective in clearing Empty Heat. It also treats malnutrition and fever in children.

Questions

1. Compare and contrast the actions and indications of Gypsum Fibrosum and Rhizoma Anemarrhenae.
2. Compare and contrast the actions and indications of Rhizoma Coptidis, Radix Scutellariae and Cortex Phellodendri. Explain their side-effects and the precautions for their use.
3. Flos Lonicerae, Fructus Forsythiae, Herba Taraxaci, Folium Isatidis, Herba Houttuyniae, Radix Pulsatillae and Cortex Fraxini are all herbs that clear Heat and Fire Poison. How do their indications differ?
4. Compare and contrast the actions and indications of Radix Gentianae, Fructus Gardeniae, Spica Prunellae and Semen Cassiae.
5. Of the herbs that clear Heat, which ones also
   a. nourish Yin?
   b. clear Empty Heat?
   c. move Blood and treat Blood Stasis?

3 *Herbs that purge and promote digestion*

A. Purgative herbs

■ RADIX ET RHIZOMA RHEI, NATRII SULFAS AND FOLIUM CASSIAE

- *Da Huang, Mang Xiao and Fan Xie Ye*

Similarities
— All are purgative and are thus indicated for constipation due to accumulation of Heat, constipation with fullness of the abdomen due to high fever, and acute abdomen. They also clear Heat and Fire.

Differences
— Radix et Rhizoma Rhei is bitter and cold in nature. It clears Heat and Fire, stops bleeding, clears Fire Poison, invigorates Blood and disperses Stasis. It is thus indicated for Fire Poison in the upper body, haemorrhagic patterns due to Blood Heat, carbuncles and furuncles due to Fire Poison, jaundice due to Damp-Heat, urinary dysfunction, amenorrhoea due to stagnation of Qi and Blood, palpable abdominal masses and contusions and sprains.

— Natrii Sulfas is salty and cold in nature and thus softens and resolves masses as well as purging. It is indicated for dry stool and mastitis. External application resolves hard lumps and inhibits lactation.
— Folium Cassiae is indicated for habitual constipation. It is also used to cleanse the intestines.

■ FRUCTUS CANNABIS AND SEMEN PRUNI

- *Huo Ma Ren and Yu Li Ren*

Similarities
— Both moisten and purge the intestines and are thus indicated for constipation due to deficiency of Fluids and Blood, and dryness of the intestines.

Differences
— Fructus Cannabis relieves constipation solely by moistening the intestines.
— Semen Pruni also promotes diuresis and relieves swelling and is thus indicated for oedema (Fig. 3.1).

Radix et Rhizoma Rhei	clears Heat and Fire Poison	purges the intestines
Natrii Sulfas	softens masses	
Folium Cassiae		
Fructus Cannabis		moistens the intestines
Semen Pruni	promotes diuresis	

Fig. 3.1 Differentiation of purgative herbs.

B. Herbs that promote digestion

■ FRUCTUS CRATAEGI, MASSA FERMENTATA, FRUCTUS HORDEI GERMINATUS, FRUCTUS ORYZAE GERMINATUS, ENDOTHELIUM CORNEUM GIGERIAE GALLI, SEMEN RAPHANI AND SEMEN ARECAE

● *Shan Zha, Shen Qu, Mai Ya, Gu Ya, Ji Nei Jin, Lai Fu Zi and Bing Long*

Similarities
— All promote digestion and are thus indicated for retention of food, with symptoms of epigastric distension, abdominal pain, belching, acid regurgitation and abnormal bowel movement.

Differences
— Fructus Crataegi promotes digestion, strengthens the Spleen and disperses Blood Stasis. It is indicated for poor digestion of meat (Fig. 3.2), lack of gastric acid, dyspepsia and stagnation of Blood.
— Massa Fermentata Medicinalis is more effective in promoting the digestion of rice, wheat flour and alcohol (Fig. 3.2). It harmonizes the Middle Burner and stops diarrhoea and is indicated for retention of food accompanied by fever, diarrhoea or dysentery.
— Fructus Hordei Germinatus and Fructus Oryzae Germinatus promote the digestion of rice and wheat flour (Fig. 3.2), assist the Stomach and harmonize the Middle Burner. Fructus Hordei Germinatus also inhibits lactation and promotes the Liver's function of regulating the free flow of Qi.
— Endothelium Corneum Gigeriae Galli astringes seminal emission and dissolves stones, and is thus indicated for spermatorrhoea, nocturnal enuresis and stones in the urinary and biliary tracts. It also promotes the function of the Stomach and is thus indicated for poor digestion due to Stomach weakness.
— Semen Raphani resolves Phlegm and regulates Qi and is thus indicated for retention of food due to Qi Stagnation and for other patterns of stagnant Qi and Phlegm.
— Semen Arecae regulates Qi and dispels parasites and is thus indicated for retention of food due to Qi Stagnation and abdominal pain due to parasites.

Questions

1. Compare and contrast the actions and indications of Radix et Rhizoma Rhei and Natrii Sulfas.
2. In addition to promoting digestion, what are the other actions of Fructus Crataegi, Fructus Hordei Germinatus, Semen Raphani and Endothelium Corneum Gigeriae Galii?

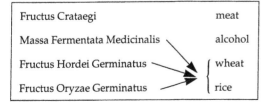

Fig. 3.2 Differentiation of digestive herbs by type of food.

4 *Herbs that resolve Phlegm and stop coughing and wheezing*

A. Herbs that resolve Phlegm

■ RHIZOMA PINELLIAE and RHIZOMA ARISAEMATIS

- *Ban Xia and Tian Nan Xing*

Similarities
— Both are pungent, warm and toxic in nature and resolve Cold Phlegm by warming or drying Dampness. They are thus indicated for patterns of Cold Phlegm or Damp Phlegm. External application relieves swelling and pain and they are used in the treatment of boils and ulcers.

Differences
— Rhizoma Pinelliae conducts Rebellious Qi downward and stops vomiting and is thus indicated for vomiting due to Rebellious Stomach Qi. It also relieves fullness and disperses lumps and is thus indicated for a distressing sensation of fullness in the epigastrium and for Plum-Stone Qi (the sensation of a foreign body in the throat).
— Rhizoma Arisaematis eliminates Wind Phlegm and stops convulsions, and is thus indicated for Wind Phlegm patterns such as dizziness and vertigo, deviation of the mouth and eye, hemiplegia and tetanus. It is bitter and cool in nature and also cools Heat.

■ RHIZOMA ARISAEMATIS AND RHIZOMA TYPHONII

- *Tian Nan Xing and Bai Fu Zi*

Similarities
— Both eliminate Wind Phlegm and stop convulsion and are thus indicated for patterns of Wind Phlegm, including tetanus and deviation of the mouth and eye.

Differences
— Rhizoma Arisaematis also dries Dampness and resolves Phlegm and is thus indicated for patterns of Damp Phlegm. Rhizoma Typhonii is mainly used for disorders of the head and face.

■ SEMEN SINAPIS ALBAE

- *Bai Jie Zi*

— This herb is similar to Rhizoma Pinelliae in resolving Cold Phlegm with warmth. It is more effective in promoting the circulation of Qi and dispersing masses and is indicated for Phlegm between the skin and muscles, retention of fluid in the hypochondrium and Yin-type jaundice.

■ RADIX PLATYCODI, RADIX PEUCEDANI, RHIZOMA CYNANCHI STAUNTONII AND FLOS INULAE

- *Jie Geng, Qian Hu, Bai Qian and Xuan Fu Hua*

Similarities
— All resolve Phlegm and stop cough and are thus indicated for cough with profuse sputum.

Differences
— Radix Platycodi and Radix Peucedani both promote the Lung's function of dispersing and are thus indicated for cough due to an impairment of the Lung's dispersing function following an invasion of the Lung by pathogenic factors. Radix Platycodi also eases the throat and drains pus and is thus indicated for sore throat and lung abscess. Radix Peucedani also conducts Rebellious Qi downward and is thus indicated for cough and wheeze when Lung Qi fails to

descend due to retention of Phlegm in the lungs.

— Rhizoma Cynanchi Stauntonii and Flos Inulae both conduct Rebellious Qi downward and resolve Phlegm. They are thus indicated for cough with profuse sputum, and wheeze due to failure of the Lung Qi to descend. Flos Inulae also sends Stomach Qi downward and is thus indicated for vomiting and hiccup due to Rebellious Stomach Qi.

■ FRUCTUS TRICHOSANTHIS AND BULBUS FRITILLARIAE

- *Gua Lou and Bei Mu*

Similarities
— Both clear Heat, resolve Phlegm and moisten the lungs and are thus indicated for patterns of Heat Phlegm and Dry Phlegm.

Differences
— Fructus Trichosanthis opens the chest, relieves stagnation, moistens the intestines and relieves constipation. It is thus indicated for patterns of Chest Bi due to stagnation arising from Deficient Yang in the chest and for constipation due to dryness of the intestines. Pericarpium Trichosanthis is more effective in opening the chest and regulating Qi. Semen Trichosanthis is more effective in moistening the lungs and intestines and relieving constipation.

— Bulbus Fritillariae is more effective than Fructus Trichosanthis in moistening the lungs and stopping cough. It also clears Heat and disperses masses and is indicated for tuberculosis of the lymph nodes, abscess and swelling. It is sweet and moist in nature and is often used in the treatment of Yin deficiency and Lung dryness due to chronic illness. Bulbus Fritillariae Thunbergii is bitter and discharging in nature and is often used in the treatment of Fire Poison patterns due to External Invasion.

■ CAULIS BAMBUSAE IN TAENIAM AND SUCCUS BAMBUSAE

- *Zhu Ru and Zhu Li*

Similarities
— Both clear Heat and resolve Phlegm and are thus indicated for cough due to Phlegm Heat.

Differences
— Caulis Bambusae in Taeniam clears Stomach Heat and stops vomiting and is thus

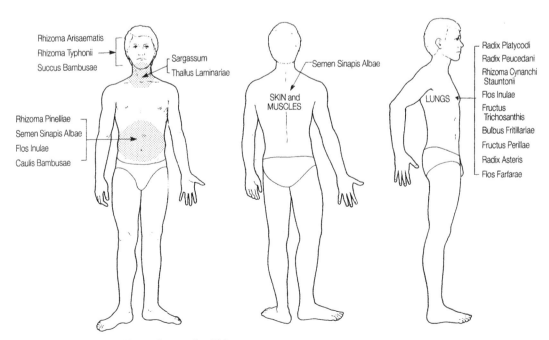

Fig. 4.1 Local actions of herbs that resolve Phlegm.

indicated for vomiting due to Stomach Heat.

— Succus Bambusae expels Phlegm and opens the orifices and is thus indicated for Wind Stroke with gurgling in the throat and unconsciousness due to Phlegm Heat.

■ SARGASSUM AND THALLUS LAMINARIAE

- *Hai Zao and Kun Bu*

Similarities

— Both resolve Phlegm and soften hard masses and are thus indicated for goitre, tuberculosis of the lymph nodes and subcutaneous nodules (Fig. 4.1). They also promote diuresis and relieve swelling and are used in the treatment of beri-beri, oedema and dysuria. They are often used in combination and can be substituted for each other. They are used in dietary therapy to treat hypertension and arteriosclerosis.

B. Herbs that stop coughing and wheezing

■ SEMEN ARMENIACAE AMARUM AND FRUCTUS PERILLAE

- *Xing Ren and Su Zi*

Similarities

— Both conduct Lung Qi downward to stop cough and wheeze and are thus indicated for cough and wheeze due to Rebellious Lung Qi. They also moisten the intestines and relieve constipation and are thus indicated for constipation due to dryness of the intestines.

Differences

— Semen Armeniacae Amarum is effective in sending Qi downward and promoting the Lung's dispersing function. It is thus an important herb for stopping cough and wheeze. It treats various kinds of cough and asthma in combination with other herbs.

— Fructus Perillae also resolves Phlegm and is thus more effective when Lung Qi fails to descend due to blockage by Cold Phlegm or Damp Phlegm.

■ RADIX STEMONAE, RADIX ASTERIS AND FLOS FARFARAE

- *Bai Bu, Zi Wan and Kuan Dong Hua*

Similarities

— All moisten the lungs and stop cough and are indicated for both acute and chronic cough.

Differences

— Radix Stemonae also kills insects and lice. It is applied externally to treat head and body lice and *Trichomonas vaginalis* and administered as an enema to treat pinworms.

— Radix Asteris and Flos Farfarae both resolve Phlegm and stop cough. The former is more effective in stopping cough and the latter more effective in resolving Phlegm. They are often used in combination.

■ FOLIUM ERIOBOTRYAE and FRUCTUS ARISTOLOCHIAE

- *Pi Pa Ye and Ma Dou Ling*

Similarities

— Both clear Lung Heat and stop cough and are thus indicated for cough due to Lung Heat.

Differences

— Folium Eriobotryae clears Stomach Heat, conducts Rebellious Qi downward and stops vomiting and is thus indicated for vomiting due to Stomach Heat.

— Fructus Aristolochiae calms the Liver and lowers blood pressure and is thus indicated for hypertension due to Liver Yang Rising.

■ CORTEX MORI RADICIS AND SEMEN LEPIDII SEU DESCURAINIAE

- *Sang Bai Pi and Ting Li Zi*

Similarities

— Both clear Lung Heat, soothe wheeze, promote diuresis and relieve swelling. They are thus indicated for cough and wheeze due to Lung Heat and for oedema.

Differences

— Cortex Mori Radicis is more effective in

clearing Heat and Fire from the lungs. Semen Lepidii seu Descurainiae is more effective in eliminating water from the Lungs and soothing asthma. This herb has a potent action and renders good therapeutic results in the treatment of pulmonary heart disease with dyspnoea and pulmonary oedema, but it is a harsh cathartic and should be used with extreme caution.

■ HERBA EPHEDRAE, SEMEN LEPIDII SEU DESCURAINIAE AND SEMEN GINKGO

● *Ma Huang, Ting Li Zi and Bai Guo*

Similarities
— All soothe asthma and are thus indicated for cough and wheeze.

Differences
— Herba Ephedrae promotes the dispersing function of the Lung and is thus indicated for asthma when the dispersing function of the Lung is impaired due to an Excess pattern.
— Semen Lepidii seu Descurainiae reduces Lung Fire and soothes asthma and is thus indicated for cough and wheeze due to Lung Fire and the retention of Phlegm Fluid.
— Semen Ginkgo astringes the lungs and soothes asthma, and is thus indicated for chronic cough and wheeze due to Lung Qi Deficiency.

Questions

1. Rhizoma Pinelliae, Rhizoma Arisaematis, Fructus Trichosanthis and Bulbus Fritillariae all resolve Phlegm. Compare and contrast their other actions and indications.
2. Compare and contrast the actions and indications of Radix Platycodi, Radix Peucedani, Rhizoma Cynanchi Stauntonii and Flos Inulae.
3. What are the differences in action of Semen Armeniacae Amarum, Fructus Perillae, Herba Ephedrae and Semen Lepidii seu Descurainiae?

5 *Herbs that eliminate Wind-Damp*

■ **RADIX ANGELICAE PUBESCENTIS, RHIZOMA SEU RADIX NOTOPTERYGII AND RADIX CLEMATIDIS**

● *Du Huo, Qiang Huo and Wei Ling Xian*

Similarities
— All are warm in nature and eliminate Wind-Damp and relieve pain. They are thus indicated for Bi syndromes involving Wind, Cold and Dampness.

Differences
— Radix Notopterygii and Radix Angelicae Pubescentis are warm and dry in nature and are more effective in eliminating Cold Damp. They are thus indicated for Bi syndromes in which Cold Damp predominates. Radix Notopterygii goes upward and is thus used for Bi syndromes involving the upper body. It also strongly Releases the Exterior and so is used for Exterior patterns complicated with Dampness. Radix Angelicae Pubescentis is less effective in Releasing the Exterior, but it strongly eliminates Wind-Damp and so is commonly used in the treatment of Bi syndromes. Its action goes downward and it is more effective for treating the lower body. If Bi syndromes affect the entire body, these herbs are used in combination.
— Radix Clematidis is more effective in eliminating Wind, removing obstructions from the channels, and relieving pain. It is thus indicated for Wandering Bi, in which pathogenic Wind predominates. It also dissolves fishbones lodged in the throat and treats oesophageal cancer.

■ **RADIX GENTIANAE MACROPHYLLAE, RADIX STEPHANIAE TETRANDRAE, HERBA SIEGESBECKIAE AND FOLIUM CLERODENDRI**

● *Qin Jiu, Fang Ji, Xi Xian Cao and Chou Wu Tong*

Similarities
— All are cold in nature and eliminate Wind Damp. They are thus indicated for Wind Damp Bi syndromes with signs of heat.

Differences
— Radix Gentianae Macrophyllae eliminates Wind Damp without drying and is thus referred to as a moist herb for eliminating Wind. It also clears Empty Heat and is thus used for Bi syndromes with heat signs due to Blood and Yin Deficiency. It also treats fever and tidal fever due to Yin Deficiency, and Damp-Heat-type jaundice.
— Radix Stephaniae Tetrandrae is more effective in eliminating Dampness and is thus indicated for Damp Bi syndromes. It also promotes diuresis and relieves swelling and thus treats oedema.
— Herba Siegesbeckia and Folium Clerodendri eliminate Wind Damp, remove obstruction from the channels and lower blood pressure. They are thus indicated for Wind Damp Bi syndromes, numbness of the limbs and body, hemiplegia and hypertension.

■ FRUCTUS CHAENOMELIS, RAMULUS MORI, CAULIS TRACHELOSPERMI AND CAULIS PIPERIS FUTOKADSURAE

- *Mu Gua, Sang Zhi, Luo Shi Teng and Hai Feng Teng*

Similarities
— All relax the muscles and tendons and remove obstruction from the channels. They are thus indicated for Wind-Damp Bi syndromes, muscle contracture and limited motion of the joints.

Differences
— Fructus Chaenomelis eliminates Dampness and harmonizes the Stomach and is indicated for beri-beri and for cholera with vomiting, diarrhoea and tenesmus.
— Ramulus Mori removes obstruction from the channels and benefits the joints of the four limbs, and is thus indicated for painful joints of the limbs.
— Caulis Trachelospermi clears heat and removes obstruction from the channels and is thus indicated for Febrile Bi syndromes.

— Caulis Piperis Futokadsurae is warm in nature. It eliminates Wind and removes obstruction from the channels and is thus indicated for Cold Bi syndromes with pathogenic Wind predominating.

■ AGKISTRODON ACUTUS AND ZAOCYS

- *Bai Hua She and Wu Shao She*

Similarities
— Both eliminate Wind, remove obstruction from the channels, relieve pain and stop convulsion and are thus indicated for stubborn Wind-Damp Bi syndromes, infantile convulsion and tetanus.

Differences
— Agkistrodon is potent and toxic and is thus used in small doses, administered as a tincture, pill or powder.
— Zaocys has a weaker action and is not toxic and is thus used in large doses, administered as a decoction or tincture.

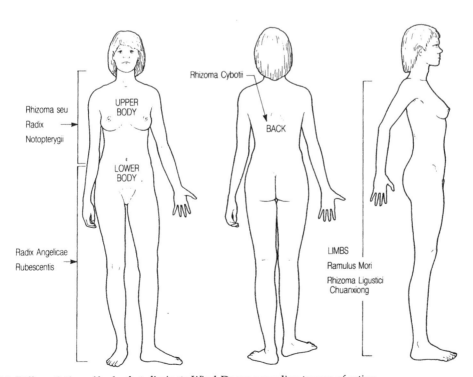

Fig. 5.1 Differentiation of herbs that eliminate Wind-Damp according to area of action.

■ RAMULUS LORANTHI, CORTEX ACANTHOPANACIS RADICIS AND RHIZOMA CIBOTII

- *Sang Ji Sheng, Wu Jia Pi and Gou Ji*

Similarities
— All eliminate Wind-Damp, tonify the Liver and Kidney and strengthen the tendons and bones, and are thus indicated for chronic Bi syndromes, weakness of the tendons and bones and lumbar pain with atrophic debility of bones.

Differences
— Ramulus Loranthi tonifies the Kidney, prevents miscarriage and lowers blood pressure and is thus used for Restless Fetus due to Kidney Deficiency and for hypertension.
— Cortex Acanthopanacis Radicis promotes diuresis and relieves swelling and is thus indicated for oedema. Acanthopanax (*Nan Wu Jia*) is more effective in eliminating Wind-Damp and strengthening the bones and tendons while Periploca Sepium (*Bai Wu Jia*) is more effective in promoting diuresis and relieving swelling.
— Rhizoma Cibotii is more effective in tonifying the Kidneys and is thus indicated for back pain (Fig. 5.1), frequent urination and leucorrhoea due to Kidney Deficiency.

Questions

1. How do Rhizoma seu Radix Notopterygii and Radix Angelicae Pubescentis differ in their actions?
2. How do Radix Gentianae Macrophyllae and Radix Stephaniae Tetrandrae differ in their actions?
3. How do Fructus Chaenomelis, Ramulus Loranthi, Ramulus Mori and Agkistrodon Acutus differ in their actions and indications?

Herbs that resolve and drain Dampness

6

A. Herbs that resolve dampness

■ RHIZOMA ATRACTYLODIS AND CORTEX MAGNOLIAE OFFICINALIS

● *Cang Zhu and Hou Po*

Similarities
— All are pungent, bitter, warm and dry in nature and thus have a drying effect on Dampness. They are indicated for patterns of Dampness invading the Spleen and Stomach, giving rise to symptoms of distension and fullness in the epigastrium and abdomen, diarrhoea and a sticky tongue coating. Because bitter and dry herbs consume Body Fluids they are contraindicated in cases of Yin Deficiency and consumption of Body Fluids.

Differences
— Rhizoma Atractylodis dries Dampness, invigorates the Spleen and eliminates Wind-Damp. It is indicated for diarrhoea and loose stools due to impairment of the Spleen's function of transportation and transformation as a result of an invasion of Dampness. It is also used for Exterior Dampness patterns and for Wind-Damp Bi syndromes.
— Cortex Magnoliae Officinalis treats Interior Dampness but also circulates Qi, conducts Rebellious Qi downward and soothes asthma. It is thus indicated for epigastric distress and abdominal distension due to stagnation of Qi and retention of Dampness in the Middle Burner, as well as for cough and wheeze due to Phlegm-Damp.

■ HERBA AGASTACHIS AND HERBA EUPATORII

● *Huo Xiang and Pei Lan*

Similarities
— Both are aromatic in nature and resolve Dampness and eliminate Summer Heat. They are indicated for retention of Dampness in the Middle Burner and for patterns of Summer Heat and Dampness.

Differences
— Herba Agastachis also Releases the Exterior and stops vomiting, and is thus indicated for Exterior patterns of Summer Heat and Dampness and for vomiting due to Turbid Damp.
— Herba Eupatorii is more effective in eliminating Summer Heat, resolving Dampness and regulating the function of the Stomach. It is thus used for poor appetite with a sweet taste and stickiness in the mouth due to Summer Heat and Dampness invading the Stomach.

■ FRUCTUS AMOMI AND SEMEN AMOMI CARDAMOMI

● *Sha Ren and Bai Dou Kou*

Similarities
— Both resolve Dampness, regulate Qi, warm the Middle Burner and stop vomiting. They are thus indicated for stagnation of Qi and Dampness giving rise to distension and pain in the epigastrium and abdomen, vomiting and a sticky tongue coating.

Differences
— Fructus Amomi is more effective in treating stagnation of Qi and Dampness in the

Middle and Lower Burners. It also invigorates the Spleen, regulates Qi and prevents miscarriage.
— Semen Amomi Cardamomi is more effective in treating stagnation of Qi and Dampness in the Middle and Upper Burners.

B. Herbs that drain dampness

■ PORIA, POLYPORUS UMBELLATUS, RHIZOMA ALISMATIS AND SEMEN COICIS

- *Fu Ling, Zhu Ling, Ze Xie and Yi Yi Ren*

Similarities
— All are bland in nature and eliminate Dampness by diuresis. They are thus indicated for oedema, dysuria, diarrhoea and retention of Phlegm and Fluid.

Differences
— Poria and Semen Coicis both invigorate the Spleen and are thus indicated for retention of Dampness due to Spleen Deficiency. Poria also calms the Mind. Semen Coicis treats Bi syndromes by draining Dampness and treats lung abscess and appendicitis by clearing Heat and draining pus. Poria peel (*Fu Ling Pi*) is more effective in promoting diuresis. Poria cum Ligno Hospite (*Fu Shen*) is more effective in calming the Mind.
— Polyporus Umbellatus and Rhizoma Alismatis strongly promote diuresis (Fig. 6.1). This is the sole action of Polyporus Umbellatus, while Rhizoma Alismatis also clears Heat from the Kidneys and Bladder and is thus used to treat Damp-Heat in the Lower Burner. It is also indicated for dizziness and vertigo due to retention of Phlegm and Fluid.

■ SEMEN PLANTAGINIS, TALCUM and CAULIS CLEMATIDIS ARMANDII

- *Che Qian Zi, Hua Shi and Chuan Mu Tong*

Similarities
— All clear heat, drain Dampness and relieve urinary disturbance and are thus indicated for urinary disturbances due to Damp-Heat in the Lower Burner.

Differences
— Semen Plantaginis clears Liver Heat and improves vision, and clears Lung Heat and resolves Phlegm. It is thus indicated for redness, swelling and pain in the eyes due to Heat and Fire in the Liver and for productive cough due to Lung Heat. This herb tends to float on the surface of a decoction and should therefore be wrapped before cooking.
— Talcum clears Summer Heat and is thus indicated for patterns of Summer Heat and Dampness. It should be wrapped before adding to a decoction to avoid making the decoction turbid.
— Caulis Clematidis Armandii clears Heart Fire, removes obstruction from the channels and promotes the secretion of milk. It is thus indicated for mouth and tongue ulcers due to Heart Fire, as well as for Febrile Bi syndromes and obstruction of milk secretion.
— Caulis Aristolochiae Manshuriensis (*Guan Mu Tong*) is toxic and it is therefore advisable not to administer it in large doses.

Warm herbs that DRY Damp

Rhizoma Atractylodis
Cortex Magnoliae Officinalis
Pericarpium Citri Reticulatae

Aromatic herbs that RESOLVE Damp

Herba Agastachis
Herba Eupatorii
Fructus Amomi
Semen Amomi Cardamomi
Pericardium Citri Reticulatae

Bland herbs that DRAIN Damp

Poria, especially the peel
Polyporus Umbellatus
Rhizoma Alismatis
Semen Coicis
Semen Plantaginis
Talcum
Caulis Clematidis Armandii
Herba Lysimachiae
Spora Lygodii
Folium Pyrrosiae

Fig. 6.1 Three ways that herbs eliminate Damp.

■ HERBA LYSIMACHIAE, SPORA LYGODII AND FOLIUM PYRROSIAE

- *Che Qian Zi, Hua Shi and Chuan Mu Tong*

Similarities
— All clear heat, drain Dampness, dissolve stones and relieve urinary disturbance and are thus indicated for urinary disturbance due to heat or complicated by stones. They are commonly used in the treatment of stones in the urinary tract.

Differences
— Herba Lysimachiae and Spora Lygodii are major herbs for stones. Herba Lysimachiae and Caulis Lygodii (*Hai Jin Sha Teng*) also clear heat, drain Dampness and relieve jaundice and are thus indicated for Damp-Heat jaundice.
— Folium Pyrrosiae also clears Lung Heat, stops cough and wheeze, cools Blood and stops bleeding. It is thus indicated for cough and wheeze due to Lung Heat, and for Blood Heat giving rise to haemoptysis, epistaxis, haematuria and uterine bleeding.

■ RHIZOMA DIOSCOREAE SEPTEMLOBAE AND HERBA ARTEMISIAE CAPILLARIS

- *Bi Xie and Yin Chen Hao*

— Herba Artemisiae Capillaris clears heat, drains Dampness and relieves jaundice. It is an important herb for jaundice.
— Rhizoma Dioscoreae Septemlobae drains Turbid Damp and is a major herb for turbid urine. It also eliminates Wind-Damp and is thus indicated for Wind-Damp Bi syndromes.

Questions

1. Compare and contrast the actions and indications of Rhizoma Atractylodis and Cortex Magnoliae Officinalis.
2. How do Herba Agastachis, Herba Eupatorii and Fructus Amomi differ in their actions?
3. How do Poria, Polyporus Umbellatus, Rhizoma Alismatis and Semen Coicis differ in their actions?
4. How do Semen Plantaginis, Caulis Clematidis Armandii, Herba Lysimachiae, Rhizoma Dioscoreae Septemlobae and Herba Artemisiae Capillaris differ in their actions and indications?

7 *Herbs that warm the Interior and regulate Qi*

A. Herbs that warm the interior

■ RADIX ACONITI PRAEPARATA, RADIX ACONITI, CORTEX CINNAMOMI AND RAMULUS CINNAMOMI

● *Fu Zi, Wu Tou, Rou Gui and Gui Zhi*

Similarities
— All warm the Interior, disperse Cold and relieve pain. They are indicated for abdominal pain due to Interior Cold and for Cold Bi syndromes.

Differences
— Radix Aconiti Praeparata and Cortex Cinnamomi both warm Kidney Yang and are thus indicated for patterns of Deficient Kidney Yang. They also warm Heart Yang and Spleen Yang and are thus indicated for pain and a cold sensation in the cardiac and abdominal regions.
— Radix Aconiti Praeparata recaptures Collapsed Yang and is a main herb for Collapse of Yang. It warms the Yang of the entire body and thus treats various patterns of Yang Deficiency.
— Cortex Cinnamomi enters the Blood. It treats abdominal pain, dysmenorrhoea and irregular menstruation due to a Cold and Deficient Lower Burner.
— Radix Aconiti Praeparata and Radix Aconiti come from the same plant. Both warm the Interior, disperse Cold and relieve pain, but Radix Aconiti is more effective in dispersing Cold, relieving pain and eliminating Wind-Damp, while Radix Aconiti Praeparata is more effective in warming Yang and

recapturing Collapsed Yang. Radix Aconiti, however, is toxic and should be administered only with caution.
— Cortex Cinnamomi and Ramulus Cinnamomi come from the same plant. Both warm the Interior and disperse Cold, warm the channels and relieve pain. Cortex Cinnamomi enters the Interior and the Lower Burner and is thus more effective in warming Kidney Yang, while Ramulus Cinnamomi goes to the Exterior and the four limbs, and is more effective in Releasing the Exterior and invigorating Yang (Fig. 7.1).

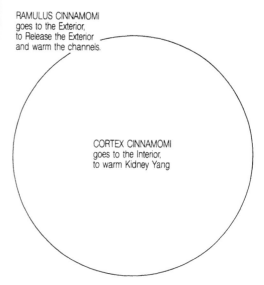

DIFFERENTIATION OF CORTEX CINNAMOMI AND RAMULUS CINNAMOMI

RAMULUS CINNAMOMI goes to the Exterior, to Release the Exterior and warm the channels.

CORTEX CINNAMOMI goes to the Interior, to warm Kidney Yang

Fig. 7.1 Differentiation of Cortex Cinnamomi and Ramulus Cinnamomi.

■ RHIZOMA ZINGIBERIS, BAKED GINGER, RHIZOMA ZINGIBERIS RECENS AND RHIZOMA ALPINIAE OFFICINALIS

● *Gan Jiang, Pao Jiang, Sheng Jiang and Gao Liang Jiang*

Similarities
— All warm the Middle Burner and disperse Cold and are thus indicated for Cold patterns of the Middle Burner.

Differences
— Rhizoma Zingiberis is a major herb to warm Spleen Yang. It also recaptures Collapsed Yang, warms the Lungs and resolves retained Fluid.
— Baked ginger is more effective in warming the channels and stopping bleeding. It is indicated for haemorrhagic patterns due to failure of the Spleen to hold the Blood within the vessels, with an underlying pattern of Spleen Yang Deficiency.
— Rhizoma Zingiberis Recens is more effective in warming the Middle Burner, stopping vomiting and Releasing the Exterior.
— Rhizoma Alpiniae Officinalis is more effective in warming the stomach and relieving pain and is thus indicated for epigastric pain due to Cold in the stomach.
— Rhizoma Zingiberis and Radix Aconiti Praeparata both recapture Collapsed Yang and warm Spleen Yang, but Radix Aconiti Praeparata is more effective in warming Kidney Yang and recapturing Collapsed Yang while Rhizoma Zingiberis is more effective in warming Spleen Yang. Rhizoma Zingiberis has the additional actions of warming the Lungs and resolving retained Fluid, warming the channels and stopping bleeding.

■ FRUCTUS EVODIAE, FRUCTUS FOENICULI, FLOS CARYOPHYLLI AND PERICARPIUM ZANTHOXYLI

● *Wu Zhu Yu, Xiao Hui Xiang, Ding Xiang and Hua Jiao*

Similarities
— All warm the Interior, disperse Cold and relieve pain and are indicated for pain in the epigastrium and abdomen due to Cold.

Differences
— Fructus Evodiae and Fructus Foeniculi both warm the Liver and disperse Cold and are indicated for periumbilical colic due to invasion by Cold. Fructus Evodiae also warms the Middle Burner and conducts Rebellious Qi downward and is thus indicated for epigastric pain and vomiting due to Cold in the stomach, and for epigastric pain and acid regurgitation due to disharmony between the Liver and Stomach. It is also used to treat Jue Yin headache with vomiting of Phlegm due to upward perversion of Liver Qi with Turbid Phlegm. Fructus Foeniculi is indicated only for periumbilical colic due to invasion of Cold.
— Flos Caryophylli and Pericarpium Zanthoxyli both warm the Middle Burner, relieve pain and stop vomiting and are thus indicated for epigastric pain and vomiting due to Cold in the Stomach. Flos Caryophylli is more effective in conducting Rebellious Qi downward, and is an important herb for vomiting and hiccup. It also warms Kidney Yang and is indicated for impotence due to Kidney Yang Deficiency (Fig. 7.2). Pericarpium Zanthoxyli also kills parasites and is thus indicated for abdominal pain due to ascariasis.

B. Herbs that regulate Qi

■ PERICARPIUM CITRI RETICULATAE AND PERICARPIUM CITRI RETICULATAE VIRIDE

● *Chen Pi and Qing Pi*

Similarities
— Both herbs come from the same plant. The first is ripe tangerine peel while the second is the unripe fruit or its green peel. Both regulate Qi and resolve Phlegm.

Differences
— Pericarpium Citri Reticulatae has a mild action in dispersing stagnation of Qi in the Spleen and Stomach but it also resolves Dampness and Phlegm. It is primarily used for patterns of Damp Phlegm.
— Pericarpium Citri Reticulatae Viride has a stronger action in promoting the smooth circulation of Liver Qi and dispersing

Exterior and channels		Ramulus Cinnamomi Baked ginger Rhizoma Zingiberis
Upper burner		Radix Aconiti Praeparata Cortex Cinnamomi Rhizoma Zingiberis
Middle burner	(Spleen/Stomach)	Radix Aconiti Praeparata Cortex Cinnamomi Rhizoma Zingiberis Rhizoma Zingiberis Recens Baked ginger Rhizoma Alpiniae Officinalis Flos Caryophylli Pericarpium Zanthoxyli
	(Liver)	Fructus Evodiae Fructus Foeniculi
Lower Burner (Kidney Yang)		Radix Aconiti Praeparata Cortex Cinnamomi Flos Caryophylli
Note that Radix Aconiti Praeparata and Cortex Cinnamomi go to all three Burners.		

Fig. 7.2 Differentiation of warming herbs by area of action.

stagnation, and it is thus indicated for abdominal masses and Food Retention patterns.

■ FRUCTUS AURANTII IMMATURUS AND FRUCTUS AURANTII

- *Zhi Shi and Zhi Qiao*

Similarities
— Both circulate Qi, resolve Phlegm and relieve stagnation and are thus indicated for stagnation of Qi and Phlegm and Retention of Food. They activate the smooth muscles of the stomach, intestines and uterus and are indicated for prolapse of the internal organs. They are administered by injection in the treatment of shock.

Differences
— Fructus Aurantii Immaturus is more effective in relieving Qi stagnation in the Middle and Lower Burners and is thus indicated for distension and pain in the epigastrium and abdomen.
— Fructus Aurantii is more effective in relieving Qi stagnation in the Middle and Upper Burners and is thus indicated for distension and fullness in the epigastrium and chest.

— Fructus Aurantii Immaturus, Fructus Aurantii and Pericarpium Citri Reticulatae all relieve stagnation in the Spleen and Stomach, but Fructus Aurantii Immaturus and Fructus Aurantii are more effective in regulating Qi than Pericarpium Citri Reticulatae. Pericarpium Citri Reticulatae is warm in nature and acts primarily to dry Dampness and resolve Phlegm while Fructus Aurantii and Fructus Aurantii Immaturus are Cold in nature and disperse Food Retention.

■ FRUCTUS CITRI SARCODACTYLIS and FRUCTUS CITRI

- *Fo Shou and Xiang Yuan*

Similarities
— Both disperse stagnation of Qi in the Liver and Stomach and resolve Phlegm and are indicated for epigastric pain due to disharmony between the Liver and Stomach.

Differences
— Fructus Citri Sarcodactylis acts gently to harmonize the Stomach and stop vomiting.
— Fructus Citri has a stronger action and is similar to Pericarpium Citri Reticulatae Viride in promoting the smooth circulation

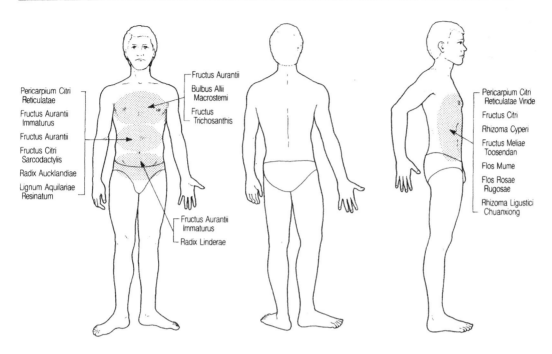

Fig. 7.3 Differentiation of herbs that regulate Qi according to areas of action.

of Liver Qi and dispersing stagnant Qi (Fig. 7.3).

■ RHIZOMA CYPERI, RADIX AUCKLANDIAE, RADIX LINDERAE AND LIGNUM AQUILARIAE RESINATUM

- *Xiang Fu, Mu Xiang, Wu Yao and Chen Xiang*

Similarities
— All are pungent and warm in nature, and regulate Qi and relieve pain. They are indicated for pain in the epigastrium and abdomen due to stagnation of Qi and Cold.

Differences
— Rhizoma Cyperi promotes the smooth circulation of Liver Qi and regulates menstruation and is an important herb for patterns of Liver Qi Stagnation, irregular menstruation and dysmenorrhoea.
— Radix Aucklandiae regulates Spleen and Stomach Qi, invigorates the Spleen and stops diarrhoea, and is thus indicated for epigastric and abdominal pain, diarrhoea and dysentery due to stagnation of Qi in the

Spleen and Stomach. It is used raw to regulate Qi and roasted to invigorate the Spleen and stop diarrhoea.
— Radix Linderae warms the Lower Burner and is indicated for pain and a cold sensation in the lower abdomen.
— Lignum Aquilariae Resinatum warms the Interior, disperses Cold, regulates Qi and conducts Rebellious Qi downward. It stops vomiting by warming the Stomach and conducting Rebellious Stomach Qi downward, and treats asthma by conducting Rebellious Lung Qi downward and warming the Kidneys so they receive the Qi. It is added to a decoction at the end of cooking or is administered as a powder.

■ FRUCTUS MELIAE TOOSENDAN and RHIZOMA CORYDALIS

- *Chuan Lian Zi and Yan Hu Suo*

Similarities
— Both regulate Qi and relieve pain and are indicated for epigastric and abdominal pain due to stagnation of Qi in the Liver and Stomach. They are often used in combination.

Differences

— Fructus Meliae Toosendan clears Liver Heat and promotes the smooth circulation of Liver Qi and is indicated for pain and a sensation of heat. It also expels parasites.
— Rhizoma Corydalis is more effective in relieving pain as it also invigorates the circulation of Blood. It is indicated for pain due to Qi and Blood Stagnation.

■ BULBUS ALLII MACROSTEMI AND FRUCTUS TRICHOSANTHIS

- *Xie Bai and Gua Lou*

Similarities

— Both regulate Qi, open the chest and invigorate Yang and are thus indicated for Chest Bi syndromes due to retention of Turbid Phlegm and hindrance of Heart Yang.

Differences

— Bulbus Allii Macrostemi is pungent and warm in nature and is more effective in invigorating Yang than Fructus Trichosanthis. It also circulates Qi and disperses stagnation and is indicated for dysentery with symptoms of abdominal pain and tenesmus.
— Fructus Trichosanthis is more effective in resolving Phlegm than Bulbus Allii Macrostemi. It also moistens the lungs and stops cough and moistens the intestines and relieves constipation.

■ FLOS MUME and FLOS ROSAE RUGOSAE

- *Lu E Mei and Mei Gui Hua*

Similarities

— Both promote the smooth circulation of Liver Qi and are indicated for stuffiness of the chest, hypochondriac pain and mental depression due to Liver Qi Stagnation. They regulate Qi without injuring Qi and Yin but do not have a strong action.

Differences

— Flos Mume is more effective in relieving depression and is thus indicated for depressive patterns.
— Flos Rosae Rugosae activates Blood circulation and regulates menstruation and is thus

indicated for irregular menstruation and dysmenorrhoea due to Qi and Blood Stagnation resulting from Stagnation of Liver Qi.

Questions

1. How do Radix Aconiti Praeparata and Radix Aconiti differ in their actions and indications?
2. How do Radix Aconiti Praeparata, Rhizoma Zingiberis and Cortex Cinnamomi differ in their actions and indications?
3. How do Rhizoma Zingiberis, Rhizoma Zingiberis Recens and Baked ginger differ in their actions and indications?
4. How do Cortex Cinnamomi and Ramulus Cinnamomi differ in their actions and indications?
5. Compare and contrast the actions of Fructus Evodiae, Rhizoma Alpiniae Officinalis and Flos Caryophylli.
6. Compare and contrast the actions and indications of Pericarpium Citri Reticulatae and Pericarpium Citri Reticulatae Viride.
7. Compare and contrast the actions and indications of Fructus Aurantii Immaturus and Fructus Aurantii.
8. Radix Aucklandiae, Rhizoma Cyperi, Radix Linderae, Lignum Aquilariae Resinatum, Fructus Meliae Toosendan and Rhizoma Corydalis all regulate Qi and relieve pain. How do they differ?

Herbs that regulate Blood **8**

A. Herbs that stop bleeding

■ HERBA SEU RADIX CIRSII JAPONICI AND HERBA CEPHALANOPLORIS

● *Da Ji and Xiao Ji*

Similarities
— Both cool Blood, stop bleeding and clear Fire Poison. They are thus indicated for bleeding due to Blood Heat and for ulcers and boils due to Fire Poison. They also lower blood pressure and are thus indicated for hypertension.

Differences
— Herba seu Radix Cirsii Japonici is more effective in treating haemoptysis and haematemesis. It has a strong action in clearing Fire Poison
— Herba Cephalanoploris is more effective in treating haematuria.

■ RADIX SANGUISORBAE AND FLOS SOPHORAE

● *Di Yu and Huai Hua*

Similarities
— Both cool Blood and stop bleeding and are indicated for bloody stool or bleeding due to haemorrhoids.

Differences
— Radix Sanguisorbae cools Blood and stops dysentery, and clears Fire Poison and acts on the skin. It is thus indicated for bloody dysentery, carbuncles, boils, ulcers and burns.
— Flos Sophorae is more effective in stopping bleeding due to haemorrhoids. It also clears Liver Fire and is indicated for headache and redness of the eyes.

■ FOLIUM CALLICARPAE, CACUMEN BIOTAE AND RADIX BOEHMERIAE

● *Zi Zhu, Ce Bai Ye and Zhu Me Gen*

Similarities
— All cool Blood and stop bleeding and are indicated for various haemorrhagic patterns due to Heat.

Differences
— Folium Callicarpae is more effective in stopping bleeding in various haemorrhagic patterns. It also clears Heat and Fire Poison and is thus indicated for carbuncles, boils, ulcers and burns.
— Cacumen Biotae is more effective in stopping bleeding in the digestive and respiratory tracts. It also resolves Phlegm and stops cough. It can be combined with herbs that warm the channels and stop bleeding to treat bleeding due to deficiency and cold.
— Radix Boehmeriae stops bleeding and prevents miscarriage and is thus indicated for uterine bleeding and threatened abortion.

■ RHIZOMA BLETILLAE, HERBA AGRIMONIAE AND NODUS NELUMBINIS RHIZOMATIS

● *Bai Ji, Xian He Cao and Ou Jie*

Similarities
— All stop bleeding by astringing and are indicated for various haemorrhagic patterns.

Differences
— Rhizoma Bletillae effectively stops bleeding in various haemorrhagic patterns. It also relieves swelling and promotes healing and is thus indicated for haemoptysis due to cavernous pulmonary tuberculosis and

for chronic festering abscesses, ulcers and boils.
— Herba Agrimoniae is indicated for pulmonary tuberculosis with cough and for Food Retention with diarrhoea, Blood Deficiency due to overwork and stress, and cancer.
— Nodus Nelumbinis Rhizomatis is used in its raw form to cool Blood, dispel Blood Stasis and stop bleeding. It is charred to stop bleeding by astringing.

■ PETIOLUS TRACHYCARPI CARBONISATUS AND CRINIS CARBONISATUS

● *Zong Lu Tan and Xue Yu Tan*

Similarities
— Both stop bleeding by astringing and are indicated for haemorrhagic patterns.

Differences
— Petiolus Trachycarpi Carbonisatus is strongly astringent and can thus aggravate Blood Stasis. It is often used in the treatment of uterine bleeding.
— Crinis Carbonisatus not only astringes to stop bleeding but also treats Blood Stasis and is thus more widely used. It is often used in the treatment of uterine bleeding, haemoptysis, haematemesis, epistaxis and bloody stool.

■ RADIX NOTOGINSENG, RADIX RUBIAE AND POLLEN TYPHAE

● *San Qi, Qian Cao and Pu Huang*

Similarities
— All treat Blood Stasis and stop bleeding and are thus used for haemorrhagic patterns. They are most effective in the treatment of bleeding complicated with Blood Stasis.

Differences
— Radix Notoginseng not only effectively stops bleeding but also resolves Blood Stasis and stops pain. It thus stops bleeding without causing Stasis and treats Stasis without injuring Upright Qi. In addition to treating haemorrhagic patterns it is a major herb for the treatment of Stagnant

Blood and pain due to trauma. It is also indicated for various patterns of Blood Stagnation in internal medicine and gynaecology.
— Radix Rubiae cools and moves Blood, stops bleeding and regulates menstruation. It is thus indicated for haemorrhagic patterns due to Blood Heat complicated with Stasis, as well as amenorrhoea and dysmenorrhoea due to Blood Stasis, contusions and sprains and Wind-Damp Bi syndromes.
— Pollen Typhae resolves Blood Stasis and promotes diuresis and is thus indicated for urinary disorders with haematuria. In its raw form it is more effective in resolving Blood Stasis and relieving pain, while its stir-baked form is more effective in stopping bleeding.

■ FOLIUM ARTEMISIAE ARGYI, BAKED YELLOW EARTH AND BAKED GINGER

● *Ai Ye, Zao Xin Tu and Pao Jiang*

Similarities
— All warm the channels and stop bleeding and are thus indicated for Deficient and Cold haemorrhagic patterns.

Differences
— Folium Artemisiae Argyi warms the uterus and regulates menstruation and is thus indicated for uterine bleeding and dysmenorrhoea due to Deficiency and Cold. It treats infertility due to Cold in the Uterus and prevents miscarriage. It also soothes asthma and is thus used in the treatment of asthma due to Cold. It is also used for moxibustion.
— Baked yellow earth warms the Middle Burner and stops bleeding and diarrhoea. It is thus indicated for bleeding due to a failure of Spleen Yang to control the Blood and for vomiting and diarrhoea due to a cold and Deficient Spleen and Stomach. Halloysitum Rubrum (*Chi Shi Zhi*) may be used as a substitute.
— Baked ginger warms the channels and stops bleeding and is a major herb in the treatment of bleeding due to a failure of Spleen Yang to control the Blood (Fig. 8.1). It also treats abdominal pain and diarrhoea due to a Cold and Deficient Middle Burner.

Cause of bleeding	What to do
Heat Blood becomes reckless and escapes from vessels	*Cool Blood:* Herba seu Radix Cirsii Japonici Herba Cephalanoploris Radix Sanguisorbae Flos Sophorae Flos Callicarpae Cacumen Biotae Radix Boehmerae
Stasis Blood cannot flow within vessels so flows outside them	*Activate circulation of Blood within the vessels:* Crinus Carbonisatus Radix Notoginseng Radix Rubiae Pollen Typhae
Deficiency The Spleen fails to hold the Blood within the vessels	*Strengthen the Spleen's function of holding the Blood; warm the channels:* Baked yellow earth Halloysitum Rubrum Baked ginger
Any cause	*Astringents will stop bleeding, but treat only the Biao:* Rhizoma Bletillae Herba Agrimoniae Nodus Nelumbinis Rhizomatis Petiolus Trachycarpi Carbonisatus Crinus Carbonisatus

Fig. 8.1 Treatment of bleeding.

B. Herbs that invigorate Blood circulation and resolve Blood Stasis

■ **RHIZOMA LIGUSTICI CHUANXIONG AND RADIX SALVIAE MILTIORRHIZAE**

● *Chuan Xiong and Dan Shen*

Similarities
— Both are important herbs to invigorate Blood circulation and resolve Blood Stasis. They relieve pain and regulate menstruation and are thus indicated for various patterns of Blood Stagnation including amenorrhoea, dysmenorrhoea, palpable masses and cardiac and abdominal pain due to Stagnation of Blood.

Differences
— Rhizoma Ligustici Chuanxiong also regulates Qi and eliminates Wind. It acts on the head and eyes and is an important herb

for headache. Because it relieves stagnation in the Middle, it is indicated for costal and hypochondriac pain and abdominal pain due to Stagnation of Qi and Blood. Because it removes obstruction from the channels and collaterals of the four limbs, it treats Wind-Damp Bi syndromes.
— Radix Salviae Miltiorrhizae cools Blood and calms the Mind and is thus indicated for restlessness and coma due to Heat at the Nutritive (Ying) level, and restlessness and insomnia following a long-term illness. It also treats carbuncles, boils and ulcers.

■ **RADIX CURCUMAE, RHIZOMA CURCUMAE LONGAE, RHIZOMA SPARGANII AND RHIZOMA ZEDOARIAE**

● *Yu Jin, Jiang Huang, San Leng and E Zhu*

Similarities
— All primarily invigorate Blood circulation

and secondarily regulate Qi and are thus indicated for patterns of Stagnant Blood and Qi.

Differences
— Radix Curcumae soothes the Liver and Gall Bladder, cools Blood, relieves Stagnation and opens the orifices. It is thus indicated for Stagnation of Liver Qi, Damp-Heat in the Liver and Gall Bladder, Phlegm and Stagnant Blood Misting the Heart and rising of Stagnant Qi and Fire with symptoms of haemoptysis and epistaxis.
— Rhizoma Curcumae Longae removes obstruction from the channels and relieves pain and is thus indicated for pain in the chest, hypochondrium and limbs and for Wind-Damp Bi syndromes.
— Rhizoma Sparganii and Rhizoma Zedoariae both break Stagnant Qi and Blood and are thus indicated for palpable abdominal masses. Rhizoma Sparganii is more effective in breaking Stagnant Blood. Rhizoma Zedoariae is more effective in moving Stagnant Qi and also treats cancer.

■ RESINA OLIBANI AND RESINA MYRRHAE

● *Ru Xiang and Mo Yao*

Similarities
— Both invigorate Blood and Qi circulation, relieve pain and swelling and promote healing. They are thus indicated for pain due to Stagnation of Qi and Blood, carbuncles, boils and ulcers, and contusions and sprains. They are important herbs in the treatment of skin diseases and trauma and are often used in combination. They should not be prescribed in large doses, especially in cases of weakness of the Spleen and Stomach.

Differences
— Resina Olibani is more effective in moving Qi while Resina Myrrhae is more effective in resolving Blood Stasis.

■ RADIX ACHYRANTHIS BIDENTATAE, RHIZOMA POLYGONI CUSPIDATI AND HERBA LEONURI

● *Niu Xi, Hu Zhang and Yi Mu Cao*

Similarities
— All invigorate Blood circulation, resolve Blood Stasis and eliminate Dampness. They are indicated for patterns of Blood Stagnation, oedema due to Dampness in the Lower Burner and urinary disorders with turbid urine.

Differences
— Radix Achyranthis Bidentatae tonifies the Liver and Kidneys, strengthens tendons and bones and conducts Fire and Blood downward. It is indicated for pain in the lower back and knees, headache, dizziness and vertigo due to rising of Fire, and haemoptysis and epistaxis.
— Rhizoma Polygoni Cuspidati eliminates Dampness, relieves jaundice and clears Heat and Fire Poison. It is indicated for jaundice, cough due to Lung Heat, burns, urinary and biliary stones, abscess and swelling due to Fire Poison, and Wind-Damp Bi syndromes.
— Herba Leonuri invigorates Blood circulation and regulates menstruation and is thus indicated for dysmenorrhoea, irregular menstruation and postpartum abdominal pain due to Blood Stagnation. It is commonly used in gynaecology.

■ SEMEN PERSICAE, FLOS CARTHAMI AND CAULIS SPATHOLOBI

● *Tao Ren, Hong Hua and Ji Xue Teng*

Similarities
— All invigorate Blood circulation and resolve Blood Stasis and are thus indicated for patterns of Stagnant Blood.

Differences
— Semen Persicae and Flos Carthami are commonly used to invigorate Blood circulation and resolve Stasis. Semen Persicae also moistens the intestines to relieve constipation and resolves abscess, and is thus indicated for both internal and external abscess and for constipation due to dry

intestines. Flos Carthami invigorates Blood circulation and regulates menstruation, and is thus often used in gynaecology.
— Caulis Spatholobi moves both Qi and Blood, nourishes Blood and relaxes the muscles and tendons, and is thus indicated for Stagnation and Deficiency of Blood, Wind-Damp Bi syndromes and numbness.

■ FAECES TROGOPTERORUM, SQUAMA MANITIS, EUPOLYPHAGA SEU STELEOPHAGA AND HIRUDO

- *Wu Ling Zhi, Chuan Shan Jia, Di Bie Chong and Shui Zhi*

Similarities
— All act strongly to invigorate Blood circulation and resolve Stasis and are thus indicated for severe Blood Stasis and palpable abdominal masses.

Differences
— Faeces Trogopterorum is more effective in resolving Stasis and relieving pain. It also stops bleeding. It is often combined with Pollen Typhae.
— Squama Manitis is effective in promoting the secretion of milk, draining pus and relieving swelling.

— Eupolyphaga seu Steleophaga promotes the healing of fractures and torn tendons and is thus an important herb in traumatology. Hirudo strongly dispels Blood Stasis. It is reported to be useful in the treatment of intracranial haematoma and thrombocytosis (Fig. 8.2).

Questions

1. In what ways do Herba Cephalanoploris, Rhizoma Bletillae, Radix Notoginseng and Folium Artemisiae stop bleeding? What are their other actions?
2. Apart from stopping bleeding, what are the actions and indications of Radix Boehmeriae, Cacumen Biotae and Herba Agrimoniae?
3. Compare and contrast the actions and indications of Rhizoma Ligustici Chuanxiong, Radix Salviae Miltiorrhizae, Semen Persicae, Flos Carthami and Radix Achyranthis Bidentatae.
4. How do Resina Olibani and Resina Myrrhae differ in their actions?
5. How do Radix Curcumae, Rhizoma Sparganii and Rhizoma Zedoariae differ in their actions?

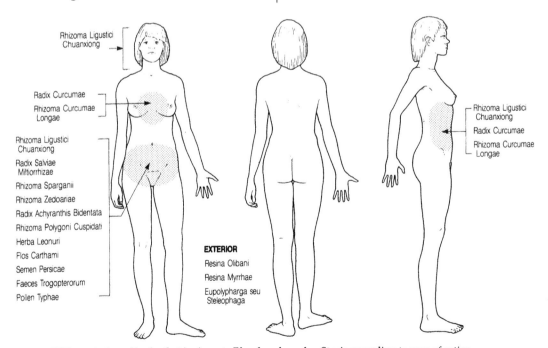

Fig. 8.2 Differentiation of herbs that invigorate Blood and resolve Stasis according to area of action.

9

Herbs that calm the Mind and the Liver and extinguish Wind

A. Herbs that calm the mind

■ CINNABARIS, MAGNETITUM, OS DRACONIS AND SUCCINUM

- *Zhu Sha, Ci Shi, Long Gu and Hu Po*

Similarities
— All soothe the Heart and calm the Mind and are thus indicated for Excess patterns giving rise to palpitations, insomnia and manic and depressive disorders.

Differences
— Cinnabaris strongly calms the Mind. It also clears Heart and Liver Fire and Fire Poison. It is thus indicated for restlessness due to Heart and Liver Fire and for carbuncles, boils, ulcers and swelling and pain in the mouth and throat due to Fire Poison. It is used to coat and dye other herbs that calm the Mind before they are decocted and to coat pills to enhance their effect in calming the Mind. It also prevents putrefaction.
— Cinnabaris is, however, toxic and should be administered only in small doses and for a short time.
— Magnetitum calms the Liver and suppresses hyperactive Yang, and assists the reception of Qi and soothes asthma. It is thus indicated for headache, dizziness, vertigo and tinnitus due to hyperactive Liver Yang and for asthma due to Kidney Deficiency.
— Os Draconis calms the Liver and suppresses hyperactive Yang, and astringes discharges. It is thus indicated for Liver Yang Rising and for spontaneous sweating, night sweating, spermatorrhoea and leucorrhoea. Succinum is most effective in calming the Mind but also resolves Blood Stasis and relieves urinary disorders. It is thus indicated for

amenorrhoea and for painful and difficult urination.

■ SEMEN ZIZIPHI SPINOSAE AND SEMEN BIOTAE

- *Suan Zao Ren and Bai Zi Ren*

Similarities
— Both nourish the Heart and calm the Mind and are thus indicated for Deficiency patterns giving rise to palpitations and insomnia.

Differences
— Semen Ziziphi Spinosae also nourishes Yin and astringes sweating and is thus indicated for night sweats due to Yin Deficiency. Semen Biotae also moistens the intestines to relieve constipation and is thus indicated for dry constipation due to Yin and Blood Deficiency.

■ RADIX POLYGALAE AND CORTEX ALBIZIAE

- *Yuan Zhi and He Huan Pi*

Similarities
— Both calm the Mind and resolve Phlegm and are indicated for insomnia due to restlessness.

Differences
— Radix Polygalae is more effective in resolving Phlegm and is thus indicated for cough with profuse sputum and for unconsciousness due to Phlegm Misting the Heart.
— Cortex Albiziae resolves Stagnation, invigorates Blood circulation and resolves abscess and is indicated for mental depression and lung abscess.

B. Herbs that calm the Liver and extinguish Wind

■ CONCHA HALIOTIDIS, CONCHA OSTREAE, MARGARITA, CONCHA MARGARITIFERA USTA AND HAEMATITUM

- *Shi Jue Ming, Mu Li, Zhen Zhu, Zhen Zhu Mu and Dai Zhe Shi*

Similarities
— All calm the Liver and suppress hyperactive Yang and are thus indicated for headache, dizziness and vertigo due to Liver Yang Rising.

Differences
— Concha Haliotidis is more effective in calming the Liver and suppressing hyperactive Yang. It also clears Liver Heat and improves vision. It is thus indicated for redness, swelling and pain of the eyes due to flaring of Liver Fire and for blurring of vision due to Deficiency of Liver Yin.
— Concha Ostreae soothes the Heart, calms the Mind, astringes discharges and softens hard masses. It is thus indicated for restlessness, spontaneous sweating, night sweats, spermatorrhoea, leucorrhoea and tuberculosis of lymph nodes.
— Margarita and Concha Margaritifera Usta both soothe the Heart, calm the Mind and improve vision. Margarita also stops convulsion and astringes ulcers and is thus indicated for infantile convulsions, epilepsy and chronic festering ulcers and boils. Concha Margaritifera Usta is more effective in soothing the Heart, calming the Mind, calming the Liver and suppressing hyperactive Yang.
— Haematitum conducts Rebellious Qi downward, stops vomiting, relieves asthma, soothes the Heart and calms the Mind. It also stops bleeding by sending Qi and Fire downward. Os Draconis and Concha Ostreae both calm the Liver and suppress hyperactive Yang, soothe the Heart and calm the Mind. Os Draconis is more effective in soothing the Heart and calming the Mind, while Concha Ostreae is more effective in calming the Liver and suppressing hyperactive Yang. Concha Ostreae also astringes discharges and softens hard masses.

■ CORNU ANTELOPIS, RAMULUS UNCARIAE CUM UNCIS AND RHIZOMA GASTRODIAE

- *Ling Yang Jiao, Gou Teng and Tian Ma*

Similarities
— All calm the Liver and extinguish Wind and are indicated for headache, dizziness and vertigo due to Liver Yang Rising and for dizziness and convulsion due to Liver Wind.

Differences
— Cornu Antelopis strongly clears Liver Fire, suppresses hyperactive Liver Yang and extinguishes Liver Wind. It also clears Liver Heat and improves vision, and clears Heat and Fire Poison.
— Ramulus Uncariae cum Uncis clears Liver Heat and extinguishes Liver Wind and is thus indicated for stirring of Liver Wind due to Heat or excessive Yang. It is added at the end of a decoction.
— Rhizoma Gastrodiae extinguishes Wind and removes obstruction from the channels and is thus indicated for Wind-Damp Bi syndromes, numbness and tetanus.

■ FRUCTUS TRIBULI AND FOLIUM APOCYNI VENETI

- *Ci Ji Li and Luo Bu Ma*

Similarities
— Both suppress hyperactive Liver Yang and extinguish Liver Wind and are thus indicated for headache, dizziness and vertigo due to Liver Yang Rising and upward stirring of Liver Wind.

Differences
— Fructus Tribuli expels External Wind, improves vision and soothes the Liver. It is thus indicated for eye disorders due to Wind-Heat and hypochondriac pain due to Stagnation of Liver Qi.
— Folium Apocyni Veneti promotes diuresis, relieves swelling and stops cough and wheeze. It is indicated for hypertension, bronchitis, oedema and heart disease with palpitations.

■ SCORPIO, SCOLOPENDRA, BOMBYX BATRYTICATUS AND LUMBRICUS

- *Quan Xie, Wu Gong, Jiang Can and Di Long*

Similarities
— All extinguish Wind and stop convulsion and are thus indicated for convulsions due to Liver Wind, Wind-Stroke due to Heat stirring Liver Wind, infantile convulsions, epilepsy and tetanus.

Differences
— Scorpio and Scolopendra have a strong action in extinguishing Liver Wind and stopping convulsion. They also remove obstruction from the channels, relieve pain, clear Fire Poison and disperse masses. They are thus indicated for stubborn Wind-Damp Bi syndromes, chronic or unilateral headache, hemiplegia, tuberculosis of the lymph nodes, carbuncles, boils, ulcers and cancer. Scorpio is more effective in extinguishing Wind while Scolopendra is more effective in clearing Fire Poison.
— Bombyx Batryticatus eliminates Wind-Heat, resolves Phlegm and disperses masses. It is thus indicated for Wind-Heat patterns with symptoms of sore throat, rubella, redness of the eyes or headache and for subcutaneous nodules or tuberculosis of the lymph nodes.
— Lumbricus clears Heat, soothes asthma, removes obstruction from the channels and promotes diuresis. It is thus indicated for asthma with sputum due to Lung Heat, Febrile Bi syndromes and dysuria and oedema due to retention of Heat in the Bladder.

Questions

1. Cinnabaris, Semen Biotae and Semen Ziziphi Spinosae all calm the Mind. In what different ways do they do this? What other actions do each of them have?
2. Compare and contrast the actions and indications of Os Draconis and Concha Ostreae.
3. Compare and contrast the actions and indications of Magnetitum and Haematitum.

Herbs that Suppress Liver Yang and/or Extinguish Liver Wind

Cinnabaris
Magnetitum
Os Draconis
Succinum
Concha Haliotidis
Concha Ostreae
Concha Margaritifera Usta
Haematitum
Cornu Antelopis
Ramulus Uncaria cum Uncis
Rhizoma Gastrodiae
Fructus Tribuli
Scorpio
Scolopendra
Bombyx Batryticatus
Lumbricus

Herbs that Nourish Heart Blood and Yin

Semen Ziziphi Spinosae
Semen Biotae

Herbs that Resolve Phlegm

Radix Polygalae
Cortex Albiziae
Bombyx Batryticatus

Herbs that Resolve Stagnation
Cortex Albiziae
Fructus Tribuli
Radix Polygalae

Fig. 9.1 Herbs that calm the Mind: a comparable table of actions.

4. Compare and contrast the actions and indications of Rhizoma Gastrodiae and Ramulus Uncariae cum Uncis.
5. Compare and contrast the actions and indications of Scorpio, Scolopendra, Bombyx Batryticatus and Lumbricus.

Tonics

10

A. Qi Tonics

■ **RADIX GINSENG, RADIX PANACIS QUINQUEFOLII, RADIX CODONOPSIS PILOSULAE, RADIX PSEUDOSTELLARIAE AND RADIX ASTRAGALI SEU HEDYSARI**

● *Ren Shen, Xi Yang Shen, Dang Shen, Tai Zi Shen and Huang Qi*

Similarities
— All tonify Spleen and Lung Qi and are thus indicated for Spleen Qi Deficiency, Lung Qi Deficiency and other patterns of Qi Deficiency. By tonifying Qi they also produce Blood and are thus indicated for Blood Deficiency.

Differences
— Radix Ginseng strongly tonifies Source (Yuan) Qi and is used to treat Collapse of Qi. It is the strongest of the Qi tonics and is an important herb for shock. It also produces Body Fluids, calms the Mind and improves intelligence and is thus indicated for thirst due to consumption of Body Fluids, Wasting and Thirsting syndromes, palpitations, poor memory and insomnia. By tonifying Qi it also controls Blood and is thus indicated for haemorrhagic patterns.
— Radix Ginseng Rubra (*Hong Shen*) is warm in nature, while Radix Ginseng Alba (*Bai Shen*) is neutral. Radix Ginseng should be decocted separately from other ingredients of a prescription by simmering.
— Radix Panacis Quinquefolii strongly nourishes Yin. It also clears Fire and is thus indicated for Empty Fire due to Lung and Stomach Yin Deficiency.
— Radix Codonopsis Pilosulae and Radix Pseudostellariae are similar to Radix Ginseng in action but are weaker. They are indicated for patterns of general Qi Deficiency. Radix Pseudostellariae is less effective in tonifying Qi than Radix Codonopsis Pilosulae, but it is neutral in nature and also produces Body Fluids and is thus indicated for patterns of combined Qi and Yin Deficiency.
— Radix Astragali seu Hedysari is similar to Radix Codonopsis Pilosulae in tonifying Qi. It also lifts Yang, promotes diuresis, consolidates the Exterior and promotes the drainage of pus and tissue regeneration. It is thus indicated for Sinking of Qi and oedema due to Spleen Deficiency, spontaneous sweating in Deficiency-type Exterior patterns, frequent invasion by External pathogenic factors due to Qi Deficiency, chronic carbuncles due to Qi and Blood Deficiency, and Fire Poison at a deep level. Its raw form goes to the surface and thus acts to consolidate the Exterior, promote diuresis and the draining of pus and speed tissue regeneration. Its treated form goes to the Interior and thus acts to tonify the Middle Burner, benefit Qi and lift Yang (Fig. 10.1).

■ **RHIZOMA ATRACTYLODIS MACROCEPHALAE, RHIZOMA DIOSCOREAE AND SEMEN DOLICHORIS**

● *Bai Zhu, Shan Yao and Bian Dou*

Similarities
— All tonify Qi and invigorate the Spleen and

Raw	Toasted
Consolidates the Exterior	Tonifies the Middle Burner
Promotes tissue regeneration	Lifts Yang

Fig. 10.1 Actions of Astragali seu Hedysari.

are thus indicated for diarrhoea, loose stools and leucorrhoea due to Spleen Qi Deficiency.

Differences
— Rhizoma Atractylodis Macrocephalae is dry in nature. It dries Dampness, promotes diuresis, stops sweating and prevents miscarriage. It is indicated for retention of fluid and Dampness due to Spleen Deficiency and for spontaneous sweating and threatened abortion. Both Rhizoma Atractylodis and Rhizoma Atractylodis Macrocephalae dry Dampness and invigorate the Spleen, but Rhizoma Atractylodis Macrocephalae is more effective in tonifying Qi and invigorating the Spleen while Rhizoma Atractylodis is more effective in drying Dampness. The latter also disperses External Dampness and Wind-Damp.
— Rhizoma Dioscoreae is moist in nature and nourishes Lung and Kidney Yin. It is thus indicated for patterns of Lung and Kidney Yin Deficiency such as diabetes.
— Semen Dolichoris eliminates Summer Heat and Dampness and is thus indicated for diarrhoea due to Summer Heat and Dampness. It is less effective in tonifying Qi and invigorating the Spleen than Rhizoma Atractylodis Macrocephalae and Rhizoma Dioscoreae.

■ **RADIX GLYCYRRHIZAE, FRUCTUS ZIZIPHI JUJUBAE, MEL AND SACCHARUM GRANORUM**

● *Gan Cao, Da Zao, Feng Mi and Yi Tang*

Similarities
— All tonify the Middle Burner and relieve spasm and are thus indicated for weakness of the Spleen and Stomach and abdominal pain due to deficiency of the Middle Burner. Because they can cause fullness and Dampness in the Middle Burner, they are contraindicated in cases of stuffiness of the chest and abdominal distension due to Stagnation of Qi and excessive Dampness.

Differences
— Radix Glycyrrhizae and Fructus Ziziphi Jujubae both regulate the Middle Burner and

harmonize the ingredients of a prescription. Radix Glycyrrhizae also tonifies Heart Qi and stops cough. Its treated form (*Zhi Gan Cao*) tonifies the Middle Burner and benefits Qi; its raw form (*Sheng Gan Cao*) clears Fire and Fire Poison. Fructus Ziziphi Jujubae tonifies the Spleen and nourishes Blood.
— Mel and Saccharum Granorum both moisten the Lung and stop cough. Mel is more effective in providing moisture; it also moistens the intestines to relieve constipation. Saccharum Granorum is more effective in tonifying the Middle Burner and relieving spasm and is thus often used in the treatment of abdominal pain due to deficiency of the Middle Burner.

B. Blood tonics

■ **RADIX ANGELICAE SINENSIS AND RADIX PAEONIAE ALBA**

● *Dang Gui and Bai Shao*

Similarities
— Both tonify Blood and are thus indicated for Deficient Blood patterns. They also tonify Qi and relieve pain and are thus indicated for abdominal pain due to deficiency of the Middle Burner. In addition, they regulate Blood and stop dysentery and are thus indicated for dysentery with bloody stool.

Differences
— Radix Angelicae Sinensis activates Blood circulation, regulates menstruation, relieves pain and moistens the intestines. It is indicated for various gynaecological patterns of Blood Deficiency, Blood Stasis, pain due to Qi and Blood Stagnation, and dry constipation.
— Radix Paeoniae Alba nourishes and astringes Yin, stops sweating, nourishes and calms the Liver and relieves spasm. It is indicated for Liver Yin Deficiency, Liver Yang Rising, spontaneous sweating, night sweats, spasmodic pain, hypochondriac pain due to Liver Blood Deficiency and constraint of Liver Qi.

■ RADIX REHMANNIAE PRAEPARATA, COLLA CORII ASINI AND RADIX POLYGONI MULTIFLORI

- *Shu Di, E Jiao and He Shou Wu*

Similarities
— All tonify Blood and Liver and Kidney Yin and are thus indicated for patterns of Blood Deficiency and Liver and Kidney Yin Deficiency.

Differences
— Radix Rehmanniae Praeparata is more effective in tonifying Liver and Kidney Yin and is a major herb for tonifying Kidney Yin.
— Radix Rehmanniae and Radix Rehmanniae Praeparata both tonify Yin. Radix Rehmanniae Praeparata is slightly warm in nature and also tonifies Blood. Radix Rehmanniae is cold in nature and cools Blood, stops bleeding, clears heat and promotes Body Fluids.
— Colla Corii Asini is an important herb for Blood tonification. It also nourishes Yin, moistens dryness and stops bleeding and is thus indicated for dryness arising from Lung and Kidney Yin Deficiency and for haemorrhagic patterns. It is either stir-baked to pearls before adding to a decoction or is melted and administered separately from other ingredients of a prescription.
— Radix Polygoni Multiflori in its treated form tonifies the Liver and Kidneys, while its raw form moistens the intestines, relieves constipation, clears Fire Poison and treats malaria.

C. Yin tonics (Fig. 10.2)

■ RADIX GLEHNIAE, RADIX ADENOPHORAE, RADIX OPHIOPOGONIS, RADIX ASPARAGI, HERBA DENDROBII, RHIZOMA POLYGONATI ODORATI AND RHIZOMA POLYGONATI

- *Bei Sha Shen, Nan Sha Shen, Mai Dong, Tian Dong, Shi Hu, Yu Zhu and Huang Jing*

Similarities
— All are sweet and cold in nature and nourish Lung and Stomach Yin and promote Body Fluids. They are thus indicated for Deficient Lung and Stomach Yin, and consumption of Body Fluids.

Differences
— Radix Glehniae is more effective in nourishing Yin while Radix Adenophorae also resolves Phlegm.
— Radix Ophiopogonis nourishes Heart Yin while Radix Asparagi nourishes Kidney Yin.
— Herba Dendrobii is more effective in nourishing Stomach Yin and promoting Body Fluids. It also improves vision and strengthens tendons and bones and is thus indicated for eye disorders due to Liver Deficiency and for muscular atrophy and motor impairment due to Kidney Deficiency.
— Rhizoma Polygonati Odorati and Rhizoma Polygonati are similar in their action of nourishing Lung and Stomach Yin, but Rhizoma Polygonati Odorati is more effective in nourishing Yin while Rhizoma Polygonati also benefits Qi and invigorates the Spleen. At present Rhizoma Polygonati Odorati is used similarly to Radix Ophiogonis in the treatment of cardiac insufficiency with symptoms of Heart Yin Deficiency.

	LUNG YIN	HEART YIN	STOMACH YIN	LIVER YIN	KIDNEY YIN
Radix Glehniae	■		■		
Radix Adenophorae	■		■		
Radix Ophiopogonis	■	■	■		
Radix Asparagi	■		■		■
Herba Dendrobii			■		
Rhizoma Polygonati Odorati	■		■		
Rhizoma Polygonati	■		■		
Fructus Corni				■	■
Fructus Lycii				■	■
Fructus Ligustri Lucidi				■	■
Herba Ecliptae				■	■
Plastrum Testudinis				■	■
Carapax Trionycis				■	■

Fig. 10.2 Yin tonics.

■ FRUCTUS CORNI, FRUCTUS LYCII, FRUCTUS LIGUSTRI LUCIDI AND HERBA ECLIPTAE

- *Shan Zhu Yu, Gou Qi Zi, Nu Zhen Zi and Mo Han Lian*

Similarities
— All nourish Liver and Kidney Yin and are thus indicated for patterns of Deficient Liver and Kidney Yin.

Differences
— Fructus Corni strongly nourishes Liver and Kidney Yin, but especially Liver Yin. It is an important astringent herb and is indicated for spermatorrhoea, nocturnal enuresis, spontaneous sweating, night sweats and shock due to excessive sweating.
— Fructus Lycii nourishes the Liver and improves vision. It is an important herb for eye disorders due to Liver Blood and Yin Deficiency.
— Fructus Ligustri Lucidi and Herba Ecliptae both have a slow action in nourishing Liver and Kidney Yin. Fructus Ligustri Lucidi is more effective in nourishing the Liver and Kidney while Herba Ecliptae also cools Blood and stops bleeding.

■ PLASTRUM TESTUDINIS AND CARAPAX TRIONYCIS

- *Gui Ban and Bie Jia*

Similarities
— Both nourish Yin, clear Empty Heat and suppress hyperactive Yang and are thus indicated for tidal fever due to Liver and Kidney Yin Deficiency, dizziness and blurring of vision due to Yin Deficiency and hyperactive Yang, tremor due to Liver Wind, and a deep red tongue.

Differences
— Plastrum Testudinis strongly nourishes Kidney Yin. It strengthens bones, consolidates the Chong and Ren channels and stops bleeding and is thus indicated for atrophic debility of bones due to Kidney Deficiency, delayed closure of fontanelles, chondropathy and uterine bleeding due to weakness of the Chong and Ren channels.
— Carapax Trionycis is more effective than

Plastrum Testudinis in clearing Empty Heat. It also softens hard masses and is thus indicated for palpable abdominal masses, and malaria with splenomegaly.

D. Yang tonics

■ CORNU CERVI PANTOTRICHUM, CORNU CERVI AND COLLA CORNUS CERVI

- *Lu Rong, Lu Jiao and Lu Jiao Jiao*

Similarities
— All tonify Kidney Yang, invigorate Yang, benefit Essence (Jing) and Blood and strengthen tendons and bones. They are indicated for Kidney Yang Deficiency, impotence, infertility, sore and weak back and knees, osteoporosis, muscular weakness and atrophy and Deficiency of Kidney Essence with resulting Blood Deficiency.

Differences
— Of the three, Cornu Cervi Pantotrichum has the strongest action and is often administered in the form of pills or powder. Cornu Cervi also has a strong action; it activates Blood circulation and reduces swelling and is indicated for Yin jaundice and swelling due to Stagnation of Blood.
— Colla Cornus Cervi is similar to Cornu Cervi and is more effective in nourishing Essence and Blood. It also stops bleeding and is thus indicated for haemorrhagic patterns due to Deficiency and Cold.

■ RADIX MORINDAE OFFICINALIS, HERBA CISTANCHIS AND HERBA CYNOMORII

- *Ba Ji Tian, Rou Cong Rong and Suo Yang*

Similarities
— All tonify Kidney Yang and are indicated for impotence and premature ejaculation due to Kidney Yang Deficiency and for infertility due to retention of Cold in the uterus.

Differences
— Radix Morindae Officinalis tonifies Yang, strengthens tendons and bones and elimi-

nates Wind-Damp. It is thus indicated for chronic Wind-Damp Bi syndromes, osteoporosis and muscular weakness and atrophy.
— Herba Cistanchis and Herba Cynomorii also moisten the intestines and are thus indicated for dry constipation complicated with Kidney Yang Deficiency.

■ RHIZOMA CURCULIGINIS AND HERBA EPIMEDII

● *Xian Mao and Yin Yang Huo*

Similarities
— Both warm the Kidneys, invigorate Yang, eliminate Cold-Damp and strengthen tendons and bones. They are indicated for impotence, infertility and urinary frequency due to Kidney Yang Deficiency and for chronic Cold-Damp Bi syndromes and weak tendons and bones.

Differences
— Rhizoma Curculiginis is warm and dry in nature and has a strong action in eliminating Cold-Damp.
— Herba Epimedii strongly tonifies Yang. It also lowers blood pressure and treats Deficiency-type asthma.

■ PENI ET TESTES CALLORHINI AND HIPPOCAMPUS

● *Hai Gou Shen and Hai Ma*

Similarities
— Both tonify the Kidneys and invigorate Yang and are indicated for impotence and lack of libido.

Differences
— Hippocampus also activates Blood circulation and resolves Blood Stasis and is thus indicated for palpable abdominal masses.

■ CORTEX EUCOMMIAE, RADIX DIPSACI AND RHIZOMA DRYNARIAE

● *Du Zhong, Xu Duan and Gu Sui Bu*

Similarities
— All tonify the Liver and Kidneys and strengthen the tendons and bones. They are

thus indicated for chronic Wind-Damp Bi syndromes, osteoporosis, muscular weakness and atrophy, and lumbago due to Kidney Deficiency.

Differences
— Cortex Eucommiae tonifies the Kidneys, prevents miscarriage and lowers blood pressure. It is thus indicated for threatened abortion or hypertension due to Kidney Deficiency.
— Radix Dipsaci is similar to Cortex Eucommiae but is more effective in treating injury to the tendons and bones. It also stops bleeding and is thus indicated for uterine bleeding or threatened abortion with bleeding.
— Rhizoma Drynariae is similar to Radix Dipsaci in treating injury to the tendons and bones, and similar to Fructus Psoraleae in tonifying the Kidneys and strengthening the lumbar region.

■ FRUCTUS PSORALEAE AND FRUCTUS ALPINIAE OXYPHYLLAE

● *Bu Gu Zhi and Yi Zhi Ren*

Similarities
— Both tonify the Kidneys, invigorate Yang, warm the Spleen and stop diarrhoea. They are indicated for diarrhoea due to Spleen and Kidney Yang Deficiency.

Differences
— Fructus Psoraleae is more effective in warming the Kidneys. It also tonifies the Kidneys and invigorates Yang, assists reception of Qi to relieve asthma and strengthens the lumbar region.
— Fructus Alpiniae Oxyphyllae is more effective in warming the Spleen and astringing discharges and is thus indicated for diarrhoea due to Spleen Deficiency and for excessive salivation and nocturnal enuresis.

■ GECKO, CORDYCEPS AND SEMEN JUGLANDIS

● *Ge Jie, Dong Chong Xia Cao and Hu Tao Rou*

Similarities
— All tonify the Kidneys and benefit the Lungs

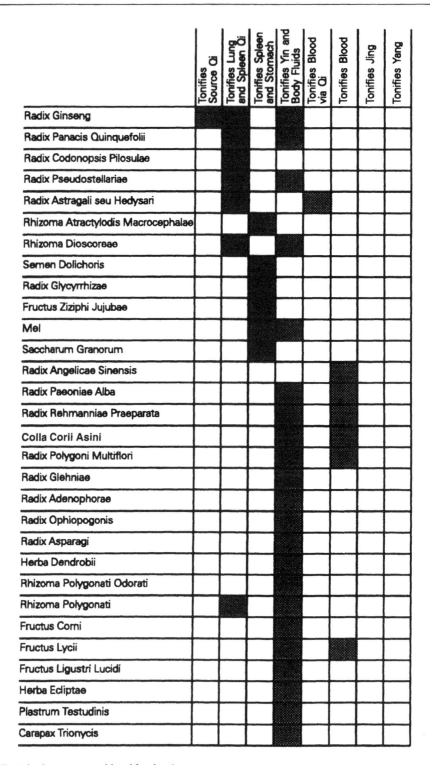

	Tonifies Source Qi	Tonifies Lung and Spleen Qi	Tonifies Spleen and Stomach	Tonifies Yin and Body Fluids	Tonifies Blood via Qi	Tonifies Blood	Tonifies Jing	Tonifies Yang
Radix Ginseng	■			■				
Radix Panacis Quinquefolii		■		■				
Radix Codonopsis Pilosulae		■						
Radix Pseudostellariae		■		■				
Radix Astragali seu Hedysari		■			■			
Rhizoma Atractylodis Macrocephalae			■					
Rhizoma Dioscoreae		■	■					
Semen Dolichoris			■					
Radix Glycyrrhizae			■					
Fructus Ziziphi Jujubae			■					
Mel			■					
Saccharum Granorum			■					
Radix Angelicae Sinensis						■		
Radix Paeoniae Alba				■		■		
Radix Rehmanniae Praeparata				■		■		
Colla Corii Asini				■		■		
Radix Polygoni Multiflori				■		■		
Radix Glehniae				■				
Radix Adenophorae				■				
Radix Ophiopogonis				■				
Radix Asparagi				■				
Herba Dendrobii				■				
Rhizoma Polygonati Odorati				■				
Rhizoma Polygonati		■		■				
Fructus Corni				■				
Fructus Lycii				■		■		
Fructus Ligustri Lucidi				■				
Herba Ecliptae				■				
Plastrum Testudinis				■				
Carapax Trionycis				■				

Fig. 10.3 Tonic herbs: a comparable table of actions.

	Tonifies Source Qi	Tonifies Lung and Spleen Qi	Tonifies Spleen and Stomach	Tonifies Yin and Body Fluids	Tonifies Blood via Qi	Tonifies Blood	Tonifies Jing	Tonifies Yang
Cornu Cervi Pantotrichum						■	■	■
Cornu Cervi						■	■	■
Colla Cornus Cervi						■	■	■
Radix Morindae Officinalis								■
Herba Cystanchis								■
Herba Cynomorii								■
Rhizoma Curculiginis								■
Herba Epimedii								■
Peni et Testes Callorhini								■
Hippocampus								■
Cortex Eucommiae								■
Radix Dipsaci								■
Rhizoma Drynariae								■
Fructus Psoralae								■
Fructus Alpiniae Oxyphyllae								■
Gecko								■
Cordyceps								■
Semen Juglandis								■
Placenta hominis						■	■	■
Umbilical cord						■	■	■
Semen Cuscutae				■			■	■
Semen Astragali Complanati				■			■	■

and thus assist reception of Qi to relieve asthma. They are indicated for Deficiency-type asthma and chronic cough due to Lung and Kidney Deficiency.

Differences
— Gecko is more effective in assisting reception of Qi to relieve asthma. It also benefits Essence and invigorates Yang and is thus indicated for impotence and spermatorrhoea.
— Cordyceps is more effective in tonifying the Lungs and is indicated for pulmonary tuberculosis. It also invigorates Yang and benefits Essence.
— Semen Juglandis also strengthens the lumbar region and moistens the intestines to relieve dry constipation.

■ PLACENTA HOMINIS AND UMBILICAL CORD

● *Zi He Che and Qi Dai*

Similarities
— Both tonify the Kidneys, benefit Essence and assist reception of Qi.

Differences
— Placenta Hominis is more effective in nourishing Essence and Blood and benefiting Qi, while umbilical cord is more effective in assisting reception of Qi to relieve asthma.

■ SEMEN CUSCUTAE AND SEMEN ASTRAGALI COMPLANATI

● *Tu Si Zi and Tong Ji Li*

Similarities
— Both tonify the Kidney, consolidate the Essence, nourish the Liver and improve vision. They tonify both Yin and Yang and are indicated for lumbago, tinnitus, spermatorrhoea and urinary frequency due to Kidney Deficiency, and for impaired vision and dizziness due to Liver and Kidney Deficiency.

Differences
— Semen Cuscutae is more effective in tonifying the Kidneys and consolidating the Essence while Semen Astragali Complanati

is more effective in nourishing the Liver and improving vision.

Questions

1. Compare and contrast the actions and indications of Radix Ginseng and Radix Astragali seu Hedysari.
2. How do the actions of Radix Ginseng and Radix Panacis Quinquefolii differ?
3. How do the actions of Radix Glehniae and Radix Adenophorae differ?
4. Compare and contrast the actions and indications of Rhizoma Atractylodis Macrocephalae and Rhizoma Atractylodis.
5. Compare and contrast the actions and indications of Rhizoma Atractylodis Macrocephalae and Rhizoma Dioscoreae.
6. How do the actions of Radix Rehmanniae Praeparata and Radix Rehmanniae differ?
7. What are the differences in the actions of Radix Angelicae Sinensis and Radix Rehmanniae Praeparata?
8. What are the differences in the actions of Radix Angelicae Sinensis and Radix Paeoniae Alba?
9. Compare and contrast the actions and indications of Radix Glycyrrhizae and Fructus Ziziphi Jujubae.
10. What are the differences in action of Radix Ophiopogonis, Radix Asparagi and Herba Dendrobii?
11. What are the differences in action of Fructus Corni, Fructus Lycii, Plastrum Testudinis and Carapax Trionycis?
12. Compare and contrast the actions of Cornu Cervi Pantotrichum, Cornu Cervi, Herba Cistanchis and Herba Epimedii.
13. Compare and contrast the actions of Cortex Eucommiae and Radix Dipsaci, and Fructus Psoraleae and Fructus Alpiniae Oxyphyllae.
14. Compare and contrast the actions of Gecko and Cordyceps, and of Semen Cuscutae and Semen Astragali Complanati.

Astringent herbs

11

■ FRUCTUS SCHISANDRAE, FRUCTUS MUME AND GALLA CHINENSIS

● *Wu Wei Zi, Wu Mei and Wu Bei Zi*

Similarities
— All astringe in various ways, e.g. they stop sweating, stop coughing by astringing the lungs and stop diarrhoea by astringing the intestines. They are thus indicated for spontaneous sweating, night sweats, chronic cough and wheeze and chronic diarrhoea and dysentery.

Differences
— Fructus Schisandrae benefits Qi and promotes Body Fluids, consolidates Essence, soothes the Heart and calms the Mind. It is thus indicated for collapse due to Qi and Yin Deficiency, thirst due to consumption of Fluids, diabetes, spermatorrhoea, nocturnal enuresis, palpitation and insomnia.
— Fructus Mume promotes Body Fluids, relieves thirst and sedates roundworm. It is indicated for thirst due to consumption of Fluids, diabetes and abdominal pain due to ascariasis.
— Galla Chinensis consolidates Essence, astringes Blood, clears Fire Poison and promotes the healing of skin eruptions. It is indicated for spermatorrhoea, nocturnal enuresis, haemorrhagic patterns, ulcerative gingivitis and carbuncles, boils and ulcers.

■ RADIX EPHEDRAE AND FRUCTUS TRITICI LEVIS

● *Ma Huang Gen and Fu Xiao Mai*

Similarities
— Both stop sweating and are thus indicated for spontaneous sweating and night sweats.

Differences
— Radix Ephedrae stops sweating only. Fructus Tritici Levis also nourishes the Heart and relieves restlessness. Normal wheat grain is similar to Fructus Tritici Levis in action; the latter stops sweating more effectively while the former is more effective in nourishing the Heart and relieving restlessness.

■ SEMEN MYRISTICAE, FRUCTUS CHEBULAE AND HALLOYSITUM RUBRUM

● *Rou Dou Kou, He Zi and Chi Shi Zhi*

Similarities
— All astringe the intestines and stop diarrhoea and are thus indicated for chronic diarrhoea and dysentery.

Differences
— Semen Myristicae warms the Middle Burner and regulates Qi and is thus indicated for Stagnation of Stomach and Spleen Qi due to Deficiency and Cold. Both Semen Cardomomi Rotundi and Semen Myristicae warm the Middle Burner and regulate Qi, but the former is more effective in resolving Dampness while the latter is more effective in astringing the intestines.
— Fructus Chebulae astringes the Lungs to stops cough and eases the throat and voice. It is indicated for chronic cough due to Lung Qi Deficiency and for sore throat and hoarseness due to Lung Fire.

■ CORTEX AILANTHI AND PERICARPIUM GRANATI

- *Chun Gen Pi and Shi Liu Pi*

Similarities
— Both astringe the intestines to stop diarrhoea, and clear Damp-Heat and dysentery. They are indicated for chronic diarrhoea and dysentery, Damp-Heat in the intestines and prolapse of the anus due to Spleen Deficiency.

Differences
— Pericarpium Granati is more effective in killing intestinal parasites while Cortex Ailanthi is more effective in astringing bleeding and leucorrhoea and is thus also indicated for uterine bleeding and leucorrhoea.

■ SEMEN EURYALES, SEMEN NELUMBINIS AND FRUCTUS ROSAE LAEVIGATAE

- *Qian Shi, Lian Zi and Jin Ying Zi*

Similarities
— All consolidate Essence, control urination and stop diarrhoea and leucorrhoea. They are indicated for spermatorrhoea and nocturnal enuresis due to Kidney Deficiency and for chronic diarrhoea and leucorrhoea due to Spleen and Kidney Deficiency.

Differences
— Semen Euryales is more effective in invigorating the Spleen to stop diarrhoea while Semen Nelumbinis is more effective in tonifying the Kidneys and nourishing the Heart.
— Fructus Rosae Laevigatae is more effective in consolidating Essence and is thus indicated for nocturnal emission and spermatorrhoea (Fig. 11.1).

■ OOTHECA MANTIDIS AND FRUCTUS RUBI

- *Sang Piao Xiao and Fu Pen Zi*

Similarities
— Both tonify and astringe the Kidneys and are thus indicated for spermatorrhoea and nocturnal enuresis due to Kidney Deficiency.

Differences
— Ootheca Mantidis invigorates Yang and is thus indicated for impotence. Fructus Rubi

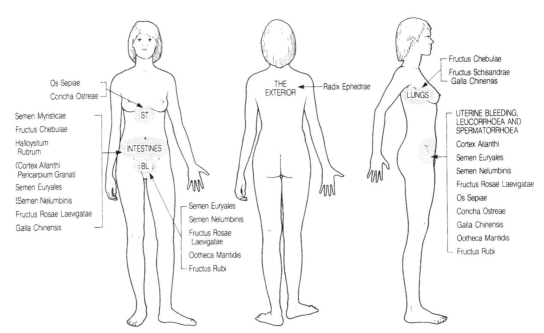

Fig. 11.1 Differentation of astringent herbs according to area of action.

improves vision and can be substituted for Fructus Corni and Fructus Lycii.

■ OS SEPIAE AND CONCHA OSTREAE

- *Wu Zei Gu and Mu Li*

Similarities
— Both are astringent, and inhibit the secretion of gastric acid. They are thus indicated for leucorrhoea and spermatorrhoea in Deficient patterns and for epigastric pain due to gastritis.

Differences
— Concha Ostreae stops sweating, calms Liver Yang and softens hard masses. Os Sepiae stops bleeding and promotes the healing of skin diseases.

Questions

1. How do Fructus Schisandrae, Fructus Mume, and Fructus Corni differ in their actions?
2. Compare and contrast the actions and indications of Radix Ephedrae, Os Draconis and Concha Ostreae.
3. How do Semen Myristicae, Semen Amomi Cardamomi and Fructus Chebulae differ in their actions?
4. Compare and contrast the actions of Halloysitum Rubrum, Cortex Ailanthi and Pericarpium Granati.
5. How do Fructus Rosae Laevigatae, Ootheca Mantidis and Os Sepiae differ in their actions?

Part 2:
Combinations of common Chinese herbs

The actions and indications of individual herbs change according to the way in which they are combined within a formula. It is essential for a practitioner of Chinese medicine to have a good command of the combination of herbs.

Herbs that release the exterior and stop cough and wheeze

12

■ HERBA EPHEDRAE AND RAMULUS CINNAMOMI

- *Ma Huang and Gui Zhi*

— Both of these herbs Release the Exterior; they induce diaphoresis, disperse Cold and relieve pain.
— In combination, these actions are potentiated. They are thus indicated for severe Exterior Wind-Cold patterns of the Excess type, i.e. marked by absence of sweating, and for Cold Bi syndromes. In treating Bi syndromes, if there is severe pain due to Cold, Radix Aconiti may be added to further strengthen the action of dispersing Cold to relieve pain.

■ RAMULUS CINNAMOMI AND RADIX PAEONIAE ALBA

- *Gui Zhi and Bai Shao*

— When combined in equal dosages, these herbs harmonize Nutrient (Ying) Qi and Defensive (Wei) Qi and regulate Yin and Yang. Ramulus Cinnamomi goes to the Defensive level and disperses Excess while Radix Paeoniae Alba goes to the Nutritive level and astringes in order to tonify Deficiency. This combination dispels pathogenic factors from the superficial muscles and reduces Heat. It is indicated for Exterior Wind-Cold patterns of the Deficient type, i.e. marked by spontaneous sweating which does not expel the pathogen.

— When the dosage of Radix Paeoniae Alba is larger than that of Ramulus Cinnamomi, this combination warms the Middle Burner and relieves pain. It is used to treat abdominal pain due to deficiency of the Middle Burner (Fig. 12.1).

■ HERBA SCHIZONEPETAE AND RADIX LEDEBOURIELLAE

- *Jing Jie and Fang Feng*

— Both of these herbs disperse Wind-Cold, relieve pain and itching, and express skin rashes, and these actions are potentiated when they are used in combination.
— The combination is indicated for invasion of Wind-Cold with symptoms of the common cold. For Wind-Cold headache, their action may be strengthened further by the addition of Radix Angelicae Dahuricae.
— They are also used in combination to expel Wind from the skin, in the treatment of pruritus, rubella and other skin rashes.

■ RHIZOMA SEU RADIX NOTOPTERYGII AND RADIX ISATIDIS OR FOLIUM ISATIDIS

- *Qiang Huo and Ban Lan Gen or Da Qing Ye*

— Together, these herbs Release the Exterior and clear Heat. Rhizoma seu Radix

Ramulus Cinnamomi = Radix Paeoniae Alba Harmonizes Nutritive and Defensive Qi	Ramulus Cinnamomi < Radix Paeoniae Alba Warms the Middle Burner and relieves pain
Indicated for Deficiency patterns of Wind-Cold (see Fig. 1.1)	Indicated for abdominal pain due to Deficiency of the Middle Burner

Fig. 12.1 Combined actions of Ramulus Cinnamomi and Radix Paeoniae Alba in different relative dosages.

Notopterygii induces diaphoresis to Release the Exterior, expel Wind and relieve pain, while Radix Isatidis clears Heat and Fire Poison. They are used in combination in the treatment of influenza with headache and fever.

■ HERBA MENTHAE AND HERBA SCHIZONEPETAE

- *Bo He and Jing Jie*

— Both Release the Exterior and express rashes. Herba Menthae is pungent and cool in nature while Herba Schizonepetae is pungent and slightly warm. When used in combination, their actions are potentiated, and they are indicated for Exterior Wind-Heat patterns and the early stages of measles and rubella.

■ FOLIUM MORI AND FLOS CHRYSANTHEMI

- *Sang Ye and Ju Hua*

— Both disperse Wind-Heat and clear Heat from the head and eyes. Folium Mori is more effective in clearing Wind-Heat from the Lung channel to stop cough while Flos Chrysanthemi is more effective in clearing Heat from the Liver and improving vision. When used in combination, their actions are potentiated and they are used to treat Exterior Wind-Heat, especially with headache and redness of the eyes, and Liver Yang Rising or Liver Heat with symptoms of headache, dizziness and vertigo, and redness of the eyes.

■ HERBA MENTHAE AND PERIOSTRACUM CICADAE

- *Bo He and Chan Tui*

— Both disperse Wind-Heat, express rashes and ease the throat and voice. They are indicated for redness of the eyes, sore throat and hoarseness due to invasion of Wind-Heat and for the early stages of measles and rubella.
— Because they also clear Heart and Liver Heat

they are calming and are used to treat night crying in children.

■ FOLIUM MORI AND SEMEN ARMENIACAE AMARUM

- *Sang Ye and Xing Ren*

— Both disperse Wind-Heat, moisten the Lung and stop cough. In combination they stimulate the descending function of Lung Qi and are thus indicated for cough due to Wind-Heat, External Dryness or Lung Yin Deficiency.

■ HERBA EPHEDRAE AND SEMEN ARMENIACAE AMARUM

- *Ma Huang and Xing Ren*

— Both stimulate the dispersing function of the Lung to stop cough and wheeze. In combination this action is potentiated and they are thus indicated for cough due to invasion of Wind-Cold. They are used in combination with Herba Asari and Rhizoma Pinelliae for cough due to retention of Cold-Phlegm, and in combination with Gypsum Fibrosum, Rhizoma Anemarrhenae and Radix Scutellariae for cough and wheeze due to Lung Heat.

■ RADIX BUPLEURI AND RADIX PUERARIAE

- *Chai Hu and Ge Gen*

— Both reduce Heat and dispel pathogenic factors from the muscles. Radix Bupleuri enters the Shao Yang Channel and treats alternating chills and fever. Radix Puerariae enters the Yang Ming Channel and treats fever, headache and neck rigidity due to External Invasion.
— In combination, their actions of reducing Heat and dispelling pathogenic factors from the muscles are potentiated and they are indicated for headache, fever, and neck rigidity due to invasion of Wind-Heat, and for persistent fever after sweating.
— Both of these herbs also raise Yang Qi and they are used in combination to treat diarrhoea and loose stools due to sinking of Spleen Qi.

■ RADIX BUPLEURI AND RADIX SCUTELLARIAE

- *Chai Hu and Huang Qin*

— Radix Bupleuri clears External Heat from Shao Yang and Radix Scutellariae clears Internal Heat from Shao Yang. In combination they thus harmonize Shao Yang and are indicated for alternating chills and fever, and fullness and discomfort in the costal and hypochondriac regions due to Shao Yang disharmony (Table 12.1).

■ HERBA ELSHOLTZIAE AND SEMEN DOLICHORIS

- *Xiang Ru and Bian Dou*

— Herba Elsholtziae is pungent and warm in nature and thus Releases the Exterior and disperses Cold, but it is also aromatic and thus dispels Summer Heat and resolves Dampness. Semen Dolichoris dispels Summer Heat and eliminates Dampness.
— In combination they are indicated for the common cold and diarrhoea due to invasion of Summer Heat, or of Dampness in the Summer and Autumn. Better therapeutic results may be obtained with the addition of Herba Agastachis and Cortex Magnoliae Officinalis.

■ RADIX STEMONAE AND RADIX PLATYCODI

- *Bai Bu and Jie Geng*

— Radix Stemonae moistens the Lung and stops cough. Radix Platycodi resolves Phlegm, stimulates the Lung's dispersing function, stops cough and eases the throat.

— They are used in combination to treat cough.

■ RADIX ASTERIS AND FLOS FARFARAE

- *Zi Wan and Kuan Dong Hua*

— Both are warm but not drying in nature and moisten the Lung, resolve Phlegm and stop cough. Radix Asteris is more effective in resolving Phlegm and benefiting Lung Qi while Flos Farfarae is more effective in stopping cough.
— Combining these herbs reinforces their actions in the treatment of productive cough.

■ SEMEN ARMENIACAE AMARUM AND RADIX PEUCEDANI

- *Xing Ren and Qian Hu*

— Both herbs stimulate the Lung's descending and dispersing functions to stop cough. Semen Armeniacae Amarum is more effective in sending Lung Qi downward while Radix Peucedani is more effective in stimulating the Lung's dispersing function. In combination their antitussive action is potentiated and they are indicated for cough and wheeze due to a failure of Lung Qi to disperse and descend.

■ SEMEN PERILLAE AND SEMEN ARMENIACAE AMARUM

- *Su Zi and Xing Ren*

— Semen Perillae stops cough and wheeze by stimulating the Lung's descending function

Table 12.1 Actions and indications of Radix Bupleuri in combination with other herbs

Radix Bupleuri + Radix Puerariae	This combination has two actions: a. it reduces Heat and dispels pathogenic factors from the muscles	Indicated for headache, fever, and neck rigidity due to invasion of Wind-Heat
	b. it raises Yang Qi	Indicated for diarrhoea and loose stool due to Sinking of Spleen Qi
Radix Bupleuri + Radix Scutellariae	This combination harmonizes Shao Yang	Indicated for alternating chills and fever, and fullness and discomfort in the costal and hypochondriac regions

Table 12.2 Actions and indications of Semen Armeniacae Amarum in combination with other herbs

Semen Armeniacae Amarum + Herba Ephedrae	This combination stimulates the dispersing function of the Lungs to stop cough and wheeze	Stops cough and wheeze due to invasion of Wind-Cold
Semen Armeniacae Amarum + Radix Peucedani	Semen Armeniacae Amarum stimulates the descending function, while Radix Peucedani stimulates the dispersing function	Stops cough and wheeze due to failure of Lung Qi to disperse and descend
Semen Armeniacae Amarum + Semen Perillae	Semen Armenicae Amarum stimulates dispersing and descending; Semen Perillae stimulates the descending function and resolves Phlegm	Stops cough and wheeze due to retention of Cold and Phlegm in the Lungs

and resolving Phlegm. Semen Armeniacae Amarum stops cough and wheeze by stimulating the Lung's dispersing and descending functions. The combination of the two is indicated for cough and wheeze due to retention of Cold and Phlegm in the Lungs (Table 12.2).

■ SEMEN PERILLAE AND SEMEN LEPIDII SEU DESCURAINIAE

● *Su Zi and Ting Li Zi*

— These herbs combine to stimulate the descending function of the Lung, clear Lung Heat and soothe wheezing. They are indicated for shortness of breath, cough and wheeze due to retention of Phlegm Fluid.

■ CORTEX MORI RADICIS AND SEMEN LEPIDII SEU DESCURAINIAE

● *Sang Bai Pi and Ting Li Zi*

— These herbs combine to clear Lung Heat and soothe wheeze and are indicated for cough and wheeze due to Phlegm Fire and pulmonary oedema.

■ CORTEX MORI RADICIS AND RADIX SCUTELLARIAE

● *Sang Bai Pi and Huang Qin*

— These herbs combine to clear Lung Heat and stop cough and are indicated for cough due to Heat or Fire in the Lung.

Table 12.3 Actions and indications of Herba Ephedrae in combination with other herbs

Herba Ephedrae + Ramulus Cinnamomi	This combination Releases the Exterior, induces diaphoresis, disperses Cold and relieves pain	Indicated for Wind-Cold invasion with absence of sweating, and for Cold Bi Syndrome
Herba Ephedrae + Semen Armeniacae Amarum	This combination stimulates the dispersing function of the Lungs	Indicated for cough due to invasion of Wind-Cold to stop cough and wheeze
Herba Ephedrae + Semen Ginkgo	Herba Ephedrae stimulates the dispersing function of the Lungs while Semen Ginkgo astringes the Lungs and resolves Phlegm	Indicated for cough, wheeze and dyspnoea
Herba Ephedrae + Lumbricus	Herba Ephedrae stimulates the dispersing function of the Lungs while Lumbricus clears Heat and resolves Phlegm	Indicated for cough and wheeze due to retention of Phlegm-Heat in the Lungs

■ HERBA EPHEDRAE AND RADIX SCUTELLARIAE

- *Ma Huang and Huang Qin*

— Herba Ephedrae is pungent and warm in nature and stops cough and wheeze by stimulating the Lung's dispersing function. Radix Scutellariae is bitter and cold in nature and stops cough by clearing Lung Heat.

— When used together, Radix Scutellariae modifies the warm nature of Herba Ephedrae and the common action of both herbs in stopping cough and wheeze is potentiated. This combination is especially appropriate for cough and wheeze when there is Exterior Cold and Interior Heat.

■ HERBA EPHEDRAE AND LUMBRICUS

- *Ma Huang and Di Long*

— In combination, these substances stimulate the Lung's dispersing function, clear Heat and resolve Phlegm. This combination is thus indicated for cough and wheeze due to Retention of Phlegm Heat in the Lung.

■ HERBA EPHEDRAE AND SEMEN GINKGO

- *Ma Huang and Bai Guo*

— Herba Ephedrae stimulates the Lung's dispersing function, while Semen Ginkgo astringes the Lung and resolves Phlegm. In combination, they are indicated for cough, wheeze and shortness of breath (Table 12.3).

13 *Herbs that clear Heat*

■ GYPSUM FIBROSUM AND RHIZOMA ANEMARRHENAE

• *Shi Gao and Zhi Mu*

— Both substances clear Full Heat from the Qi level. Gypsum Fibrosum is extremely cold in nature. It clears Heat and Fire, particularly from the Lung and Stomach, and relieves restlessness. Rhizoma Anemarrhenae not only clears Heat and Fire but also nourishes Yin and promotes Body Fluids. When combined, their action of clearing Heat from the Qi level is potentiated and they are indicated for:
1. pathogenic Heat at the Qi level with symptoms of high fever, restlessness, thirst and profuse sweating
2. cough and wheeze due to Full Heat in the Lungs
3. toothache, haematemesis and epistaxis due to Stomach Heat or Fire
4. consumption of Body Fluids due to Full Heat in the Lung and Stomach with symptoms of thirst, a desire to drink large quantities and loss of body weight.

■ GYPSUM FIBROSUM, HERBA ASARI AND RADIX ANGELICAE DAHURICAE

• *Shi Gao, Xi Xin and Bai Zhi*

— Gypsum Fibrosum clears Stomach Heat and Fire. Herba Asari and Radix Angelicae Dahuricae are pungent and scattering in nature and relieve pain. The three substances in combination relieve pain due to Heat or Fire in the Stomach. They are indicated for toothache and headache due to Stomach Heat and Fire.

■ GYPSUM FIBROSUM AND RHIZOMA CIMICIFUGAE

• *Shi Gao and Sheng Ma*

— Gypsum Fibrosum clears Stomach Fire. Rhizoma Cimicifugae clears Fire and Fire Poison. In combination they are indicated for painful and swollen gums or mouth ulcers due to Stomach Fire.

■ RHIZOMA ANEMARRHENAE AND BULBUS FRITILLARIAE

• *Zhi Mu and Bei Mu*

— Both herbs clear Lung Heat; Bulbus Fritillariae also moistens dryness, resolves Phlegm and stops cough. In combination they are indicated for cough due to Lung Heat or Yin Deficiency with Empty Heat.

■ RHIZOMA ANEMARRHENAE AND CORTEX PHELLODENDRI

• *Zhi Mu and Huang Bai*

— Rhizoma Anemarrhenae nourishes Yin and clears Fire while Cortex Phellodendri clears Empty Fire. In combination they are indicated for spermatorrhoea and tidal fever due to Kidney Yin Deficiency with Empty Fire.
— With the addition of Cortex Cinnamomi, this combination nourishes the Kidneys, stimulates the transformation of Water and promotes diuresis and is thus indicated for urinary dysfunction and oedema.

■ **RHIZOMA COPTIDIS AND RADIX SCUTELLARIAE**

• *Huang Lian and Huang Qin*

— Both herbs clear Heat, Fire, Fire Poison and Damp-Heat. Radix Scutellariae works on the Upper Burner while Rhizoma Coptidis works on the Middle Burner. They are often used in combination to treat retention of Heat and Fire in the Upper and Middle Burners, Retention of Damp-Heat in the intestines and retention of Fire Poison.

■ **RHIZOMA COPTIDIS AND RADIX AUCKLANDIA**

• *Huang Lian and Mu Xiang*

— Rhizoma Coptidis clears Heat, dries Dampness and stops dysentery while Radix Aucklandia regulates Qi, relieves pain and stops dysentery. In combination the action of clearing Heat from the intestines and stopping dysentery is potentiated and they are indicated for dysentery and abdominal pain due to retention of Damp-Heat in the intestines.

■ **RHIZOMA COPTIDIS AND CORTEX CINNAMOMI**

• *Huang Lian and Rou Gui*

— Rhizoma Coptidis clears Heart Fire while Cortex Cinnamomi warms Kidney Yang and conducts Ming Men Fire to its source. In combination they harmonize the Heart and Kidneys and are indicated for insomnia due to disharmony between the Heart and Kidneys.

■ **RHIZOMA COPTIDIS AND FRUCTUS EVODIAE**

• *Huang Lian and Wu Zhu Yu*

— Rhizoma Coptidis is bitter and cold in nature; it clears Stomach Heat and stops vomiting. Fructus Evodiae is pungent and hot in nature; it enters the Liver Channel and conducts Rebellious Qi downward to stop vomiting. This combination is indicated for vomiting due to Stomach Heat and for epigastric pain and acid regurgitation due to disharmony between the Liver and Stomach.

■ **RADIX SCUTELLARIAE AND RADIX PAEONIAE ALBA**

• *Huang Qin and Bai Shao*

— Radix Scutellariae clears Heat from the intestines to stop diarrhoea and dysentery while Radix Paeoniae Alba harmonizes the Blood and relaxes spasm. In combination they are indicated for abdominal pain and dysentery, especially with blood in the stool.

■ **RADIX SCUTELLARIAE AND RHIZOMA ATRACTYLODIS MACROCEPHALAE**

• *Huang Qin and Bai Zhu*

— Radix Scutellariae clears Heat and prevents miscarriage while Rhizoma Atractylodis Macrocephalae tonifies Qi, invigorates the Spleen and prevents miscarriage. In combination their action of preventing miscarriage is potentiated and they are thus indicated for threatened abortion.

■ **CORTEX PHELLODENDRI AND FRUCTUS GARDENIAE**

• *Huang Bai and Zhi Zi*

— Both herbs clear Damp-Heat and relieve jaundice. Cortex Phellodendri strongly clears Heat and dries Dampness while Fructus Gardeniae drains Dampness and relieves urinary disturbance. In combination they are indicated for jaundice due to retention of Damp-Heat and for urinary disturbance with turbid urine due to Damp-Heat in the Lower Burner.

■ **RADIX GENTIANAE, FRUCTUS GARDENIAE AND RADIX REHMANNIAE**

• *Long Dan Cao, Zhi Zi and Sheng Di*

— Radix Gentianae and Fructus Gardeniae clear Liver Fire. Radix Rehmanniae not only clears Heat but also nourishes Yin, thus preventing the first two herbs from damaging the Yin. This combination is indicated for Liver Fire with symptoms of headache, red eyes, hypochondriac pain and jaundice and for Damp-Heat in the Lower Burner with symptoms of leucorrhoea and urinary disturbance with turbid urine.

■ CORTEX MOUTAN RADICIS AND FRUCTUS GARDENIAE

- *Dan Pi and Zhi Zi*

— Both of these herbs clear Liver Fire and cool Blood. This combination is thus indicated for Liver Qi Stagnation turning to Fire, or retention of Heat in the Liver Channel, with symptoms of hypochondriac pain, a bitter taste in the mouth, red eyes and headache, and for Heat in the Blood with symptoms of haematemesis and epistaxis.

■ SPICA PRUNELLAE AND FLOS CHRYSANTHEMI

- *Xia Ku Cao and Ju Hua*

— Both herbs clear Liver Heat, pacify the Liver and improve vision. This combination is thus indicated for Liver Fire with symptoms of headache and eye disease, or Liver Yang Rising with symptoms of headache, dizziness and vertigo.

■ SPICA PRUNELLAE, RADIX SCROPHULARIAE, BULBUS FRITILLARIAE, SARGASSUM AND THALLUS LAMINARIAE SEU ECKLONIAE

- *Xia Ku Cao, Xuan Shen, Bei Mu, Hai Zao and Kun Bu*

— Spica Prunellae clears Liver Fire and disperses masses. Radix Scrophulariae nourishes Yin and clears Fire and Poison. Bulbus Fritillariae, Sargassum and Thallus Laminariae seu Eckloniae resolve Phlegm and soften hard masses. The combination of these herbs is indicated for tuberculosis of the lymph nodes, goitre and tumours.

■ FLOS LONICERAE AND FRUCTUS FORSYTHIAE

- *Jin Yin Hua and Lian Qiao*

— Both herbs clear Heat and Fire Poison and this action is potentiated when they are used in combination. They are indicated for Heat and Fire Poison at the Defensive (Wei) and Qi levels and for carbuncles, boils and ulcers.

■ FOLIUM ISATIDIS OR RADIX ISATIDIS AND RADIX GENTIANAE

- *Da Qing Ye or Ban Lan Gen and Long Dan Cao*

— Folium and Radix Isatidis clear Heat and Fire Poison and are antiviral. Radix Gentianae clears Heat and Fire and stops convulsion. This combination is indicated for febrile diseases with Fire Poison, headache, convulsion and spasm due to high fever.

■ HERBA VIOLAE AND HERBA TARAXACI

- *Zi Hua Di Ding and Pu Gong Ying*

— Both clear Heat and Fire Poison and are thus indicated for sores and ulcers due to Fire Poison and for various infections.

■ CAULIS SARGENTODOXAE AND HERBA PATRUBIAE, AND RADIX ET RHIZOMA RHEI AND CORTEX MOUTAN RADICIS

- *Hong Teng and Bai Jiang Cai, and Da Huang and Dan Pi*

— These combinations clear Heat and Poison. They are indicated for acute appendicitis and pelvic inflammation.

■ RADIX PULSATILLAE, CORTEX FRAXINI AND RHIZOMA COPTIDIS

- *Bai Tou Weng, Qin Pi and Huang Lian*

— This combination clears Heat and Fire Poison from the intestines, cools Blood and stops dysentery. It is indicated for dysentery

Table 13.1 Actions and indications of Rhizoma Coptidis, in combination with other herbs

Rhizoma Coptidis + Radix Scutellariae	Rhizoma Coptidis clears Heat from the Middle Burner; Radix Scutellariae clears Heat from the Upper Burner	Indicated for Heat in the Upper and Middle Burners, Damp-Heat in the intestines and Fire Poison
Rhizoma Coptidis + Radix Aucklandiae	Rhizoma Coptidis clears Heat and Damp; Radix Aucklandiae regulates Qi and relieves pain; both treat dysentery	Indicated for dysentery or abdominal pain due to Damp-Heat in the intestines
Rhizoma Coptidis + Cortex Cinnamomi	Rhizoma Coptidis clears Heart Fire; Cortex Cinnamomi warms Kidney Yang and conducts Ming Men Fire back to its source	Indicated for insomnia due to disharmony between the Heart and Kidneys
Rhizoma Coptidis + Fructus Evodiae	Rhizoma Coptidis clears Stomach Heat and stops vomiting; Fructus Evodiae enters the Liver and regulates Rebellious Qi	Indicated for vomiting due to Stomach Heat, epigastric pain and acid reflux due to disharmony between the Liver and Stomach
Rhizoma Coptidis + Radix Pulsatillae + Cortex Fraxini	All three herbs cool Blood, and clear Heat and Fire Poison from the intestines	Indicated for dysentery with bloody stool due to Fire Poison
Rhizoma Coptidis + Cortex Magnoliae Officinalis	Both herbs clear Heat and Damp	Indicated for epigastric and abdominal distension and pain due to Damp-Heat and for Damp-Heat febrile disease

with blood in the stool due to Fire Poison (Table 13.1).

■ INDIGO NATURALIS AND POWDER OF CONCHA MERETRICIS SEU CYLINAE

● *Qing Dai and Ge Fen*

— Indigo Naturalis clears Liver Fire and cools Blood. Powder of Concha Meretricis seu Cylinae clears Phlegm Heat. In combination they clear Lung Heat and Liver Fire and cool Blood to stop bleeding. This combination is indicated for cough and haemoptysis due to invasion of the Lung by Liver Fire.

■ CORNU RHINOCERI ASIATICI AND RADIX REHMANNIAE

● *Xi Jiao and Sheng Di*

— This combination clears Heat and cools Blood and is thus indicated for febrile disease at the Blood level and for haematemesis and epistaxis due to Heat in the Blood. Its action is further strengthened by the addition of Cortex Moutan Radicis and Radix Paeoniae Rubra.

■ RADIX REHMANNIAE AND RADIX SCROPHULARIAE

● *Sheng Di and Xuan Shen*

— This combination clears Heat, cools Blood, nourishes Yin and promotes Body Fluids. It is thus indicated for febrile disease at the Nutritive (*Ying*) and Blood levels and for constipation due to Liver and Kidney Yin Deficiency.

■ HERBA ARTEMISIAE CHINGHAO AND CARAPAX TRIONYCIS

● *Qing Hao and Bie Jia*

— This combination nourishes Yin and clears Heat and is thus indicated for tidal fever and night sweats due to Yin Deficiency with Empty Heat.

■ HERBA ARTEMISIAE CHINGHAO AND RADIX SCUTELLARIAE

● *Qing Hao and Huang Qin*

— This combination clears Heat and harmonizes Shao Yang and is indicated for alternating fever and chills, severe fever and mild chills, or fever without chills.

■ RADIX STELLARIAE AND CORTEX LYCII RADICIS

- *Yin Chai Hu and Di Gu Pi*

— This combination clears Empty Heat and is thus indicated for Yin Deficiency with Empty Heat and tidal fever.

■ RADIX GENTIANAE MACROPHYLLAE AND CARAPAX TRIONYCIS

- *Qin Jiao and Bie Jia*

— Both herbs clear Empty Heat and this action is potentiated when the two are used in combination. In addition, Radix Gentianae Macrophyllae eliminates Wind-Damp, and Carapax Trionycis nourishes Yin. This combination is indicated for Yin or Blood Deficiency with Empty Heat, tidal fever and painful joints due to Wind and Dampness.

Purgative and digestive herbs **14**

■ **RADIX ET RHIZOMA RHEI AND NATRII SULFAS**

● *Da Huang and Mang Xiao*

— Radix et Rhizoma Rhei clears Heat and Fire and purges accumulation. Natrii Sulfas softens hardness and promotes the discharge of dry faeces. Their mutual action of clearing Heat and relieving constipation is potentiated when they are used in combination.

— This combination is indicated for febrile disease with high fever and constipation due to retention of Heat in the intestines. These two herbs are also applied externally in the form of a powder to treat appendicitis, carbuncles, boils and ulcers.

■ **RADIX ET RHIZOMA RHEI AND RADIX ACONITI PRAEPARATA**

● *Da Huang and Fu Zi*

— Rhei purges stagnation while Aconiti warms the Interior and disperses Cold. Combining

the two changes the action of Rhei from purging by Cold to purging by Warmth. The combination is thus indicated for constipation due to stagnation of Cold.

■ **RADIX ET RHIZOMA RHEI, SEMEN PERSICAE AND CORTEX MOUTAN RADICIS**

● *Da Huang, Tao Ren and Dan Pi*

— These herbs combine to invigorate Blood circulation and resolve Blood Stasis. This combination is thus indicated for various patterns of Blood Stagnation, including appendicitis, pain due to trauma and abdominal pain due to stagnation of Qi and Blood.

■ **RADIX ET RHIZOMA RHEI AND EUPOLYPHAGA SEU STELEOPHAGA**

● *Da Huang and Di Bie Chong*

— Both substances invigorate Blood circulation and resolve Blood Stasis in the collaterals.

Table 14.1 Actions and indications of Radix et Rhizoma Rhei in combination with other herbs

Radix et Rhizoma Rhei + Natrii Sulfas	Radix et Rhizoma Rhei clears Heat and purges accumulation; Natrii Sulfas softens hardness and promotes discharge of faeces	Indicated for febrile disease with constipation due to retention of Heat in the intestines
Radix et Rhizoma Rhei + Radix Aconiti Praeparata	Radix et Rhizoma Rhei purges stagnation; Radix Aconiti Praeparata warms the Interior and disperses Cold	Indicated for constipation due to stagnation of Cold
Radix et Rhizoma Rhei + Semen Persicae + Cortex Moutan Radicis	All three herbs invigorate Blood and resolve Stasis	Indicated for various patterns of Blood Stagnation, especially in the Lower Burner
Radix et Rhizoma Rhei + Eupolyphaga seu Steleophaga	Eupolyphaga seu Steleophaga resolves Blood Stasis and promotes the healing of sprains and fractures; Radix et Rhizoma Rhei invigorates Blood and resolves Stasis	Indicated for amenorrhoea and palpable abdominal masses and for traumatic injury

Eupolyphaga seu Steleophaga also promotes the healing of sprains and fractures and disperses palpable masses due to Blood Stasis.

— This combination is indicated for amenorrhoea and palpable abdominal masses due to Blood Stasis and for swelling and pain due to stagnation of Blood following traumatic injury (Table 14.1).

■ FRUCTUS CANNABIS, SEMEN PRUNI, RADIX ANGELICAE SINENSIS AND RADIX REHMANNIAE

● *Huo Ma Ren, Yu Li Ren, Dang Gui and Sheng Di*

— Fructus Cannabis, Semen Pruni and Radix Angelicae Sinensis moisten the intestines and relieve constipation; Radix Angelicae Sinensis and Radix Rehmanniae nourish Blood and Yin and moisten dryness. Their action of moistening the intestines to relieve constipation is potentiated when they are used in combination.

— This combination is indicated for dry constipation due to old age, weak constitution and deficiency of Blood and Body Fluids. If constipation is caused by weakness in transmission due to Spleen Qi Deficiency, add large doses of Rhizoma Atractylodis Macrocephalae.

■ FRUCTUS ORYZAE GERMINATUS AND FRUCTUS HORDEI GERMINATUS

● *Gu Ya and Mai Ya*

— These herbs combine to promote digestion and harmonize the Stomach and are thus indicated for poor appetite, Retention of Food and dyspepsia.

■ FRUCTUS CRATAEGI, MASSA FERMENTATA AND FRUCTUS HORDEI GERMINATUS

● *Shan Zha, Shen Qu and Mai Ya*

— Fructus Crataegi promotes the digestion of meat, invigorates the Stomach and stops dysentery. Massa Fermentata and Fructus Hordei Germinatus promote the digestion of rice and wheat. Massa Fermentata also harmonizes the Stomach, stops diarrhoea and clears Heat.

— This combination promotes digestion and harmonizes the Middle Burner and is indicated for Retention of Food with symptoms of diarrhoea, dysentery, epigastric distension, abdominal pain, foul belching and fever.

■ RADIX AUCKLANDIAE, SEMEN ARECAE AND FRUCTUS AURANTII IMMATURUS

● *Mu Xiang, Bing Long and Zhi Shi*

— Radix Aucklandiae regulates Qi while Semen Arecae and Fructus Aurantii Immaturus promote digestion and resolve Stagnation. This combination is indicated for Retention of Food and Stagnation of Qi marked by abdominal distention and pain, and dysentery.

Herbs that relieve Bi syndromes **15**

■ RHIZOMA SEU RADIX NOTOPTERYGII
AND RADIX ANGELICAE
PUBESCENTIS

● *Qiang Huo and Du Huo*

— Both herbs Release the Exterior, expel Wind
and disperse Cold and Dampness. Rhizoma
seu Radix Notopterygii is more effective in
treating Bi syndromes of the upper body
while Radix Angelicae Pubescentis is more
effective in treating Bi syndromes of the
lower body. When used in combination their
effectiveness in treating Bi syndromes is
enhanced.
— This combination is indicated for Cold-
Damp Bi. It is also combined with herbs that
Release the Exterior to treat Exterior patterns
complicated with Dampness, and headache
due to invasion of Wind, Cold and
Dampness.

■ RADIX GENTIANAE MACROPHYLLAE
AND RADIX CLEMATIDIS

● *Qin Jiao and Wei Ling Xian*

— This combination removes obstruction in the
collaterals and stops pain and is indicated
for Wandering Bi syndromes.

■ RADIX GENTIANAE MACROPHYLLAE,
RADIX STEPHANIAE TETRANDRAE,
RADIX REHMANNIAE AND RAMULUS
LORANTHI

● *Qin Jiao, Fang Ji, Sheng Di and Sang Ji
Sheng*

— This combination treats Bi syndrome and
clears Heat and is thus indicated for Febrile
Bi. A stronger therapeutic effect will be
obtained with the addition of Lumbricus
and Rhizoma Anemarrhenae.

■ RAMULUS CINNAMOMI, RADIX
PAEONIAE ALBA AND RHIZOMA
ANEMARRHENAE

● *Gui Zhi, Bai Shao and Zhi Mu*

— This combination clears Heat, removes
obstruction from the channels and relieves
pain. It is thus indicated for Febrile Bi. If
Heat is severe, add Gypsum Fibrosum and
Cortex Phellodendri. If both Heat and Cold
are combined, add Radix Aconiti
Kusnezoffii (*Chuan Cao Wu*) and Herba
Ephedrae.

■ FRUCTUS CHAENOMELIS AND RADIX
ACHYRANTHIS BIDENTATAE

● *Mu Gua and Niu Xi*

— This combination relaxes the tendons,
activates Qi and Blood circulation and eliminates Dampness. It is indicated for Bi
syndrome affecting the lower limbs.

■ RADIX LEDEBOURIELLAE AND RADIX
STEPHANIAE TETRANDRAE

● *Fang Feng and Fang Ji*

— Radix Ledebouriellae expels Wind and
relieves pain while Stephandrae Tetrandrae
expels Dampness and relieves joint pain.
This combination is indicated for Wind-
Damp Bi syndromes.

■ HERBA SIEGESBECKIAE AND FOLIUM
CLERODENDRI TRICHOTOMI

● *Xi Xian Cao and Chou Wu Tong*

— This combination treats Bi syndrome and
lowers blood pressure. It is indicated for
Damp Bi syndrome and for hypertension,

headache, dizziness and vertigo, numbness of the limbs and hemiplegia.

■ ZAOCYS AND SCOLOPENDRA

- *Wu Shao She and Wu Gong*

— This combination expels Wind and removes obstruction from the channels. It is indicated for chronic and stubborn Bi syndromes. A stronger action will be obtained if Bungarus Parvus (*Bai Hua She*) is substituted for Zaocys. Scorpio, Eupolyphaga seu Steleophaga and Lumbricus may be substituted for Scolopendra.

■ RADIX ANGELICAE PUBESCENTIS AND RAMULUS LORANTHI

- *Du Huo and Sang Ji Sheng*

— This combination treats lower back pain and chronic Bi syndrome complicated with deficiency of Defensive (*Wei*) Qi. The therapeutic action is strengthened by the addition of Radix Dipsaci, Rhizoma Cibotii and Cortex Acanthopanacis Radicis. For concurrent Qi and Blood Deficiency, add Radix Astragali seu Hedysari and Radix Angelicae Sinensis.

■ RADIX ANGELICAE PUBESCENTIS, RAMULUS LORANTHI, ZAOCYS AND SCOLOPENDRA

- *Du Huo, Sang Ji Sheng, Wu Shao She and Wu Gong*

— This combination tonifies the Liver and Kidneys, strengthens tendons and bones, removes obstruction from the channels and eases the joints. It is indicated for chronic Bi syndromes with deficiency of Defensive (*Wei*) Qi and for rheumatoid arthritis with deformity of the joints.

■ RADIX GENTIANAE MACROPHYLLAE, RAMULUS CINNAMOMI AND RAMULUS MORI

- *Qin Jiao, Gui Zhi and Sang Zhi*

— This combination goes to the four limbs, removes obstruction from the channels and relieves pain. It is indicated for Bi syndromes

of the limbs and particularly the upper limbs.

Herbs that resolve and drain Dampness

16

■ **HERBA AGASTACHIS AND HERBA EUPATORII**

● *Huo Xiang and Pei Lan*

— This combination fragrantly resolves Summer Heat and Dampness, and is thus indicated for Summer Heat, Dampness and Damp-Heat patterns.

■ **RHIZOMA ATRACTYLODIS AND CORTEX MAGNOLIAE OFFICINALIS**

● *Cang Zhu and Hou Po*

— The bitter, warm and dry nature of this combination dries Dampness, invigorates the Spleen and relieves distension and fullness. It is indicated for fullness and distending pain in the epigastrium and abdomen and for diarrhoea due to invasion of the Middle Burner by External Dampness.

■ **RHIZOMA ATRACTYLODIS AND CORTEX PHELLODENDRI**

● *Cang Zhu and Huang Bai*

— Rhizoma Actractylodis dries Dampness;

Cortex Phellodendri dries Dampness and clears Heat, especially from the Lower Burner. This combination is indicated for all Damp-Heat patterns of the Lower Burner, including flaccidity and motor impairment of the lower limbs, Damp-Heat Bi syndrome, Damp-Heat leucorrhoea, suppurating skin infections and eczema on the lower body.

■ **RHIZOMA ATRACTYLODIS, GYPSUM FIBROSUM AND RHIZOMA ANEMARRHENAE**

● *Cang Zhu, Shi Gao and Zhi Mu*

— Rhizoma Atractylodis dries Dampness and treats Bi syndrome; Gypsum Fibrosum and Rhizoma Anemarrhenae clear Heat and Fire. This combination is indicated for Damp-Heat febrile diseases and Damp-Heat Bi syndromes (Table 16.1).

■ **CORTEX MAGNOLIAE OFFICINALIS AND RHIZOMA COPTIDIS**

● *Hou Po and Huang Lian*

— This combination clears Heat and dries

Table 16.1 Actions and indications of Rhizoma Atractylodis in combination with other herbs

Rhizoma Atractylodis + Cortex Magnoliae Officinalis	Both herbs dry Damp, invigorate the Spleen and relieve fullness and distension	Indicated for epigastric and abdominal fullness, and diarrhoea due to External Damp invading the Middle Burner
Rhizoma Atractylodis + Cortex Phellodendri	Rhizoma Atractylodis works on the Middle Burner and dries Damp; Cortex Phellodendri works on the Lower Burner and clears Heat and Damp	Indicated for Damp-Heat patterns of the Lower Burner
Rhizoma Atractylodis + Gypsum Fibrosum + Rhizoma Anemarrhenae	Rhizoma Atractylodis dries Damp; Gypsum Fibrosum and Rhizoma Anemarrhenae clear Heat	Indicated for febrile disease or Bi Syndromes due to Damp-Heat

Dampness. It is indicated for distension and discomfort in the epigastrium and abdomen, epigastric pain due to Damp-Heat and Damp-Heat febrile disease.

■ SEMEN BENINCASAE AND SEMEN COICIS

- *Deng Gua Ren and Yi Yi Ren*

— This combination drains Dampness and Fire Poison. It is indicated for carbuncles, lung abscess and appendicitis.

■ SEMEN PLANTAGINIS AND RADIX ACHYRANTHIS BIDENTATAE

- *Che Qian Zi and Niu Xi*

— This combination promotes diuresis and relieves swelling. It is indicated for oedema and dysuria.

■ POLYPORUS UMBELLATUS, PORIA AND RHIZOMA ATRACTYLODIS MACROCEPHALAE

- *Zhu Ling, Fu Ling and Bai Zhu*

— This combination promotes diuresis and relieves swelling. It is indicated for oedema and dysuria.

■ PORIA, RHIZOMA ATRACTYLODIS MACROCEPHALAE AND RAMULUS CINNAMOMI

- *Fu Ling, Bai Zhu and Gui Zhi*

— Poria promotes diuresis and drains retained Water; Rhizoma Atractylodis Macrocephalae promotes diuresis and invigorates the Spleen; and Ramulus Cinnamomi promotes diuresis, drains retained Water and warms the Yang. This combination is indicated for oedema and retention of Water and Phlegm.

■ GYPSUM FIBROSUM AND RADIX GLYCYRRHIZAE

- *Hua Shi and Gan Cao*

— This combination clears Summer Heat and drains Dampness. It is indicated for

patterns of Heat, Dampness and Summer Heat with a sensation of heat and deep yellow urine.

■ CAULIS AKEBIAE, RADIX REHMANNIAE AND HERBA LOPHATHERI

- *MuTong, Sheng Di and Zhu Ye*

— Caulis Akebiae clears Heat and Fire, promotes diuresis and opens the urinary passages; Herba Lophatheri clears Heat and promotes diuresis; and Radix Rehmanniae nourishes the Yin, thus preventing Caulis Akebiae from damaging Body Fluids. This combination is indicated for painful urination with scanty deep yellow urine and restlessness, and for mouth and tongue ulcers due to Heat in the Heart, Small Intestine and Bladder.

■ HERBA LYSIMACHIAE, SPORA LYGODII AND ENDOTHELIUM CORNEUM GIGERIAE GALLI

- *Jin Qian Cao, Hai Jin Sha and Ji Nei Jin*

— This combination resolves stones and open the urinary passages. It is indicated for stones in the urinary and biliary tracts.

■ HERBA ARTEMISIAE SCOPARIAE, FRUCTUS GARDENIAE, RADIX BUPLEURI AND RHIZOMA POLYGONI CUSPIDATI

- *Yin Che Hao, Zhi Zi, Chai Hu and Hu Zhang*

— Herba Artemisiae Scopariae clears Damp-Heat, soothes the Gall Bladder and relieves jaundice; Fructus Gardeniae clears Heat and Dampness and relieves jaundice; Radix Bupleuri enters the Liver and Gall Bladder and soothes the Liver; and Rhizoma Polygoni Cuspidati clears Heat and Fire Poison, drains Dampness and relieves jaundice.

— This combination is indicated for Damp-Heat jaundice.

■ **RHIZOMA DIOSCOREAE SEPTEMLOBAE, PORIA, FRUCTUS ALPINIAE OXYPHYLLAE AND RADIX LINDERAE**

● *Bi Xie, Fu Ling, Yi Zhi Ren and Wu Yao*

— Rhizoma Dioscoreae Septemlobae drains Turbid Dampness and separates the clear from the turbid; Fructus Alpiniae Oxyphyllae warms Kidney Yang; Radix Linderae strengthens the Bladder's function of controlling urine.
— This combination is indicated for turbid urine due to Yang Deficiency, as in chyluria. If turbid urine is due to Damp-Heat, replace Fructus Alpiniae Oxyphyllae with Cortex Phellodendri, Semen Plantaginis and Gypsum Fibrosum.

17 *Herbs that resolve Phlegm*

■ RHIZOMA PINELLIAE AND PERICARPIUM CITRI RETICULATAE

- *Ban Xia and Chen Pi*

— Rhizoma Pinelliae dries Dampness, resolves Phlegm and conducts Rebellious Qi downward to stop vomiting; Pericarpum Citri Reticulatae dries Dampness, resolves Phlegm, regulates Qi and harmonizes the Stomach.
— This combination is indicated for all Damp Phlegm patterns and for epigastric pain, vomiting and belching due to retention of Dampness and Stagnation of Qi.

■ RHIZOMA PINELLIAE AND RHIZOMA ARISAEMATIS

- *Ban Xia and Tian Nan Xing*

— This combination dries Dampness and resolves Phlegm. It is indicated for Closed Wind-Stroke due to Wind Phlegm. When combined with Fructus Aurantii Immaturus,

Succus Bambusae or Caulis Bambusae in Taeniam it is indicated for patterns of Damp Phlegm and Cold Phlegm.

■ RHIZOMA PINELLIAE, RHIZOMA GASTRODIAE AND RHIZOMA ATRACTYLODIS MACROCEPHALAE

- *Ban Xia, Tian Ma and Bai Zhu*

— Rhizoma Pinelliae dries Dampness and resolves Phlegm; Rhizoma Gastrodiae calms Liver Wind; Rhizoma Atractylodis Macrocephalae invigorates the Spleen. This combination is indicated for dizziness and vertigo due to Damp Phlegm.

■ RHIZOMA PINELLIAE AND BULBUS FRITILLARIAE

- *Ban Xia and Bei Mu*

— Rhizoma Pinelliae dries Dampness and resolves Phlegm; Bulbus Fritillariae

Table 17.1 Actions and indications of Rhizoma Pinelliae in combination with other herbs

Rhizoma Pinelliae + Pericarpium Citri Reticulatae	Both herbs dry Damp and resolve Phlegm; Rhizoma Pinelliae regulates Rebellious Qi, while Pericarpium Citri Reticulatae moves Qi and harmonizes the Stomach	Indicated for all Damp-Phlegm patterns and for epigastric pain, vomiting and belching due to retention of Damp and stagnation of Qi
Rhizoma Pinelliae + Rhizoma Arisaematis	Both herbs dry Damp and resolve Phlegm	Indicated for Wind-Stroke due to Wind-Phlegm
Rhizoma Pinelliae + Rhizoma Gastrodiae + Rhizoma Atractylodis Macrocephalae	Rhizoma Pinelliae dries Damp and resolves Phlegm; Rhizoma Gastrodiae calms Liver Wind; Rhizoma Atractylodis Macrocephalae invigorates the Spleen	Indicated for dizziness and vertigo due to Damp-Phlegm
Rhizoma Pinelliae + Bulbus Fritillariae	Rhizoma Pinelliae dries Damp and resolves Phlegm; Bulbus Fritillariae moistens the Lungs, resolves Phlegm and stops cough	Indicated for cough with profuse sputum

moistens the Lungs, resolves Phlegm and stops cough. Combining these herbs treats the Lungs and Spleen concurrently and potentiates the action of both herbs in resolving Phlegm to stop cough.

— This combination is thus indicated for cough with profuse sputum (Table 17.1).

■ RHIZOMA ARISAEMATIS AND RHIZOMA TYPHONII

● *Tian Nan Xing and Bai Fu Zi*

— This combination resolves Wind-Phlegm and stops convulsion. It is indicated for tetanus and for deviation of the mouth and eye due to invasion by Wind-Phlegm. A stronger therapeutic action will be obtained with the addition of Radix Ledebouriellae and Scorpio.

■ BULBUS FRITILLARIAE AND FRUCTUS TRICHOSANTHIS

● *Bei Mu and Gua Lou*

Both herbs clear Heat Phlegm, moisten the Lungs and stop cough, and these actions are potentiated when the herbs are combined. This combination is indicated for patterns of Heat Phlegm and Dry Phlegm, including cough with thick yellow sputum, chronic dry cough and tuberculosis of the lymph nodes.

■ SARGASSUM AND THALLUS LAMINARIAE SEU ECKLONIAE

● *Hai Zao and Kun Bu*

— This combination resolves Phlegm and softens hard masses. It is indicated for goitre, soft masses and tuberculosis of the lymph nodes.

■ ALUMEN AND RADIX CURCURMAE

● *Bai Fan and Yu Jin*

— Alumen resolves Phlegm while Radix Curcumae resolves Stagnation and opens the orifices. This combination is indicated for manic-depressive disorders due to Turbid Phlegm Misting the Mind. It also soothes the Gall Bladder and resolves stones.

■ SEMEN SINAPIS ALBAE, FRUCTUS PERILLAE AND SEMEN RAPHANI

● *Bai Jie Zi, Su Zi and Lai Fu Zi*

— This combination resolves Phlegm and conducts Rebellious Qi downward. It is indicated for cough and dyspnoea due to Cold Phlegm.

■ SEMEN SINAPIS ALBAE, RADIX EUPHORBIAE KANSUI AND RADIX EUPHORBIAE PEKINENSIS

● *Bai Jie Zi, Gan Sui and Da Ji*

— Semen Sinapis Albae resolves Phlegm between the skin and the muscles; Radix Euphorbiae Kansui and Radix Euphorbiae Pekinensis resolve retained Water. This combination is indicated for retained Water in the hypochondrium (pleural effusion). It is administered in the form of powder or pills.

■ SEMEN SINAPIS ALBAE AND RAMULUS CINNAMOMI

● *Bai Jie Zi and Gui Zhi*

— This combination resolves Phlegm, warms the channels and removes obstruction from the collaterals. It is indicated for painful joints and numbness of the limbs and body due to stagnation of Cold Phlegm.

18 *Herbs that subdue Wind and calm the Mind*

■ **CONCHA HALIOTIDIS AND CONCHA OSTREAE**

- *Shi Jue Ming and Mu Li*

— Both substances are shells that subdue hyperactive Liver Yang and this action is potentiated when they are used in combination. They are indicated for Liver Yang Rising giving rise to headache, dizziness and vertigo, or Liver Wind.

■ **CORNU ANTELOPIS AND RAMULUS UNCARIAE CUM UNCIS**

- *Ling Yang Jiao and Gou Teng*

— Cornu Antelopis clears Heat, calms and cools the Liver and subdues Wind; these actions are potentiated when it is combined with Ramulus Uncariae cum Uncis.
— This combination is indicated for convulsion, dizziness and vertigo, headache and red eyes due to Liver Fire, Liver Yang Rising and Liver Wind.

■ **RHIZOMA GASTRODIAE AND RAMULUS UNCARIAE CUM UNCIS**

- *Tian Ma and Gou Teng*

— This combination calms the Liver and subdues Wind. It is indicated for headache, dizziness and vertigo due to Liver Yang Rising and for convulsion, dizziness and vertigo due to Liver Wind.

■ **SCORPIO, SCOLOPENDRA AND BOMBYX BATRYTICATUS**

- *Quan Xie, Wu Gong and Jiang Can*

— All of these substances are insects that subdue Wind, and their actions of stopping

convulsion, removing obstruction from the collaterals and relieving pain are potentiated when they are used in combination.
— This combination is indicated for Excess-type Liver Wind, giving rise to convulsions, as in tetanus, Wind-Stroke and infantile convulsion.
— For Deficiency-type Liver Wind, decrease the dosage and add tonics to the prescription. If Liver Wind is due to Yin Deficiency, add herbs that nourish the Yin. For chronic convulsion in children due to Spleen Deficiency, add herbs that tonify and invigorate the Spleen.

■ **FRUCTUS LYCII AND FLOS CHRYSANTHEMI**

- *Gou Qi Zi and Ju Hua*

— Fructus Lycii nourishes Liver and Kidney Yin and improves vision. Flos Chrysanthemi clears Wind-Heat and Liver Heat, calms the Liver and improves vision.
— This combination is indicated for eye disorders due to Liver and Kidney Yin Deficiency and for headache, dizziness and vertigo due to Kidney and Liver Yin Deficiency leading to Liver Yang Rising and Liver Wind.

■ **CONCHA OSTREAE, PLASTRUM TESTUDINIS, CARAPAX TRIONYCIS, RADIX REHMANNIAE AND RADIX PAEONIAE ALBA**

- *Mu Li, Gui Ban, Bie Jia, Sheng Di and Bai Shao*

— Ostreae, Plastrum Testudinis and Carapax Trionycis are three shells that subdue hyperactive Yang. Plastrum Testudinis and Carapax Trionycis are salty and cold in nature and nourish the Yin; this action is

potentiated when they are combined with Radix Rehmanniae and Radix Paeoniae Alba.
— This combination is indicated for consumption of Body Fluids at the late stage of febrile disease and for tremor of the hands and feet due to Yin Deficiency leading to Liver Wind.

■ RHIZOMA GASTRODIAE, CORTEX EUCOMMIAE AND RAMULUS LORANTHI

- *Tian Ma, Du Zhong and Sang Ji Sheng*

— Rhizoma Gastrodiae not only calms the Liver and subdues Wind but also removes obstruction from the collaterals and treats Bi syndromes. Cortex Eucommiae and Ramulus Loranthi tonify the Liver and Kidneys, strengthen the lower back and knees and lower blood pressure.
— This combination is indicated for sore and weak lower back and knees, Bi syndromes, and hypertension due to Kidney Deficiency with symptoms of lumbar soreness, dizziness and vertigo, and numbness of the limbs and body (Table 18.1).

■ CORNU ANTELOPIS, RADIX GENTIANAE AND CONCHA HALIOTIDIS

- *Ling Yang Jiao, Long Dan Cao and Shi Jue Ming*

— This combination clears Liver Heat and

Fire and improves vision. It is indicated for red eyes and headache due to Liver Fire.

■ CORNU ANTELOPIS, FRUCTUS LYCII AND HERBA DENDROBII

- *Ling Yang Jiao, Gou Qi Zi and Shi Hu*

— This combination nourishes Yin, clears Liver Heat and improves vision. It is indicated for blurred vision and other eye disorders due to Liver and Kidney Yin Deficiency with Empty Heat.

■ HAEMATITUM, CONCHA OSTREAE AND RADIX ACHYRANTHIS BIDENTATAE

- *Zhe Shi, Mu Li and Niu Xi*

— Haematitum and Concha Ostreae calm the Liver and subdue hyperactive Liver Yang and Liver Wind. Radix Achyranthis Bidentatae assists Haematitum to conduct Fire downward.
— This combination is indicated for headache, dizziness and vertigo, burning pain in the head, tinnitus, redness of the face and restlessness due to Yin Deficiency, Liver Yang and Liver Wind. A stronger therapeutic action will be obtained with the addition of Magnetitum and Radix Paeoniae Alba.

Table 18.1 Actions and indications of Rhizoma Gastrodiae in combination with other herbs

Rhizoma Gastrodiae + Rhizoma Pinelliae + Rhizoma Atractylodis Macrocephalae	Rhizoma Pinelliae dries Damp and resolves Phlegm; Rhizoma Gastrodiae calms Liver Wind. Rhizoma Atractylodis Macrocephalae invigorates the Spleen	Indicated for dizziness and vertigo due to Damp-Phlegm
Rhizoma Gastrodiae + Ramulus Uncariae cum Uncis	Both herbs calm the Liver and subdue Liver Wind	Indicated for headache, dizziness and vertigo due to Liver Yang Rising; and for convulsion, dizziness and vertigo due to Liver Wind
Rhizoma Gastrodiae + Cortex Eucommiae + Ramulus Loranthi	Rhizoma Gastrodiae calms the Liver and subdues Wind, and removes obstruction from the collaterals; Cortex Eucommiae tonifies the Liver and Kidneys	Indicated for sore and weak lower back and knees, Bi syndromes and hypertension due to Kidney Deficiency

■ OS DRACONIS AND CONCHA OSTREAE

- *Long Gu and Mu Li*

— This combination astringes discharges, calms the Liver and subdues hyperactive Yang. It is indicated for spontaneous sweating, night sweats and thin leucorrhoea, and for headache, dizziness and vertigo, palpitations and insomnia due to Liver Yang Rising.

■ CINNABARIS AND MAGNETITUM

- *Zhu Sha and Ci Shi*

— This combination soothes the Heart and calms the Mind. It is indicated for insomnia, dream-disturbed sleep, absent-mindedness, manic-depressive disorders and red eyes and tinnitus due to Liver Fire.

■ SEMEN ZIZIPHI SPINOSAE AND SEMEN BIOTAE

- *Suan Zao Ren and Bai Zi Ren*

— This combination nourishes the Heart and calms the Mind. It is indicated for palpitations and insomnia. A stronger therapeutic action will be obtained with the addition of Poria cum Ligno Hospite (*Fu Shen*) and Os Draconis.

■ RADIX GLYCYRRHIZAE, WHEAT AND FRUCTUS ZIZIPHI

- *Gan Cao, Fu Xiao Mai and Da Zao*

— All three are sweet herbs that relax the Liver; wheat also nourishes the Heart and relieves restlessness. This combination is indicated for hysteria, neurosis and schizophrenia. Its actions of nourishing Heart Yin, clearing Heart Fire, resolving Stagnation and calming the Mind can be strengthened by the addition of Radix Ophiopogonis and Cortex Albiziae.

Tonics and astringents

19

■ **RADIX GINSENG AND RADIX
ASTRAGALI SEU HEDYARI**

● *Ren Shen and Huang Qi*

— This combination strongly tonifies Source
(*Yuan*) Qi; it also tonifies Qi generally
and thus stimulates the production of
Blood. Both herbs are important Qi tonics
and their action of tonifying Qi is
potentiated when they are used in combination.
— This combination is indicated for
Deficiency of Defensive (*Wei*) Qi, weakness
of Source Qi and Deficiency of both Qi and
Blood.

■ **RADIX GINSENG AND RADIX
ACONITI PRAEPARATA**

● *Ren Shen and Fu Zi*

— Radix Ginseng strongly tonifies Source Qi
and also tonifies Qi generally and treats
Collapse of Qi. Radix Aconiti Praeparata
restores devastated Yang and treats Collapse
of Yang.
— This combination tonifies Qi and recaptures
Yang and is indicated for Collapse of Yang.
In small doses it also treats general patterns
of Qi and Yang Deficiency.

■ **RADIX GINSENG, RADIX
OPHIOPOGONIS AND FRUCTUS
SCHISANDRAE**

● *Ren Shen, Mai Dong and Wu Wei Zi*

— Radix Ginseng tonifies Qi and treats
Collapse of Qi, Radix Ophiopogonis
nourishes Yin and Fructus Schisandrae
astringes and treats patterns of Collapse.
— This combination tonifies Qi, nourishes Yin
and treats patterns of Collapse. It is

indicated for Collapse of Yin. In small doses
it treats deficiency of Qi and Yin with
symptoms of thirst, profuse sweating, lassitude, chronic cough, shortness of breath, a
red tongue and a thready and weak
pulse due to consumption of Qi and Yin by
Heat.

■ **RADIX GINSENG AND RADIX
REHMANNIAE PRAEPARATA**

● *Ren Shen and Shu Di*

— Radix Ginseng tonifies Source Qi; it also
tonifies Qi generally and stimulates the
production of Blood. Radix Rehmanniae
Praeparata nourishes Blood and Yin.
— This combination strongly tonifies Qi and
Blood and is indicated for severe weakness
of Essential (*Jing*) Qi and Deficiency of Qi
and Blood.

■ **RADIX GINSENG AND RADIX
POLYGONI MULTIFLORI**

● *Ren Shen and Shou Wu*

— Radix Ginseng tonifies Qi; Radix Polygoni
Multiflori tonifies the Liver and Kidneys and
nourishes Yin and Blood.
— This combination tonifies Qi, Blood and
Yin and is indicated for patterns of
concurrent Qi and Yin Deficiency, Qi and
Blood Deficiency, senility and chronic
malaria marked by deficiency of Defensive
Qi.

■ **RADIX GINSENG AND GECKO OR
SEMEN JUGLANDIS**

● *Ren Shen and Ge Jie or Hu Tao Rou*

— This combination tonifies the Lungs and

Kidneys and stimulates the reception of Qi. It is indicated for chronic cough and dyspnoea due to deficiency of both the Lungs and Kidneys marked by failure of the Kidneys to grasp the Qi.

■ RADIX GINSENG AND CORNU CERVI PANTOTRICHUM

● *Ren Shen and Lu Rong*

— Radix Ginseng strongly tonifies Source Qi; Cornu Cervi Pantotrichum warms and tonifies Kidney Yang and benefits Essence and Blood.
— This combination tonifies Source Qi and benefits Essence and Blood and is indicated for Deficiency patterns of Kidney Yang, Essence, Blood and Qi and Blood concurrently. It can be taken during the winter as a general tonic by elderly

people with deficiency of Yang and Qi (Table 19.1).

■ RADIX CODONOPSIS PILOSULAE AND RHIZOMA ATRACTYLODIS MACROCEPHALAE

● *Dang Shen and Bai Zhu*

— This combination tonifies Qi and invigorates the Spleen. It is indicated for Spleen Qi Deficiency.

■ RHIZOMA ATRACTYLODIS MACROCEPHALAE AND PORIA

● *Bai Zhu and Fu Ling*

— This combination tonifies Qi, invigorates the Spleen and resolves Dampness. It is indicated for Spleen Qi Deficiency with or without oedema and diarrhoea.

Table 19.1 Actions and indications of Radix Ginseng, in combination with other herbs

Radix Ginseng + Radix Astragali seu Hedysari	This combination tonifies Source Qi, and Qi generally	Indicated for deficiency of Source Qi, Defensive Qi or Qi and Blood.
Radix Ginseng + Radix Aconiti Praeparata	Radix Ginseng tonifies Qi and treats Collapse of Qi; Radix Aconiti Praeparata treats Collapse of Yang	Indicated for Collapse of Yang
Radix Ginseng + Fructus Schisandrae + Radix Ophiopogonis	Radix Ginseng treats Collapse of Qi; Fructus Schisandrae astringes and treats patterns of Collapse; Radix Ophiopogonis nourishes Yin	Indicated for Collapse of Yin
Radix Ginseng + Radix Rehmanniae Praeparata	Radix Ginseng tonifies Qi and stimulates the production of Blood. Radix Rehmanniae Praeparata nourishes Blood and Yin	Indicated for deficiency of Essential Qi or of Qi and Blood
Radix Ginseng + Polygoni Multiflori	Radix Ginseng tonifies Qi; Polygoni Multiflori nourishes Yin and Blood	Indicated for deficiency of Qi and Blood or of Qi and Yin
Radix Ginseng + Gecko or Semen Juglandis	Radix Ginseng tonifies Qi; Gecko and Semen Judlandis stimulate reception of Qi	Indicated for chronic cough and dyspnoea due to Lung and Kidney Qi Deficiency
Radix Ginseng + Cornu Cervi Pantotrichum	Radix Ginseng tonifies Source Qi; Cornu Cervi Pantotrichum warms and tonifies Kidney Yang	Indicated for Deficiency patterns of Kidney Yang, Essence, Qi and Blood

■ RHIZOMA ATRACTYLODIS MACROCEPHALAE AND RHIZOMA DIOSCOREAE

- *Bai Zhu and Shan Yao*

— This combination tonifies Qi and invigorates the Spleen. It is indicated for diarrhoea and leucorrhoea due to Spleen Deficiency.

■ RHIZOMA ATRACTYLODIS MACROCEPHALAE AND FRUCTUS AURANTII IMMATURUS

- *Bai Zhu and Zhi Shi*

— This combination tonifies Qi, invigorates the Spleen, regulates Qi and relieves fullness. It is indicated for poor appetite and for distension and pain in the epigastrium and abdomen due to deficiency of the Middle Burner with stagnation of Qi.

■ RADIX ASTRAGALI SEU HEDYSARI, RHIZOMA CIMICIFUGAE AND RADIX BUPLEURI

- *Huang Qi, Sheng Ma and Chai Hu*

— Radix Astragali seu Hedysari tonifies Qi and lifts Yang; Rhizoma Cimicifugae and Radix Bupleuri lift the Qi of the Middle Burner.
— This combination tonifies Qi and lifts Yang. It is indicated for prolapse of the internal organs or anus and for chronic diarrhoea due to Sinking of Spleen Qi. The therapeutic action is strengthened by the addition of Fructus Aurantii Immaturus.

■ RADIX ASTRAGALI SEU HEDYSARI AND RADIX LEDEBOURIELLAE

- *Huang Qi and Fang Feng*

— Radix Ledebouriellae assists Radix Astragali seu Hedysari to go to the surface of the body

to tonify Qi and consolidate the Exterior. Radix Astragali seu Hedysari assists Radix Ledebouriellae to tonify Qi, Release the Exterior and expel Wind.
— In combination they tonify Qi, consolidate the Exterior and stop sweating. With a relatively large dose of Radix Astragali seu Hedysari the combination is indicated for spontaneous sweating due to Qi Deficiency. With a relatively large dosage of Radix Ledebouriellae the combination is indicated for Qi Deficiency complicated with External Invasion (Fig 19.1).

■ RADIX ASTRAGALI SEU HEDYSARI AND RADIX ACONITI PRAEPARATA

- *Huang Qi and Fu Zi*

— Radix Astragali seu Hedysari tonifies Qi and stops sweating; Radix Aconiti Praeparata warms the Yang.
— This combination tonifies Qi and Yang and stops sweating. It is indicated for spontaneous sweating and lassitude due to Qi and Yang Deficiency.

■ RADIX ASTRAGALI SEU HEDYSARI AND CONCHA OSTREAE

- *Huang Qi and Mu Li*

— Radix Astragali tonifies Qi, consolidates the Exterior and stops sweating. Concha Ostreae stops sweating by astringing.
— This combination tonifies Qi and stops sweating. It is indicated for spontaneous sweating due to Qi Deficiency.

■ RADIX ASTRAGALI SEU HEDYSARI AND RADIX ANGELICAE SINENSIS

- *Huang Qi and Dang Gui*

— Radix Angelicae Sinensis tonifies Blood;

Radix Astragalus Seu Hedysari > Radix Ledebouriellae	Radix Ledebouriellae > Radix Astragalus seu Hedysari
Primary function of this combination is Qi tonification	Primary function of this combination is elimination of External Wind
It is indicated for spontaneous sweating due to Qi Deficiency	It is indicated for external invasion due to Qi Deficiency

Fig. 19.1 Dose-related differences in the actions of Radix Astragali seu Hedysari and Radix Ledebouriellae.

Radix Astragali seu Hedysari tonifies Qi and thus indirectly stimulates the production and control of Blood.

— This combination tonifies Qi and Blood. It is indicated for Blood Deficiency, Qi and Blood Deficiency and haemorrhagic patterns due to failure of the Qi to control Blood (Table 19.2).

— For numbness of the limbs and body and systemic painful joints due to failure of the Blood to nourish the tendons, add Ramulus Cinnamomi and Caulis Spatholobi.

— For haemorrhagic patterns due to failure of the Qi to control Blood, add Rhizoma Zingiberis (baked), Arillus Longan and Radix Ginseng.

■ RADIX ANGELICAE SINENSIS AND RADIX PAEONIAE ALBA

● *Dang Gui and Bai Shao*

— Radix Angelicae Sinensis tonifies and moves Blood; Radix Paeoniae Alba tonifies Blood and nourishes Yin.

— This combination tonifies Blood and is indicated for patterns of Blood Deficiency and disorders of menstruation and labour. With the addition of Ramulus Cinnamomi, it treats abdominal pain due to deficiency of the Middle Burner.

■ RADIX PAEONIAE ALBA AND RADIX GLYCYRRHIZAE

● *Bai Shao and Gan Cao*

— Radix Paeoniae Alba is sour in nature; it astringes, nourishes Yin, eases the Liver and relieves pain. Radix Glycyrrhizae is sweet in nature; it relaxes spasm and relieves pain.

— This combination produces Fluids by its combination of the sweet and sour tastes; it also harmonizes the Blood, relaxes spasm and relieves pain. It is indicated for cramping abdominal pain, hypochondriac pain due to Liver Deficiency, spasm of musculus gastrocnemius and spontaneous and night sweats due to Yin Deficiency.

■ RADIX REHMANNIAE PRAEPARATA AND FRUCTUS CORNI

● *Shu Di and Shan Yu Rou*

— This combination tonifies Liver and Kidney Yin and is thus indicated for Liver and Kidney Yin Deficiency.

Table 19.2 Actions and indications of Radix Astragali seu Hedysari in combination with other herbs

Radix Astragali seu Hedysari + Radix Ginseng	Both herbs tonify Qi	Indicated for Qi Deficiency or Qi and Blood Deficiency
Radix Astragali seu Hedysari + Rhizoma Cimicifugae + Radix Bupleuri	Radix Astragali seu Hedysari tonifies Qi and lifts Yang; Rhizoma Cimicifugae and Radix Bupleuri lift the Qi of the Middle Burner	Indicated for Spleen Qi Sinking
Radix Astragali seu Hedysari + Radix Ledebouriellae	Radix Astragali seu Hedysari consolidates the Exterior; Radix Ledebouriellae expels Wind	Indicated for deficiency of Defensive Qi
Radix Astragali seu Hedysari + Radix Aconiti Praeparata	Radix Astragali seu Hedysari tonifies Qi and stops sweating; Radix Aconiti Praeparata warms the Yang	Indicated for spontaneous sweating and lassitude due to Qi and Yang Deficiency
Radix Astragali seu Hedysari + Concha Ostreae	Radix Astragali seu Hedysari stops sweating by tonifying Qi; Concha Ostreae stops sweating by astringing	Indicated for spontaneous sweating due to Qi Deficiency
Radix Astragali seu Hedysari + Radix Angelicae Sinensis	Radix Astragali seu Hedysari tonifies Qi and stimulates the production and control of Blood. Radix Angelicae Sinensis tonifies Blood	Indicated for bleeding due to Qi and Blood Deficiency

■ **RADIX REHMANNIAE PRAEPARATA AND FRUCTUS AMOMI**

● *Shu Di and Sha Ren*

— Radix Rehmanniae Praeparata nourishes Yin and Blood but is sticky in nature and can impair the function of the Stomach. Fructus Amomi regulates Qi and invigorates the Spleen and Stomach to modify the sticky nature of Radix Rehmanniae Praeparata.
— This combination thus nourishes Yin and Blood without impairing the function of the Stomach and is indicated for Yin and Blood Deficiency complicated with poor appetite.

■ **RADIX GLEHNIAE AND RADIX OPHIOPOGONIS**

● *Bei Sha Shen and Mai Dong*

— Both herbs nourish Yin and produce Body Fluids and this action is potentiated when they are used together. This combination is indicated for:
1. Cough due to Lung Yin Deficiency
2. Stomach Yin Deficiency giving rise to thirst, an empty and uncomfortable sensation in the Stomach and dull burning pain in the epigastrium
3. Lung and Stomach Heat with consumption of Body Fluids (diabetes), with symptoms of a desire to drink large quantities and loss of weight.

■ **RADIX OPHIOPOGONIS AND RADIX ASPARAGI**

● *Mai Dong and Tian Dong*

— Both herbs nourish Yin, moisten the Lungs and stop cough, and these actions are potentiated when they are used together.
— This combination is indicated for chronic non-productive cough due to Lung Yin Deficiency or Lung and Kidney Yin Deficiency.

■ **RADIX OPHIOPOGONIS, RADIX REHMANNIAE AND SEMEN ZIZIPHI SPINOSAE**

● *Mai Dong, Sheng Di and Suan Zao Ren*

— This combination nourishes Heart Yin and calms the Mind. It is indicated for restlessness, insomnia and palpitations due to Yin Deficiency with Empty Fire.

■ **RADIX OPHIOPOGONIS, RADIX REHMANNIAE AND RHIZOMA COPTIDIS**

● *Mai Dong, Sheng Di and Huang Lian*

— This combination nourishes Heart Yin and clears Heart Fire. It is indicated for febrile disease with high fever, irritability and coma and for Flaring of Heart Fire with mouth and tongue ulcers.

■ **HERBA DENDROBII AND RADIX OPHIOPOGONIS**

● *Shi Hu and Mai Dong*

— This combination nourishes the Stomach and stimulates the production of Body Fluids. It is indicated for consumption of Stomach Yin due to febrile disease, with symptoms of low grade fever, thirst and dryness of the tongue, and for Stomach Yin Deficiency with symptoms of retching, dull burning stomach pain and an empty uncomfortable feeling of the stomach.

■ **HERBA DENDROBII, FRUCTUS LYCII AND FLOS CHRYSANTHEMI**

● *Shi Hu, Gou Qi Zi and Ju Hua*

— This combination nourishes the Liver and improves vision. It is indicated for blurred vision due to Liver and Kidney Yin Deficiency and for chronic eye disorders due to Yin Deficiency.

■ **FRUCTUS LIGUSTRI LUCIDI AND HERBA ECLIPTAE**

● *Nu Zhen Zi and Han Lian Cao*

— Both herbs tonify Liver and Kidney Yin, but Fructus Ligustri Lucidi is more effective in tonifying Kidney Yin while Herba Ecliptae is more effective in tonifying Liver Yin. Herba Ecliptae also cools Blood and stops bleeding.
— This combination is indicated for patterns of Liver and Kidney Yin Deficiency and for haemorrhagic patterns due to Yin Deficiency.

■ RHIZOMA CURCULIGINIS AND HERBA EPIMEDII

● *Xian Mao and Yin Yang Huo*

— This combination warms and tonifies Kidney Yang, disperses Cold Damp and relieves Bi syndromes. It is indicated for:
  1. Kidney Yang Deficiency with symptoms of impotence and infertility
  2. chronic Cold Damp Bi syndrome with a cold sensation and pain in the lumbar region and knees
  3. menopausal hypertension.
— With the addition of Rhizoma Anemarrhenae, Cortex Phellodendri and Radix Angelicae Sinensis, these herbs lower blood pressure by regulating Yin and Yang.

■ HERBA EPIMEDII AND RAMULUS LORANTHI

● *Yin Yang Huo and Sang Ji Sheng*

— Herba Epimedii warms Kidney Yang, disperses Cold and Dampness and removes obstruction from the channels. Ramulus Loranthi tonifies the Liver and Kidneys, strengthens the tendons and bones and relieves Bi syndrome.
— This combination tonifies the Liver and Kidneys, strengthens tendons and bones and relieves paralysis and Bi syndrome. It is indicated for chronic Bi syndrome, Wei syndrome and infantile paralysis.

■ CORTEX EUCOMMIAE AND RADIX DIPSACI

● *Du Zhong and Xu Duan*

— This combination tonifies the Liver and Kidneys, strengthens the lower back and knees, promotes the healing of sprains and fractures and prevents miscarriage. It is indicated for lower back pain due to Kidney Deficiency, chronic Bi syndrome, osteoporosis, contusions and sprains and threatened abortion.

■ PLASTRUM TESTUDINIS AND CORNU CERVI

● *Gui Ban and Lu Jiao*

— Plastrum Testudinis is salty, sweet and cold in nature; it strongly tonifies Kidney Yin, nourishes Yin generally and reinforces the Ren channel. Cornu Cervi is sweet, salty and warm in nature; it warms the Kidney, tonifies Yang, benefits Essence and Blood and reinforces the Du channel.
— This combination thus tonifies both Yin and Yang and reinforces the Ren and Du channels as well as the other Extraordinary channels. It is indicated for deficiency of both Yin and Yang, and of Essence and Blood, and for severe Deficiency patterns due to Emptiness of the eight Extraordinary channels. It is often administered in the form of a liquid extract.

■ FRUCTUS ALPINIAE OXYPHYLLAE AND RADIX LINDERAE

● *Yi Zhi Ren and Wu Yao*

— Fructus Alpiniae Oxyphyllae warms and astringes the Kidneys while Radix Linderae warms the Lower Burner and eliminates Cold from the Bladder.
— This combination thus warms the Kidneys, eliminates Cold and astringes urine. It is indicated for urinary frequency or incontinence, or enuresis due to Kidney Deficiency, and for weakness of the Bladder with stagnation of Cold.

■ FRUCTUS PSORALEAE AND SEMEN MYRISTICAE

● *Bu Gu Zhi and Rou Dou Kou*

— Fructus Psoraleae warms Kidney Yang and tonifies Ming Men Fire, while Semen Myristicae warms the Spleen, regulates Qi and astringes the intestines to stop diarrhoea.
— This combination warms both the Spleen and Kidneys and astringes the intestines to stop diarrhoea. It is indicated for chronic diarrhoea and dysentery due to Spleen and Kidney Yang Deficiency.

■ FRUCTUS ROSAE LAEVIGATAE AND SEMEN EURYALES

● *Jin Ying Zi and Qian Shi*

— Rosae Laevigatae is sour and astringent in nature; it consolidates Essence and stops diarrhoea and leucorrhoea. Euryales is sweet, neutral and astringent in nature; it primarily invigorates the Spleen and tonifies the Kidneys, but also consolidates Essence to stop diarrhoea and leucorrhoea.

— When they are used together, their mutual action of astringing the Essence is strengthened and this combination is thus indicated for spermatorrhoea, enuresis, leucorrhoea and diarrhoea.

■ RADIX EPHEDRAE AND FRUCTUS TRITICI LEVIS

● *Ma Huang Gen and Fu Xiao Mai*

— This combination stops sweating and is thus indicated for spontaneous sweating and night sweats. For Yin Deficiency, add Yin tonics such as Radix Ophiopogonis and Radix Paeoniae Alba. For Qi Deficiency, add Qi tonics such as Radix Astragali seu Hedysari and Rhizoma Atractylodis Macrocephalae.

20 *Herbs that warm the Interior and regulate Qi*

■ **RADIX ACONITI PRAEPARATA AND RHIZOMA ZINGIBERIS**

• *Fu Zi and Gan Jiang*

— Rhizoma Zingiberis strengthens the action of Radix Aconiti Praeparata in restoring Collapsed Yang and moderates its toxicity.
— This combination restores Collapsed Yang, warms the Interior and disperses Cold. It is indicated for Collapse of Yang, and Yang Deficiency with Internal Cold.
— For abdominal pain and diarrhoea due to Spleen Yang Deficiency, add Radix Codonopsis Pilosulae and Rhizoma Atractylodis Macrocephalae.

■ **RADIX ACONITI PRAEPARATA AND CORTEX CINNAMOMI**

• *Fu Zi and Rou Gui*

— This combination warms Kidney Yang. It is indicated for soreness of the lower back and knees, cold limbs due to Kidney Yang Deficiency, and decline of Ming Men Fire. The action of tonifying Yang is strengthened by the addition of herbs that tonify Kidney Yin. To tonify both Yin and Yang, add Radix Rehmanniae Praeparata and Fructus Corni.

■ **RHIZOMA ATRACTYLODIS MACRO-CEPHALAE AND RADIX ACONITI PRAEPARATA**

• *Bai Zhu and Fu Zi*

— Rhizoma Atractylodis Macrocephalae invigorates the Spleen and dries Dampness. Radix Aconiti Praeparata warms Yang, disperses Cold and relieves pain.
— This combination warms Yang, disperses Cold, invigorates the Spleen and eliminates Dampness. It is indicated for abdominal distension and loose stools due to Spleen Yang Deficiency with retention of Cold Damp and for general aching due to invasion by Cold Damp.

■ **FRUCTUS EVODIAE AND RHIZOMA ZINGIBERIS RECENS**

• *Wu Zhu Yu and Sheng Jiang*

— This combination warms the Middle Burner, relieves pain and conducts Rebellious Qi downward to stop vomiting. It is indicated for pain, retching and spitting of saliva due to retention of Cold in the Stomach and for hiccup.

■ **FLOS CARYOPHYLLI AND CORTEX CINNAMOMI**

• *Ding Xiang and Rou Gui*

— Both herbs are pungent, aromatic and warm in nature and combine to warm the Middle Burner and relieve pain.
— This combination is indicated for a cold sensation and pain in the heart and abdomen. It is administered by mouth or ground to a powder and applied to the umbilicus as a medicinal plaster.

■ **CORTEX CINNAMOMI AND RADIX ET RHIZOMA RHEI**

• *Rou Gui and Da Huang*

— Cortex Cinnamomi warms the Interior and disperses Cold. Radix et Rhizoma Rhei activates Blood circulation, clears Poison and stops dysentery
— This combination disperses Cold and stops dysentery. It is indicated for chronic

Table 20.1 Actions and indications of Cortex Cinnamomi in combination with other herbs

Cortex Cinnamomi + Radix Aconiti Praeparata	Both herbs warm Kidney Yang	Indicated for Kidney Yang Deficiency
Cortex Connamomi + Flos Caryophylli	Both herbs warm the Middle Burner and move Qi to relieve pain	Indicated for a cold sensation and pain in the heart and abdomen
Cortex Cinnamomi + Radix et Rhizoma Rhei	Cortex Cinnamomi warms the Interior and disperses Cold; Radix et Rhizoma Rhei purges the intestines	Indicated for chronic dysentery due to Spleen Yang Deficiency

dysentery due to Spleen Yang Deficiency (Table 20.1).

■ RHIZOMA ALPINIAE OFFICINALIS AND RHIZOMA CYPERI

● *Gao Liang Jiang and Xiang Fu*

— Rhizoma Alpiniae Officinalis warms the Stomach and disperses Cold. Rhizoma Cyperi regulates Qi and relieves pain
— This combination warms the Stomach and regulates Qi. It is indicated for epigastric pain due to stagnation of Qi and Cold.

■ FLOS CARYOPHYLLI AND CALYX KAKI

● *Ding Xiang and Shi Di*

— Both herbs warm the Middle Burner, conduct Rebellious Qi downward and stop vomiting and hiccup, and these actions are potentiated when they are used together.
— This combination is indicated for hiccup and vomiting due to stagnation of Cold in the Stomach.

■ RHIZOMA ZINGIBERIS, HERBA ASARI AND FRUCTUS SCHISANDRA

● *Gan Jiang, Xi Xin and Wu Wei Zi*

— Rhizoma Zingiberis and Herba Asari are pungent and hot in nature; they warm the Lungs to resolve retained Water. Fructus Schisandrae is sour in nature and astringes the Lungs to stop cough.
— This combination warms the Lungs, resolves retained Water and stimulates the Lungs' function of governing respiration. It is thus indicated for chronic cough and dyspnoea due to retention of Cold and Water in the Lungs.

■ RHIZOMA ZINGIBERIS (BAKED) AND FOLIUM ARTEMISIAE ARGYI

● *Pao Jiang and Ai Ye*

— Both herbs stop bleeding. In addition, Baked Rhizoma Zingiberis warms the Spleen while Folium Artemisiae Argyi warms the uterus.
— This combination warms the channels and stops bleeding. It is indicated for bloody stools and uterine bleeding due to Deficiency with stagnation of Cold.
— If bleeding is caused by a failure of Qi to control Blood, add herbs that tonify Qi and control Blood, such as Radix Astragali seu Hedysari.

■ RHIZOMA CYPERI AND FOLIUM ARTEMISIAE ARGYI

● *Xiang Fu and Ai Ye*

— Rhizoma Cyperi regulates Qi and menstruation while Folium Artemisiae Argyi disperses Cold and warms the channels and uterus.
— This combination warms the uterus and regulates Qi and menstruation. It is indicated for dysmenorrhoea due to stagnation of Qi and Cold and for irregular menstruation and infertility due to retention of Cold in the uterus.

■ PERICARPIUM CITRI RETICULATAE VIRIDE AND PERICARPIUM CITRI RETICULATAE

● *Qing Pi and Chen Pi*

— Pericarpium Citri Reticulatae Viride harmonizes the Liver, breaks Qi stagnation and resolves masses. Pericarpium Citri Reticulatae regulates Qi and harmonizes the

Stomach. Their action of regulating Qi and relieving pain is potentiated when they are used together.

— This combination harmonizes the Liver and the Stomach and regulates Qi. It is indicated for distension and pain in the epigastrium and hypochondrium due to stagnation of Qi in the Liver and Stomach.

■ FRUCTUS MELIAE TOOSENDAN AND RHIZOMA CORYDALIS

● *Chuan Lian Zi and Yan Hu Suo*

— Fructus Meliae Toosendan harmonizes the Liver and clears Heat while Rhizoma Corydalis activates Qi and Blood circulation and relieves pain.

— Their actions of harmonizing the Liver, regulating Qi and relieving pain are potentiated when they are used together and this combination is thus indicated for pain due to Qi Stagnation or Liver Qi Stagnation turning to Heat.

■ FRUCTUS TRICHOSANTHIS AND BULBUS ALLII MACROSTEMI

● *Gua Lou and Xie Bai*

— Both herbs open the chest. In addition, Fructus Trichosanthis resolves Phlegm while Bulbus Allii Macrostemi regulates Qi, invigorates Yang and disperses masses.

— This combination invigorates Yang, resolves Phlegm, regulates Qi and relieves pain. It is indicated for obstruction of Qi in the chest marked by chest pain due to deficiency of Yang and retention of Turbid Phlegm.

■ RHIZOMA CYPERI AND FLOS INULAE

● *Xiang Fu and Xuan Fu Hua*

— Rhizoma Cyperi regulates Qi and relieves stagnation while Flos Inulae resolves Phlegm, disperses masses and harmonizes the collaterals.

— This combination regulates Qi, harmonizes the collaterals and relieves pain. It is indicated for costal and hypochondriac pain and stuffiness in the chest.

■ RADIX AUCKLANDIAE AND FRUCTUS AMOMI

● *Mu Xiang and Sha Ren*

— Radix Aucklandiae regulates Qi, invigorates the Spleen, warms the Middle Burner, relieves pain and stops diarrhoea. Fructus Amomi promotes the circulation of Qi, resolves Dampness and conducts Rebellious Qi downward to stop vomiting.

— This combination regulates Qi and harmonizes the Stomach. It is indicated for patterns of stagnation of Stomach and Spleen Qi.

■ FRUCTUS AURANTII AND RADIX PLATYCODI

● *Zhi Qiao and Jie Geng*

— Fructus Aurantii regulates Qi and conducts Rebellious Qi downward while Radix Platycodi stimulates the Lungs' dispersing function and lifts Sinking Qi.

— This combination is indicated for discomfort and stuffiness in the chest and epigastrium due to stagnation of Lung and Stomach Qi.

Herbs that activate Blood circulation and stop bleeding

21

■ RADIX ANGELICAE SINENSIS AND RHIZOMA LIGUSTICI CHUANXIONG

- *Dang Gui and Chuang Xiong*

— Both herbs activates Blood circulation. In addition, Radix Angelicae Sinensis tonifies Blood, while Rhizoma Ligustici Chuanxiong activates Qi circulation.
— This combination tonifies Blood, activates Blood circulation, regulates menstruation and relieves pain. It is indicated for disorders of menstruation and labour due to Blood Deficiency and Blood Stagnation and for patterns of Stagnant Qi and Blood.

■ RHIZOMA LIGUSTICI CHUANXIONG AND RADIX ANGELICAE DAHURICAE

- *Chuan Xiong and Bai Zhi*

— Both herbs eliminate Wind and relieve pain; in addition, Rhizoma Ligustici Chuanxiong activates Blood circulation.
— This combination eliminates Wind and relieves pain and is indicated for chronic intermittent headache due to Wind in the head.

■ RHIZOMA SPARGANII AND RHIZOMA ZEDOARIAE

- *San Leng and E Zhu*

— Both herbs break stagnation of Qi and Blood, but Rhizoma Sparganii is more effective in breaking Blood Stagnation while Rhizoma Zedoariae is more effective in breaking Qi Stagnation. Their action of breaking Stasis and resolving Stagnation is strengthened when they are used together.
— This combination breaks Qi and Blood Stagnation, relieves pain and disperses palpable abdominal masses. It is indicated for pain and palpable abdominal masses due to stagnation of Qi and Blood.

■ SEMEN PERSICAE AND FLOS CARTHAMI

- *Tao Ren and Hong Hua*

— Semen Persicae breaks Blood Stasis while Flos Carthami activates Blood circulation and regulates menstruation.
— This combination breaks Blood Stasis and activates Blood circulation. It is indicated for patterns of Blood Stagnation such as dysmenorrhoea, amenorrhoea, postpartum abdominal pain, Bi syndrome, abscess, swelling and pain due to trauma, and abdominal pain due to stagnation of Blood.

■ HERBA LEONURI AND HERBA LYCOPI

- *Yi Mu Cao and Ze Lan*

— Both herbs activate Blood circulation, regulate menstruation, promote diuresis and relieve swelling, and these actions are strengthened when they are used together.
— This combination is indicated for amenorrhoea due to stagnation of Blood and for oedema due to retention of Water and stagnant Blood.

■ RESINA OLIBANI AND RESINA MYRRHAE

- *Ru Xiang and Mo Yao*

— Both herbs resolve Blood Stasis and relieve pain, but Resina Olibani is more effective in circulating Qi while Resina Myrrhae is more effective in dispersing stagnant Blood.

— This combination is indicated for pain due to stagnation of Qi and Blood and for non-healing carbuncles, boils and ulcers.

■ RADIX SALVIAE MILTIORRHIZAE, LIGNUM SANTALI AND RHIZOMA LIGUSTICI CHUANXIONG

● *Dan Shen, Tan Xiang and Chuan Xiong*

— Radix Salviae Miltiorrhizae activates Blood circulation; Lignum Santali circulates Qi and opens the chest; Rhizoma Ligustici Chuanxiong activates the circulation of both Qi and Blood.
— This combination activates Qi and Blood circulation and relieves pain. It is indicated for stabbing pain and a feeling of suffocation in the heart and chest due to stagnant Qi and Blood obstructing the vessels of the heart.

■ POLLEN TYPHAE AND FAECES TROGOPTERORUM

● *Pu Huang and Wu Ling Zhi*

— Both substances resolve Blood Stasis, stop bleeding and relieve pain, but Pollen Typhae is more effective stopping bleeding while Faeces Trogopterorum is more effective in relieving pain.
— Their actions of resolving Blood Stasis, stopping bleeding and relieving pain are potentiated when they are used together. This combination is indicated for patterns of pain due to stagnation of Blood, such as dysmenorrhoea, postpartum abdominal pain, cardiac pain and abdominal pain, and for haemorrhagic patterns due to stagnation of Blood.

■ COLLA CORII ASINI AND POLLEN TYPHAE

● *A Jiao and Pu Huang*

— Colla Corii Asini nourishes and astringes Blood to stop bleeding while Pollen Typhae enters the Lower Burner, cools Blood and resolves Blood Stasis.
— Together, these substances nourish Blood and stop bleeding, and this combination is thus indicated for uterine bleeding, menorrhagia and haematuria.

■ COLLA CORII ASINI AND POWDER OF CONCHA MERETRICIS SEU CYCLINAE

● *A Jiao and Ge Fen Colla Corii*

— Colla Corii Asini nourishes Yin and stops bleeding while Concha Meretricis seu Cyclinae clears Lung Heat and resolves Phlegm.
— This combination nourishes Yin, clears Empty Fire and Lung Heat and stops bleeding. It is indicated for haemoptysis due to Lung Yin Deficiency with Empty Fire.

■ RADIX SANGUISORBAE AND FLOS SOPHORAE

● *Di Yu and Huai Hua*

— This combination cools Blood, stops bleeding and clears heat from the intestines. It is indicated for bloody stool and for bleeding due to haemorrhoids.

■ RADIX SANGUISORBAE AND CACUMEN BIOTAE

● *Di Yu and Ce Bai Ye*

— This combination cools Blood and stops bleeding. It is indicated for bleeding from the digestive tract due to Heat.

■ CACUMEN BIOTAE AND RHIZOMA ZINGIBERIS (BAKED)

● *Ce Bai Ye and Pao Jiang*

— This combination warms the channels and stops bleeding. It is indicated for Deficient and Cold patterns with bloody stools due to failure of the Spleen to control Blood.

■ HERBA CEPHALANOPLORIS AND RHIZOMA IMPERATAE

● *Xiao Ji and Bai Mao Gen*

— This combination cools Blood and stops bleeding and is indicated for haematuria and epistaxis.

Table 21.1 Types of blood disorder and combinations of herbs that treat them

Menstrual disorders due to Blood Deficiency and Stagnation	Radix Angelicae Sinensis Rhizoma Ligustici Chuanxiong
Uterine bleeding or haematuria due to Blood deficiency and Stagnation	Colla Corii Asini Pollen Typhae
Bloody stool due to Spleen not controlling Blood	Cacumen Biotae Baked ginger
Menstrual disorders, postpartum pain, Bi syndrome, abdominal pain or traumatic injury involving Blood Stasis	Semen Persicae Flos Carthami
Amennorhoea and oedema due to Stagnant Blood	Herba Leonuri Herba Lycopi
Cardiac or abdominal pain due to stagnation of Blood	Pollen Typhae Faeces Trogopterorum
Haematemesis or haemoptysis due to Stasis	Rhizoma Bletilla Radix Notoginseng
Palpable abdominal masses due to Qi and Blood Stagnation	Rhizoma Sparganii Rhizoma Zedoariae
Non-healing carbuncles, boils and ulcers due to stagnation of Qi and Blood	Resina Olibani Resina Myrrhae
Stabbing pain and feeling of suffocation in the chest due to stagnation of Qi and Blood	Radix Salviae Miltiorrhizae Lignum Santali Rhizoma Ligustici Chuanxiong
Haemoptysis due to Lung Empty Fire	Colla Corii Asini Concha Meretricis seu Cyclinae
Haemorrhoids or bloody stool due to Heat	Radix Sanguisorbae Flos Sophorae
Bleeding from gastrointestinal tract due to Heat	Radix Sanguisorbae Cacumen Biotae
Haematuria or epistaxis due to Heat	Herba Cephalanoploris Rhizoma Imperatae

■ RHIZOMA BLETILLAE AND RADIX NOTOGINSENG

- *Bai Ji and San Qi*

— Rhizoma Bletillae stops bleeding by astringing the Blood and promotes healing. Radix Notoginseng stops bleeding by resolving Blood Stasis and relieves pain.
— When used together, the haemostatic action of these herbs is potentiated, but without producing Blood Stagnation. This combination is indicated for haemoptysis and haematemesis.

Part 3:
Application of herbs on the basis of the differentiation of patterns of the Zang Fu

The differentiation of Zang Fu patterns is the most important method of dealing with disorders arising from internal imbalance. It is necessary for the practitioner to have a good command of the selection of the appropriate herbs when a diagnosis based on Zang Fu patterns has been made.

This section is focussed on the classification of herbs in terms of Zang Fu patterns, explaining their actions, characteristics and indications. It also covers the interaction and therapeutic combination of herbs acting on the same organs.

The Lungs

22

A. Actions, characteristics and indications of common herbs

1. HERBS THAT STIMULATE THE DISPERSING FUNCTION OF THE LUNGS

— Most of these herbs are pungent and either warm or cool in nature. They are indicated for retention of pathogenic factors in the Lungs with symptoms of cough and wheeze. Representative herbs include:

Herba Ephedrae	*Ma Huang*
Radix Platycodi	*Jie Geng*
Radix Peucedani	*Qian Hu*
Semen Armeniacae Amarum	*Xing Ren*

2. HERBS THAT CLEAR LUNG HEAT

— These herbs are often cold and either bitter or sweet in nature. They are indicated for retention of Heat in the Lungs with symptoms of cough, dyspnoea, fever, a yellow tongue coating and a rapid pulse. Commonly used herbs include:

Radix Scutellariae	*Huang Qin*
Gypsum Fibrosum	*Shi Gao*
Rhizoma Anemarrhenae	*Zhi Mu*
Cortex Mori Radicis	*Sang Bai Pi*
Cortex Lycii Radicis	*Di Gu Pi*
Herba Houttuyniae	*Yu XingCao*
Flos Lonicerae	*Jin Yin Hua*
Fructus Forsythiae	*Lian Qiao*
Rhizoma Phragmitis	*LuGen*

3. HERBS THAT MOISTEN THE LUNGS

— Most of these herbs are sweet, cold and moistening in nature. They are indicated for dryness of the Lungs and damage to Body Fluids generally.

— Herbs which are effective in moistening the Lungs and stopping cough include:

Bulbus Fritillariae	*Bei Mu*
Fructus Trichosanthis	*Gua Lou*
Mel	*Feng Mi*

— Other herbs not only moisten the Lungs but also nourish Yin and promote Body Fluids, and are thus more suitable for dryness of the Lungs complicated with consumption of Body Fluids. These include:

Colla Corii Asini	*A Jiao*
Radix Glehniae	*Bei Sha Shen*
Radix Adenophorae	*Nan Sha Shen*
Radix Ophiopogonis	*Mai Dong*
Radix Asparagi	*Tian Dong*

4. HERBS THAT PURGE THE LUNGS

— These herbs are usually bitter and cold in nature and have a strong therapeutic action. They are indicated for Lung Fire and retention of Water in the Lungs. Representative herbs include:

Radix Scutellariae	*Huang Qin*
Semen Lepidii seu Descurainiae	*Ting Li Zi*
Cortex Mori Radicis	*Sang Bai Pi*
Cortex Lycii Radicis	*Di Gu Pi*

— Radix Scutellariae is more effective in purging Lung Fire while Semen Lepidii is more effective in purging Water from the Lungs. Cortex Mori Radicis and Cortex Lycii Radicis are applicable in both conditions but have a milder action.

5. HERBS THAT STIMULATE THE DESCENDING FUNCTION OF THE LUNGS

— These herbs are descending in nature and conduct Rebellious Lung Qi downward. They are indicated for cough and dyspnoea due to upward perversion of Lung Qi. Representative herbs include:

Cortex Magnoliae Officinalis	*Hou Po*
Lignum Aquilariae Resinatum	*Chen Xiang*
Semen Armeniacae Amarum	*Xing Ren*
Flos Inulae	*Xuan Fu Hua*
Rhizoma Cynanchi Stauntonii	*Bai Qian*
Fructus Perillae	*Su Zi*

6. HERBS THAT WARM THE LUNGS

— These herbs are pungent, and warm or hot in nature. They are indicated for retention of Cold in the Lungs and for retention of Cold Damp in the Lungs with symptoms of cough, watery white sputum and a pale tongue with a white coating. Commonly used herbs include:

Rhizoma Zingiberis	*Gan Jiang*
Herba Asari	*Xi Xin*
Ramulus Cinnamomi	*Gui Zhi*

7. HERBS THAT RESOLVE PHLEGM AND STOP COUGH AND WHEEZE

— These herbs are either pungent and warm or cool and moist in nature.
— Herbs that resolve Phlegm and are pungent, warm and dry in nature are indicated for retention of Cold and Phlegm in the Lungs, characterized by profuse white sputum. Commonly used herbs of this type include:

Rhizoma Pinelliae	*Ban Xia*
Rhizoma Arisaematis	*Tian Nan Xing*
Semen Sinapis Albae	*Bai Jie Zi*
Pericarpium Citri	*Chen Pi*

— Herbs that are cold or cool and moist in nature are indicated for Phlegm Heat characterized by thick yellow sputum. Representative herbs of this type include:

Bulbus Fritillariae	*Bei Mu*
Fructus Trichosanthis	*Gua Lou*
Succus Bambusae	*Zhu Li*

— Herbs that primarily stop cough and relieve dyspnoea and secondarily resolve Phlegm include:

Radix Asteris	*Zi Wan*
Flos Farfarae	*Kuan Dong Hua*

Rhizoma Cynanchi Stauntonii	*Bai Qian*
Radix Peucedani	*Qian Hu*
Radix Polygalae	*Yuan Zhi*

— Herbs that stop cough and wheeze include:

Semen Armeniacae Amarum	*Xing Ren*
Radix Stemonae	*Bai Bu*
Herba Ephedrae	*Ma Huang*
Semen Lepidii seu Descurainiae	*Ting Li Zi*
Semen Ginkgo	*Bei Guo*

8. HERBS THAT TONIFY LUNG QI

— These herbs are sweet and warm in nature and are indicated for deficiency of Lung Qi with symptoms of dyspnoea, lassitude and a low and feeble voice. Commonly used herbs include:

Radix Ginseng	*Ren Shen*
Radix Codonopsis Pilosulae	*Dang Shen*
Radix Astragali seu Hedysari	*Huang Qi*
Rhizoma Polygonati	*Huang Jing*
Radix Panacis Quinquefolii	*Xi Yang Shen*
Bulbus Lilii	*Bai He*

9. HERBS THAT TONIFY LUNG YIN

— These herbs are sweet and cold in nature and are indicated for deficiency of Lung Yin with symptoms of malar flush, tidal fever, night sweats, cough and haemoptysis. Commonly used herbs include:

Radix Panacis Quinquefolii	*Xi Yang Shen*
Radix Glehniae	*Bei Sha Shen*
Radix Adenophorae	*Nan Sha Shen*
Radix Ophiopogonis	*Mai Dong*
Radix Asparagi	*Tian Dong*
Rhizoma Polygonati Odorati	*Yu Zhu*
Rhizoma Polygonati	*Huang Jing*
Bulbus Lilii	*Bai He*

10. HERBS THAT ASTRINGE THE LUNGS

— These herbs are sour and astringent in nature. They are indicated when Lung Qi is scattered and attenuated by chronic cough and wheeze. Representative herbs include:

Fructus Schisandrae	*Wu Wei Zi*
Fructus Mume	*Wu Mei*
Fructus Chebulae	*He Zi*
Galla Chinensis	*Wu Bei Zi*
Pericarpium Papaveris	*Ying Su Ke*

B. Interactions and combinations of herbs

1. HERBS THAT CLEAR LUNG HEAT, MOISTEN THE LUNGS AND NOURISH LUNG YIN

— Herbs that clear Lung Heat are indicated for retention of Heat or Fire in the Lung, presenting with a Full Heat pattern. Herbs that moisten the Lungs and nourish Lung Yin are indicated for dryness and/or deficiency of the Lungs, presenting with Deficiency patterns. Since pathogenic dryness and Heat tend to consume Body Fluids and damage Yin, these patterns often exist concurrently.

— Where Lung Dryness due to invasion by pathogenic dryness and Heat is complicated with symptoms of consumption of Body Fluids and Yin Deficiency, herbs that clear Lung Heat are combined with herbs that moisten the Lungs and tonify Lung Yin. For example, Folium Mori, Cortex Mori Radicis and Rhizoma Anemarrhenae are combined with Bulbus Fritillariae, Radix Glehniae, Radix Adenophorae and Radix Ophiopogonis.

— Where the Yin has been damaged by febrile disease, or in cases of Yin Deficiency with Empty Fire, with symptoms of tidal fever, night sweats, cough, malar flush and haemoptysis, herbs that nourish Yin are combined with herbs that clear Lung Heat (Fig. 22.1).

2. HERBS THAT TONIFY LUNG QI, ASTRINGE THE LUNGS, WARM THE LUNGS AND NOURISH LUNG YIN

— Herbs that astringe the Lungs are indicated for chronic cough and wheeze due to excessive scattering of Lung Qi. However, these herbs do not tonify, and thus treat the Biao without treating the Ben.

— To treat both Biao and Ben, herbs that astringe the Lungs are combined with herbs that tonify Lung Qi, e.g. Radix Ginseng and Radix Astragali seu Hedysari are combined with Fructus Schisandrae, Fructus Mume and Semen Ginkgo.

— Clinically, patterns of Lung Qi Deficiency often appear concurrently with patterns of Lung Yin Deficiency and thus Lung Qi tonics are often combined with Lung Yin tonics, e.g. Radix Ginseng and Rhizoma Polygonati are combined with Radix Adenophorae, Radix Ophiopogonis and Radix Glehniae.

— Lung Qi Deficiency may lead to Lung Yang Deficiency, resulting in retention of Phlegm Fluid in the Lungs. For this pattern, herbs that tonify Lung Qi are combined with herbs that warm the Lungs and resolve retained Water, e.g. Radix Astragali seu Hedysari and Radix Codonopsis Pilosulae are combined with Ramulus Cinnamomi, Rhizoma Zingiberis, Herba Asari, Poria, Radix Asteris and Flos Farfarae (Fig. 22.2).

3. HERBS THAT RESOLVE PHLEGM AND STOP COUGH AND WHEEZE, AND OTHER TYPES OF HERBS

a. Herbs that stimulate the dispersing function of the Lungs and herbs that resolve Phlegm

— This combination is indicated when Phlegm blocks the Lungs' dispersing function. Herba Ephedrae, Semen Armeniacae Amarum and Radix Platycodi are often combined with Radix Peucedani, Rhizoma Pinelliae and Radix Stemonae.

b. Herbs that clear Lung Heat and herbs that resolve Phlegm

— This combination is indicated for retention

| Pathological (Full) Heat in Lungs | ⟶ | Damage to Lung Yin |
| Lung Yin Deficiency | ⟶ | Lung Empty Heat |

In either case, combine:
herbs that clear Lung Heat   +   herbs that nourish Lung Yin, and moisten the Lungs

Fig. 22.1 Patterns of combined Lung Heat and Lung Yin Deficiency.

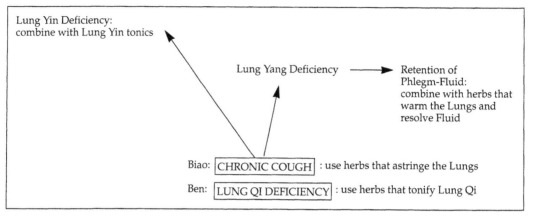

Fig. 22.2 Complications of chronic cough.

of Phlegm Heat in the Lungs. Radix Scutellariae, Cortex Mori Radicis and Rhizoma Anemarrhenae are often combined with Bulbus Fritillariae and Fructus Trichosanthis.

c. Herbs that warm the Lung and herbs that resolve Phlegm

— This combination is indicated for retention of Phlegm Fluid, Cold Phlegm or Phlegm Damp in the Lungs. Herba Ephedrae, Herba Asari and Rhizoma Zingiberis are often combined with Rhizoma Pinelliae, Fructus Perillae and Semen Sinapis Albae.

d. Herbs that stimulate the descending function of the Lung and herbs that resolve Phlegm

— This combination is indicated for Turbid Phlegm blocking the Lungs with a resulting failure of Lung Qi to descend.
— For Cold Phlegm, Fructus Perillae, Semen Armenicae Amarum and Cortex Magnoliae are combined with Rhizoma Pinelliae, Pericarpium Citri Reticulatae and Rhizoma Cynanchi Stauntonii.
— For Phlegm Heat, Semen Lepidii seu Descurainiae, Cortex Mori Radicis and Folium Eriobotryae are combined with Bulbus Fritillariae and Fructus Trichosanthis.

Questions

1. Herba Ephedrae, Fructus Perillae, Semen Lepidii seu Descurainiae and Semen Ginkgo all resolve wheeze. How do they differ in their actions and indications?
2. Herba Ephedrae, Radix Scutellariae, Radix Glehniae and Radix Adenophorae all stop cough. How do they differ in their natures, actions and indications?
3. What is the relationship between herbs that clear Lung Heat, herbs that nourish Lung Yin and herbs that resolve Phlegm? How are they combined clinically?
4. What are the differences and similarities between herbs that tonify Lung Qi, herbs that warm the Lung and herbs that resolve Phlegm?

The Heart

23

A. Actions, characteristics and indications of common herbs

1. HERBS THAT TONIFY HEART QI

— Most of these herbs are sweet and warm in nature and are indicated for Heart Qi Deficiency with symptoms of palpitations and shortness of breath. Commonly used herbs include:

Radix Ginseng	*Ren Shen*
Radix Codonopsis Pilosulae	*Dang Shen*
Radix Pseudostellariae	*Tai Zi Shen*
Radix Astragali seu Hedysari	*Huang Qi*
Radix Glycyrrhizae	*Zhi Gan Cao*

2. HERBS THAT WARM HEART YANG

— These herbs are pungent and warm or hot in nature. They are indicated for Heart Yang Deficiency, with symptoms of palpitations, cold limbs, sweating with a cold sensation of the body, cyanosis and a pulse that is feeble, thready and fading, deep and hidden, or knotted. Commonly used herbs include:

Radix Aconiti Praeparata	*Fu Zi*
Rhizoma Zingiberis	*Gan Jiang*
Ramulus Cinnamomi	*Gui Zhi*

3. HERBS THAT TONIFY HEART BLOOD

— These herbs are sweet, nourishing and sticky in nature; they may be warm, neutral or cold. They are indicated for deficiency of Heart Blood with symptoms of dizziness and vertigo, palpitations, a pale tongue and a thready pulse. Commonly used herbs include:

Radix Angelicae Sinensis	*Dang Gui*
Radix Rehmanniae Praeparata	*Shu Di*
Radix Rehmanniae	*Sheng Di*
Colla Corii Asini	*A Jiao*
Arillus Longan	*Long Yan Rou*

4. HERBS THAT TONIFY HEART YIN

— Most of these herbs are sweet and cold in nature. They are indicated for Heart Yin Deficiency with symptoms of palpitations, a red tongue and a thready and rapid pulse. Commonly used herbs include:

Radix Rehmanniae	*Sheng Di*
Radix Ophiopogonis	*Mai Dong*
Colla Corii Asini	*A Jiao*
Rhizoma Polygonati Odorati	*Yu Zhu*

5. HERBS THAT CLEAR HEART FIRE

— These herbs are primarily bitter and cold and secondarily sweet in nature. They are indicated for Heart Fire Blazing with symptoms of restlessness, mouth and tongue ulcers, coma and a red tongue tip. Representative herbs include:

Radix Coptidis	*Huang Lian*
Fructus Forsythiae	*Lian Qiao*
Fructus Gardeniae	*Zhi Zi*
Calculus Bovis	*Niu Huang*
Radix Rehmanniae	*Sheng Di*
Herba Lophatheri	*Zhu Ye*
Caulis Akebiae	*Mu Tong*
Plumula Nelumbinis	*Lian Xin*
Cortex Moutan Radicis	*Dan Pi*

6. SUBSTANCES THAT SOOTHE THE HEART AND CALM THE MIND

— Substances which strongly settle and calm the Mind are mostly minerals or fossils, while those which calm the Mind by nourishing the Heart are mostly seeds. Both types of medicinal are indicated for restlessness, insomnia, palpitations, irritability, depression and mania. Commonly used substances which settle and calm the Mind include:

Cinnabaris	*Zhu Sha*
Os Draconis	*Long Gu*
Magnetitum	*Ci Shi*
Margarita	*Zhen Zhu*
Concha Margaritifera Usta	*Zhen Zhu Mu*
Succinum	*Hu Po*
Haematitum	*Zhe Shi*
Concha Ostreae	*Mu Li*

— Herbs that calm the Mind by nourishing the Heart include:

Semen Biotae	*Bai Zi Ren*
Semen Ziziphi Spinosae	*Suan Zao Ren*
Caulis Polygoni Multiflori	*Ye Jiao Teng*
Radix Polygalae	*Yuan Zhi*
Cortex Albiziae	*He Huan Pi*
Poria cum Ligno Hospite	*Fu Shen*

7. SUBSTANCES THAT OPEN THE ORIFICES

— These substances are aromatic, pungent and penetrating in nature. They are indicated for delirium or coma due to high fever, or sudden collapse and syncope in Wind Stroke, convulsion or epilepsy. Commonly used substances include:

Moschus	*She Xiang*
Borneolum Syntheticum	*Bing Pian*
Calculus Bovis	*Niu Huang*
Rhizoma Acori Graminei	*Shi Chang Pu*
Styrax Liquidus	*Su He Xiang*
Benzoinum	*An Xi Xiang*
Radix Curcumae	*Yu Jin*
Radix Polygalae	*Yuan Zhi*
Venenum Bufonis	*Chan Su*

— With the exception of Rhizoma Acori Graminei, Radix Curcumae and Radix Polygalae, all of these substances are administered in the form of pills or powders for first aid, e.g.:

Bolus of Calculus Bovis	Niu Huang Wan
Bolus of Precious Drugs	Zhi Bao Dan
Bolus of Styrax	Su He Xiang Wan

8. HERBS THAT ACTIVATE BLOOD CIRCULATION AND RESOLVE BLOOD STASIS IN THE VESSELS

— These herbs are pungent or bitter in nature and are indicated for stagnation of Heart Blood with symptoms of cardiac pain, palpitations and oppression of the chest. Commonly used herbs include:

Radix Salviae Miltiorrhizae	*Dan Shen*
Rhizoma Ligustici Chuanxiong	*Chuan Xiong*
Ramulus Cinnamomi	*Gui Zhi*
Semen Persicae	*Tao Ren*
Flos Carthami	*Hong Hua*
Radix Paeoniae Rubra	*Chi Shao*
Eupolyphaga seu Steleeophaga	*Di Bie Chong*
Hirudo	*Shui Zhi*

B. Interactions and combinations of herbs

1. HERBS THAT TONIFY HEART QI AND HERBS THAT WARM HEART YANG

— Heart Yang Deficiency is often complicated with Heart Qi Deficiency, and herbs that warm Heart Yang are thus often used in combination with herbs that tonify Heart Qi. For example, Radix Ginseng is combined with Radix Aconiti Praeparata, and Ramulus Cinnamomi is combined with treated Radix Glycyrrhizae.

2. HERBS THAT TONIFY HEART BLOOD AND HERBS THAT NOURISH HEART YIN

— With the exception of Radix Angelicae Sinensis and Arillus Longan, the herbs that tonify Heart Blood also nourish Heart Yin. Some of the herbs that nourish Heart Yin – such as Radix Rehmanniae, Radix Rehmanniae Praeparata and Colla Corii Asini – also tonify Heart Blood.
— Since deficiency of Heart Blood and Heart Yin often appear concurrently, these categories of herbs are often used in combination.

3. HERBS THAT TONIFY HEART QI AND HERBS THAT NOURISH HEART BLOOD AND HEART YIN

— In patterns of Heart pathology, it is quite common that both Qi and Blood, or both Qi and Yin, are deficient.

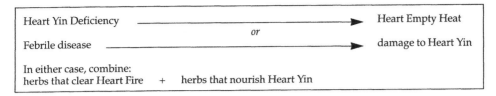

Fig. 23.1 Patterns of combined Heart Heat and Heart Yin Deficiency.

— Herbs that tonify Heart Qi are thus often used in combination with herbs that nourish Heart Blood or Heart Yin.

---

4. COMBINATIONS OF HERBS FOR MIXED CONDITIONS OF EXCESS AND DEFICIENCY

a. Herbs that nourish Heart Yin and clear Heart Fire

— Heart Yin Deficiency is likely to lead to Empty Heat in the Heart; on the other hand, febrile disease at the Nutritive (*Ying*) level may damage Heart Yin.
— Herbs that nourish Heart Yin are thus often combined with herbs that clear Heart Fire. For example, Colla Corii Asini and Radix Ophiopogonis are combined with Rhizoma Coptidis and Fructus Forsythiae (Fig. 23.1).

b. Herbs that tonify Heart Blood and Yin and herbs that calm the Mind

— When Heart Blood and Yin are deficient, the Heart is not nourished; this leads to restlessness from Deficiency. In this case, herbs that calm the Mind are combined with herbs that tonify Heart Blood and Yin. For example, Semen Biotae, Semen Ziziphi Spinosae, Os Draconis and Cinnabaris-coated Poria cum Ligno Hospite are combined with Radix

Angelicae Sinensis, Radix Ophiopogonis and Colla Corii Asini.

c. Herbs that clear Heart Fire, resolve Phlegm and open the orifices

— Mental disturbance due to obstruction of the Heart orifices can arise either from Turbid Phlegm or from exterior Heat invading the Pericardium. Since these two conditions may coexist, herbs that clear Heart Heat are often combined with herbs that open the orifices (Fig. 23.2).
— For example, Rhizoma Coptidis, Fructus Forsythiae, Cornu Rhinoceri Asiatici and Calculus Bovis are combined with Moschus, Borneolum Syntheticum, Rhizoma Acori Graminei and Radix Curcumae.
— Similarly, herbs that resolve Phlegm are combined with herbs that open the orifices. For example, Radix Polygalae, Succus Bambusae and Bulbus Fritillariae are combined with Rhizoma Acori Graminei, Radix Curcumae and Borneolum Syntheticum.
— For restlessness with insomnia due to Heart Fire Blazing with Phlegm-Fire harassing the Heart, herbs that clear Heart Fire are used in combination with herbs that clear Phlegm and herbs that calm the Mind. For example, Rhizoma Coptidis and Caulis Bambusae in Taeniam are combined with Cinnabaris-

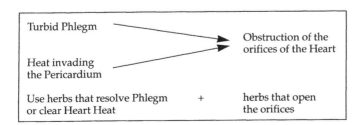

Fig. 23.2 Patterns of obstruction of the orifices of the Heart.

coated Poria cum Ligno Hospite, Semen Biotae and Os Draconis.

Questions

1. Compare and contrast herbs that tonify Heart Qi and herbs that warm Heart Yang. How do they interrelate?
2. Compare and contrast herbs that nourish Heart Yin, herbs that clear Heart Fire and herbs that calm the Mind. How do they interrelate?

The Spleen, Stomach and Large Intestines

24

A. Actions, characteristics and indications of common herbs

1. HERBS THAT TONIFY SPLEEN AND STOMACH QI

— These herbs are sweet and warm in nature and are indicated for Spleen and Stomach Qi Deficiency with symptoms of poor appetite, loose stools and lassitude. Commonly used herbs include:

Radix Ginseng	*Ren Shen*
Radix Codonopsis Pilosulae	*Dang Shen*
Radix Astragali seu Hedysari	*Huang Qi*
Rhizoma Atractylodis Macrocephalae	*Bai Zhu*
Rhizoma Dioscoreae	*Shan Yao*
Radix Glycyrrhizae	*Zhi Gan Cao*

2. HERBS THAT WARM SPLEEN YANG

— These herbs are pungent and warm or hot. They are indicated for Spleen Yang Deficiency with symptoms of poor appetite, loose stools, cold limbs and a cold sensation and pain in the epigastrium and abdomen. Commonly used herbs include:

Rhizoma Zingiberis	*Gan Jiang*
Radix Aconiti Praeparata	*Fu Zi*
Cortex Cinnamomi	*Rou Gui*
Ramulus Cinnamomi	*Gui Zhi*
Fructus Alpiniae Oxyphyllae	*Yi Zhi Ren*

3. HERBS THAT RAISE CENTRAL QI

— These herbs are ascending in nature and are indicated for patterns of Spleen Qi Sinking with symptoms of chronic diarrhoea, or prolapse of the anus or internal organs. Commonly used herbs include:

Radix Astragali seu Hedysari	*Huang Qi*
Rhizoma Cimicifugae	*Sheng Ma*
Radix Bupleuri	*Chai Hu*
Radix Puerariae	*Ge Gen*

4. HERBS THAT RESOLVE DAMPNESS

— These herbs are pungent, bitter, warm, dry and aromatic in nature. They are indicated for retention of Dampness in the Middle Burner with symptoms of epigastric and abdominal distension and fullness and a sticky tongue coating. Commonly used herbs include:

Rhizoma Atractylodis	*Cang Zhu*
Cortex Magnoliae Officinalis	*Hou Po*
Herba Agastachis	*Huo Xiang*
Herba Eupatorii	*Pei Lan*
Fructus Amomi	*Sha Ren*
Fructus Amomi Cardamomi	*Bai Dou Kou*
Herba Elsholtziae	*Xiang Ru*
Rhizoma Acori Graminei	*Shi Chang Pu*

5. HERBS THAT REGULATE SPLEEN AND STOMACH QI

— These herbs are pungent, warm and aromatic in nature. They are indicated for stagnation of Spleen and Stomach Qi with symptoms of distension and pain in the epigastrium and abdomen. Commonly used herbs include:

Radix Aucklandiae	*Mu Xiang*
Pericarpium Citri Reticulatae	*Chen Pi*
Fructus Aurantii Immaturus	*Zhi Shi*
Fructus Aurantii	*Zhi Ke*
Cortex Magnoliae Officinalis	*Hou Po*
Caulis Perillae	*Su Geng*
Fructus Amomi	*Sha Ren*
Pericarpium Arecae	*Da Fu Pi*

6. HERBS THAT CLEAR STOMACH FIRE

— These herbs are cold and either bitter or sweet in nature. They are indicated for Stomach Heat or Fire with symptoms of thirst, vomiting, burning epigastric pain, haematemesis and swelling and pain of the gums. Commonly used herbs include:

Rhizoma Coptidis	*Huang Lian*
Gypsum Fibrosum	*Shi Gao*
Rhizoma Anemarrhenae	*Zhi Mu*
Radix et Rhizoma Rhei	*Da Huang*
Rhizoma Phragmitis	*Lu Gen*

— For high fever and thirst due to Full Heat in the Stomach, Gypsum Fibrosum and Rhizoma Anemarrhenae are most effective.
— For vomiting and haematemesis due to Stomach Fire, Rhizoma Coptidis and Radix et Rhizoma Rhei should be used.

7. HERBS THAT NOURISH STOMACH YIN

— These herbs are sweet and cold in nature and are indicated for Stomach Yin Deficiency with symptoms of retching, an uncomfortable and empty sensation in the Stomach and a red tongue with scanty coating. Commonly used herbs include:

Herba Dendrobii	*Shi Hu*
Radix Ophiopogonis	*Mai Dong*
Radix GlehniaeBei	*Sha Shen*
Radix Adenophorae	*Nan Sha Shen*
Rhizoma Polygonati Odorati	*Yu Zhu*
Rhizoma Dioscoreae	*Shan Yao*

8. HERBS THAT DISPERSE COLD FROM THE SPLEEN AND STOMACH

— These herbs are pungent and hot or warm in nature. They are indicated for retention of Cold in the Middle Burner with symptoms of a cold sensation and pain in the epigastrium and abdomen. Commonly used herbs include:

Rhizoma Alpiniae Officinalis	*Gao Liang Jiang*
Rhizoma Zingiberis Recens	*Sheng Jiang*
Rhizoma Zingiberis	*Gan Jiang*
Ramulus Cinnamomi	*Gui Zhi*
Flos Caryophylli	*Ding Xiang*
Pericarpium Zanthoxyli	*Huang Jiao*
Fructus Evodiae	*Wu Zhu Yu*

9. HERBS THAT CONDUCT REBELLIOUS STOMACH QI DOWNWARD

— These herbs are descending, pungent and warm, or bitter and cold, or sweet and cold in nature. They are indicated for upward disturbance of Stomach Qi with symptoms of vomiting and hiccup. Commonly used herbs that warm the Stomach and conduct Rebellious Qi downward include:

Rhizoma Zingiberis Recens	*Sheng Jiang*
Flos Caryophylli	*Ding Xiang*
Lignum Aquilariae Resinatum	*Chen Xiang*
Rhizoma Pinelliae	*Ban Xia*
Fructus Evodiae	*Wu Zhu Yu*

— Herbs that clear Stomach Heat and conduct Rebellious Qi downward include:

Rhizoma Coptidis	*Huang Lian*
Caulis Bambusae in Taeniam	*Zhu Ru*
Rhizoma Phragmitis	*Lu Gen*

— Herbs that conduct Rebellious Qi downward and stop vomiting include:

Haematitum	*Zhe Shi*
Flos Inulae	*Xuan Fu Hua*

10. HERBS THAT ASSIST DIGESTION AND INVIGORATE THE STOMACH

— These herbs relieve Food Retention, assist digestion and invigorate the Stomach. They are indicated for Retention of Food with symptoms of distending epigastric and abdominal pain, vomiting, diarrhoea, poor appetite and indigestion. Commonly used herbs include:

Fructus Crataegi	*Shan Zha*
Fructus Oryzae Germinatus	*Gu Ya*
Fructus Hordei Germinatus	*Mai Ya*
Massa Fermentata Medicinalis	*Shen Qu*
Endothelium Corneum Gigeriae Galli	*Ji Nei Jin*
Semen Raphani	*Lai Fu Zi*

11. SUBSTANCES THAT MODERATE ACID SECRETION

— These herbs neutralize or stop acid secretion and are thus indicated for hyperacidity with symptoms of epigastric pain and acid regurgitation. Commonly used substances include:

Os Sepiellae seu Sepiae	*Wu Zei Gu*

Concha Arcae	*Wa Leng Zi*
Concha Ostreae	*Mu Li*

12. PURGATIVE HERBS

— These herbs resolve obstruction in the intestines and promote the discharge of faeces. They are divided into three types:

1. herbs that purge by eliminating pathogenic factors
2. herbs that purge by moistening
3. harsh cathartics that dispel retained Water.

— Herbs that purge by eliminating pathogenic factors are bitter and cold in nature. They are indicated for stagnation in the intestinal tract, high fever, constipation with abdominal distension and fullness, and acute abdomen. Commonly used herbs include:

Radix et Rhizoma Rhei	*Da Huang*
Natrii Sulfas	*Mang Xiao*
Folium Cassiae	*Fan Xie Ye*

— Herbs that purge by moistening are sweet and neutral, moist and oily in nature. They are indicated for constipation due to deficiency of Body Fluids and Blood. Commonly used herbs include:

Fructus Cannabis	*Huo Ma Ren*
Semen Pruni	*Yu Li Ren*
Fructus Trichosanthis	*Gua Lou Ren*
Semen Armeniacae Amarum	*Xing Ren*
Radix Angelicae Sinensis	*Dang Gui*
Herba Cistanchis	*Rou Cong Rong*

— Harsh cathartics that dispel retained Water are toxic and purge very strongly; they should therefore be used with extreme caution. They are indicated for patterns of Retention of Water in the chest and abdomen characterized by excessive pathogenic factors and strong Zheng Qi. Commonly used herbs include:

Radix Euphorbiae Kansui	*Gan Sui*
Radix Euphorbiae Pekinensis	*Da Ji*
Flos Genkwa	*Yuan Hua*
Semen Pharbitidis	*Qian Niu Zi*

13. HERBS THAT CLEAR DAMP-HEAT FROM THE LARGE INTESTINE

— These herbs are bitter and cold in nature and are indicated for diarrhoea, dysentery and haemorrhoids due to retention of Damp-Heat in the Large Intestine. Commonly used herbs include:

Rhizoma Coptidis	*Huang Lian*
Radix Scutellariae	*Huang Qin*
Cortex Phellodendri	*Huang Bai*
Cortex Fraxini	*Qin Pi*
Radix Pulsatillae	*Bai Tou Weng*
Herba Portulacae	*Ma Chi Xian*
Fructus Bruceae	*Ya Dan Zi*
Radix Sophorae Flavescentis	*Ku Shen*

— For bleeding haemorrhoids due to Heat in the Large Intestine, use Radix Sanguisorbae and Flos Sophorae.

14. HERBS THAT ASTRINGE THE INTESTINES TO STOP DIARRHOEA

— These herbs are sour and astringent in nature and are indicated for chronic diarrhoea and dysentery due to deficiency of Large Intestine Qi. Commonly used herbs include:

Fructus Mume	*Wu Mei*
Fructus Schisandrae	*Wu Wei Zi*
Semen Myristicae	*Rou Dou Kou*
Semen Euryales	*Qian Shi*
Semen Nelumbinis	*Lian Zi*
Fructus Chebulae	*He Zi*
Pericarpium Granati	*Shi Liu Pi*
Cortex Ailanthi	*Chun Gen Pi*
Halloysitum Rubrum	*Chi Shi Zhi*
Limonitum	*Yu Yu Liang*

B. Mutual interaction and combinations of herbs

1. HERBS THAT TONIFY SPLEEN QI, HERBS THAT WARM SPLEEN YANG AND HERBS THAT LIFT CENTRAL QI

— Spleen Yang Deficiency is often complicated with a general deficiency of Qi. Herbs that warm Spleen Yang are thus often combined with herbs that tonify Spleen Qi. For example, Radix Codonopsis Pilosulae and Rhizoma Atractylodis Macrocephalae are combined with Rhizoma Zingiberis and Radix Aconiti Praeparata in the treatment of deficiency of the Middle Burner with stagnation of Cold.

— Sinking of Central Qi is essentially a

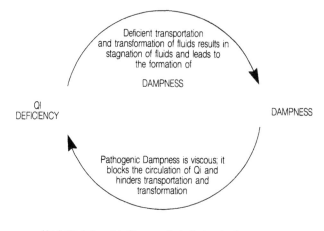

Fig. 24.1 The relationship between Qi circulation and Dampness.

manifestation of Spleen Qi Deficiency. Thus in the treatment of Sinking of Central Qi, herbs that lift the Qi such as Rhizoma Cimicifugae and Radix Bupleuri are combined with herbs that tonify Spleen Qi such as Radix Astragali seu Hedysari and Radix Codonopsis Pilosulae.

2. HERBS THAT RESOLVE DAMPNESS AND HERBS THAT REGULATE QI

— Pathogenic Dampness is characterized by viscosity and stagnation and thus tends to obstruct the circulation of Qi. Stagnation of Spleen and Stomach Qi with weakness of transportation and transformation (*Yun Hua*) results in the stagnation of Internal Dampness. Retention of Dampness leads to further Qi Stagnation; conversely, free circulation of Qi resolves Dampness. Hence

Dampness and Qi Stagnation are closely related pathological patterns (Fig. 24.1).
— Herbs that resolve Dampness and herbs that regulate Qi are similar in nature, being pungent, warm and aromatic. Some herbs that resolve Dampness also regulate Qi, such as Cortex Magnoliae Officinalis and Fructus Amomi.

3. HERBS THAT REGULATE QI AND HERBS THAT TONIFY QI

— Herbs that regulate Qi are indicated for stagnation of Spleen and Stomach Qi, which is an Excess pattern. Herbs that tonify Qi are indicated for Spleen and Stomach Qi Deficiency, which is a Deficiency pattern. These patterns often appear concurrently, as stagnation results from a weakness of the circulatory function of Qi (Fig. 24.2).

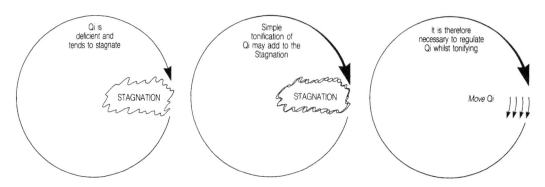

Fig. 24.2 The relationship between Qi tonification and Qi regulation.

— However, herbs that tonify Qi are like to aggravate Qi Stagnation in patients with weakness of the Middle Burner. To provide tonification without worsening stagnation, Qi tonics are combined with a small dose of herbs that regulate Qi. For example, Radix Codonopsis Pilosulae, Radix Astragali, Rhizoma Atractylodis Macrocephalae and treated Radix Glycyrrhizae may be combined with Radix Aucklandiae, Fructus Amomi and Pericarpium Citri Reticulatae.

4. HERBS THAT NOURISH STOMACH YIN AND CLEAR STOMACH FIRE

— Herbs that nourish Stomach Yin are indicated for Stomach Yin Deficiency. Herbs that clear Stomach Fire are indicated for Stomach Heat or Fire. These patterns often occur concurrently as Heat and Fire tend to damage Body Fluids, while Yin Deficiency can lead to Empty Heat. These two types of herb are thus often used together.

5. DIFFERENTIATION OF HERBS FOR THE SPLEEN AND HERBS FOR THE STOMACH

— Qi Deficiency, Yang Deficiency and Qi Stagnation often affect both the Spleen and Stomach. However, the Spleen is a Yin organ; it likes Dryness and dislikes Dampness. Conversely, the Stomach is a Yang organ; it like moisture and dislikes Dryness. When the Spleen functions properly, Spleen Qi ascends; when the Stomach functions properly, Stomach Qi descends.
— Disorders of the Spleen are treated by the methods of tonifying Qi, lifting Qi, warming Yang and resolving Dampness with bitter and dry herbs. Disorders of the Stomach are treated by the methods of nourishing Yin, moistening dryness and promoting Body Fluids with sweet and cold herbs, and of conducting Rebellious Qi downward and relieving constipation.

6. HERBS THAT CLEAR DAMP-HEAT FROM THE LARGE INTESTINE AND HERBS THAT RESOLVE DAMPNESS IN THE SPLEEN AND STOMACH

— Similar herbs are used for retention of Damp-Heat in the Large Intestine and retention of Dampness in the Spleen and Stomach. In the treatment of chronic diarrhoea and dysentery due to deficiency of the Large Intestine, herbs that stop diarrhoea by astringing the Large Intestine are combined with herbs that invigorate the Spleen and warm Spleen Yang. For example, Radix Codonopsis Pilosulae, Rhizoma Atractylodis Macrocephalae, Rhizoma Dioscoreae, Fructus Alpiniae Oxyphyllae and Rhizoma Zingiberis are often used together.

Questions

1. Rhizoma Atractylodis Macrocephalae, Rhizoma Coptidis, Rhizoma Zingiberis and Fructus Mume are all indicated for diarrhoea. How do they differ in nature, actions and indications?
2. What is the clinical relationship between herbs that tonify Spleen Qi, herbs that warm Spleen Yang, herbs that resolve Dampness in the Spleen and Stomach and herbs that regulate Spleen and Stomach Qi?
3. Compare and contrast herbs for disorders of the Spleen and those for disorders of the Stomach.

25 The Liver and Gall Bladder

A. Actions, characteristics and indications of common herbs

1. HERBS THAT CLEAR LIVER HEAT

— These herbs are bitter and cold in nature and are indicated for Liver Heat and Liver Fire with symptoms of headache, red eyes, irritability or mania and a red tongue with a yellow coating. Commonly used herbs include:

Radix Gentianae	Long Dan Cao
Spica Prunellae	Xia Ku Cao
Rhizoma Coptidis	Huang Lian
Fructus Gardeniae	Zhi Zi
Radix Scutellariae	Huang Qin
Cortex Moutan Radicis	Dan Pi
Indigo Naturalis	Qing Dai
Flos Chrysanthemi	Ju Hua
Semen Cassiae	Jue Ming Zi

2. SUBSTANCES THAT SUPPRESS HYPERACTIVE LIVER YANG

— These substances are shells, minerals, or herbs which are cold and descending in nature. They are indicated for Liver Yang Rising with symptoms of headache, dizziness and vertigo, flushed face, irritability and dream-disturbed sleep. Commonly used substances include:

Shells

Concha Haliotidis	Shi Jue Ming
Concha Ostreae	Mu Li
Concha Margaritifera Usta	Zhen Zhu Mu
Plastrum Testudinis	Gui Ban
Carapax Trionycis	Bie Jia

Minerals

Os Draconis	Long Gu
Haematitum	Zhe Shi
Magnetitum	Ci Shi

Herbs

Ramulus Uncariae cum Uncis	Gou Teng
Rhizoma Gastrodiae	Tian Ma
Folium Apocyni Veneti	Luo Bu Ma

3. HERBS THAT CALM LIVER WIND

— These herbs are indicated for Stirring of Liver Wind with symptoms of spasm, convulsions, dizziness, numbness of the limbs and hemiplegia. Commonly used herbs include:

Cornu Antelopis	Ling Yang Jiao
Rhizoma Gastrodiae	Tian Ma
Ramulus Uncariae cum Uncis	Gou Teng
Fructus Tribuli	Ci Ji Li
Scorpio	Quan Xie
Scolopendra	Wu Gong
Lumbricus	Di Long
Bombyx Batryticatus	Jiang Can

4. HERBS THAT NOURISH LIVER YIN

— These herbs are sweet, cold or slightly warm, nourishing and sticky in nature. They are indicated for Liver Yin Deficiency with symptoms of dizziness, blurred vision and a dry red tongue with scanty coating. Commonly used herbs include:

Radix Rehmanniae	Sheng Di
Radix Rehmanniae Praeparata	Shu Di
Fructus Lycii	Gou Qi Zi
Radix Paeoniae Alba	Bai Shao
Fructus Corni	Shan Zhu Yu
Radix Polygoni Multiflori	He Shou Wu
Carapax Trionycis	Bie Jia

5. HERBS THAT TONIFY LIVER BLOOD

— These herbs are sweet and slightly warm, and nourishing and sticky in nature. They are indicated for Liver Blood Deficiency with symptoms of dizziness, blurred vision, pale complexion, irregular menstruation with a scanty flow of pale blood, or amenorrhoea. Commonly used herbs include:

Radix Angelicae Sinensis	*Dang Gui*
Radix Rehmanniae Praeparata	*Shu Di*
Radix Paeoniae Alba	*Bai Shao*
Colla Corii Asini	*A Jiao*
Radix Polygoni Multiflori	*He Shou Wu*
Fructus Corni	*Gou Qi Zi*

6. HERBS THAT HARMONIZE THE LIVER

— These herbs are pungent and dispersing in nature and are indicated for stagnation of Liver Qi with symptoms of distending hypochondriac pain, mental depression or irritability and irregular menstruation. Commonly used herbs include:

Radix Bupleuri	*Chai Hu*
Rhizoma Cyperi	*Xiang Fu*
Pericarpium Citri Reticulatae Viride	*Qing Pi*
Fructus Meliae Toosendan	*Chuan Lian Zi*
Radix Curcumae	*Yu Jin*
Rhizoma Ligustici Chuanxiong	*Chuan Xiong*
Fructus Citri	*Xiang Yuan*
Fructus Citri Sarcodactylis	*Fu Shou*
Flos Mume Albus	*Lu E Mei*
Flos Rosae Rugosae	*Mei Gui Hua*

7. HERBS THAT WARM THE LIVER

— These herbs are pungent and hot or warm in nature. They are indicated for retention of Cold in the Liver channel with abdominal pain. Commonly used herbs include:

Fructus Evodiae	*Wu Zhu Yu*
Fructus Foeniculi	*Xiao Hui Xiang*
Semen Litchi	*Li Zhi He*
Fructus Litseae	*Bi Cheng Qie*
Lignum Aquilariae Resinatum	*Chen Xiang*
Radix Linderae	*Wu Yao*
Cortex Cinnamomi	*Rou Gui*
Herba Asari	*Xi Xin*

8. HERBS THAT ACTIVATE BLOOD CIRCULATION AND RESOLVE BLOOD STASIS

— These herbs are bitter, pungent and dispersing in nature. They are indicated for stagnation of Liver Blood with symptoms of palpable abdominal masses, stabbing pain, amenorrhoea, dysmenorrhoea and a purple tongue. Commonly used herbs include:

Radix Salviae Miltiorrhizae	*Dan Shen*
Rhizoma Ligustici Chuanxiong	*Chuan Xiong*
Radix Angelicae Sinensis	*Dang Gui*
Flos Carthami	*Hong Hua*
Semen Persicae	*Tao Ren*
Rhizoma Sparganii	*San Leng*
Rhizoma Zedoariae	*E Zhu*
Herba Leonuri	*Yi Mu Cao*
Radix Paeoniae Rubra	*Chi Shao*
Radix et Rhizoma Rhei	*Da Huang*
Cortex Moutan Radicis	*Dan Pi*
Resina Olibani	*Ru Xiang*
Resina Myrrhae	*Mo Yao*
Eupolyphaga seu Steleophaga	*Di Bie Chong*
Hirudo	*Shui Zhi*

9. HERBS THAT CLEAR HEAT FROM THE GALL BLADDER

— These herbs are bitter and cold in nature. They are indicated for retention of Heat in the Gall Bladder channel with symptoms of hypochondriac pain, alternating chills and fever, and jaundice. Commonly used herbs include:

Radix Gentianae	*Long Dan Cao*
Radix Scutellariae	*Huang Qin*
Fructus Gardeniae	*Zhi Zi*
Herba Artemisiae Chinghao	*Qing Hao*
Herba Artemisiae Scopariae	*Yin Chen Hao*
Rhizoma Polygoni Cuspidati	*Hu Zhang*
Herba Taraxaci	*Pu Gong Ying*

10. HERBS THAT BENEFIT THE GALL BLADDER

— These herbs are bitter and cold in nature and are indicated for patterns of Gall Bladder Damp-Heat with symptoms of jaundice, hypochondriac pain, cholecystitis and cholelithiasis. Commonly used herbs include:

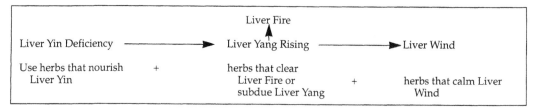

Fig. 25.1 Complications of Liver Yin Deficiency.

Herba Artemisiae Scopariae	*Yin Chen Hao*
Fructus Gardeniae	*Zhi Zi*
Radix Curcumae	*Yu Jin*
Radix Scutellariae	*Huang Qin*
Herba Lysimachiae	*Jin Qian Cao*
Spora Lygodii	*Hai Jin Sha*
Radix et Rhizoma Rhei	*Da Huang*
Natrii Sulfas	*Mang Xiao*
Endothelium Corneum	*Ji Nei Jin*
Gigeriae Galli	

B. Interactions and combinations of herbs

1. HERBS THAT CLEAR HEAT FROM THE LIVER AND GALL BLADDER

— The Gall Bladder is closely associated with the Liver. Herbs that clear Liver Heat also clear Gall Bladder Heat. The therapeutic effect of these herbs may be enhanced by combining them with herbs that harmonize the Liver and herbs that benefit the Gall Bladder.

2. HERBS THAT CLEAR LIVER HEAT AND LIVER FIRE

— Clearing Liver Heat is essentially the same as purging Liver Fire, and both categories of herbs are applicable in the treatment of patterns of Fire or Heat in the Liver channel.
— Herbs which strongly clear Liver Heat — such as Radix Gentianae and Fructus Gardeniae — will also purge Liver Fire.

— For Liver Heat without Fire, less powerful herbs such as Flos Chrysanthemi, Folium Mori and Concha Haliotidis are indicated.

3. HERBS THAT NOURISH LIVER YIN, CLEAR LIVER HEAT, SUPPRESS LIVER YANG AND CALM LIVER WIND

— Liver Yin Deficiency can lead to Liver Yang Rising, Liver Fire and the development of Liver Wind. Herbs that nourish Liver Yin are thus often combined with herbs that clear Liver Fire, suppress Liver Yang and calm Liver Wind (Fig. 25.1).

4. HERBS THAT HARMONIZE THE LIVER AND HERBS THAT COOL OR WARM THE LIVER

— When Stagnant Liver Qi turns to Heat and Fire, herbs that harmonize the Liver are combined with herbs that clear Liver Heat and Fire (Fig. 25.2).
— If retention of Cold in the Liver channel produces stagnation of Qi, herbs that warm the Liver are combined with herbs that harmonize the Liver and regulate Qi (Fig. 25.3).

Questions

1. What are the indications for herbs that nourish Liver Yin, herbs that suppress Liver

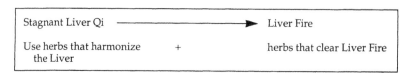

Fig. 25.2 Combination of herbs to treat Liver Fire.

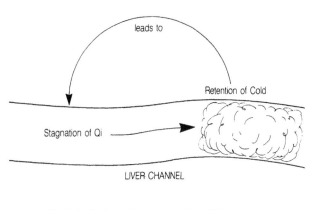

Fig. 25.3 Combination of herbs to treat Stagnation of Cold in the Liver Channel.

Yang and herbs that calm Liver Wind? How do these categories of herbs interrelate?
2. Compare and contrast herbs that harmonize the Liver, herbs that benefit the Gall Bladder and herbs that clear Heat from the Liver and Gall Bladder.

26 *The Kidneys and Bladder*

A. Actions, characteristics and indications of common herbs

1. HERBS THAT TONIFY KIDNEY YANG

— These herbs are pungent and hot, or sweet, salty and warm in nature. They consist of:

a. Herbs that warm the Kidneys and strengthen Yang

— These herbs are indicated for Kidney Yang Deficiency with symptoms of cold limbs, lower back pain, impotence, spermatorrhoea and lack of libido. Commonly used herbs include:

Radix Aconiti Praeparata	*Fu Zi*
Cortex Cinnamomi	*Rou Gui*
Cornu Cervi Pantotrichum	*Lu Rong*
Cornu Cervi	*Lu Jiao*
Rhizoma Curculiginis	*Xian Mao*
Herba Epimedii	*Yin Yang Huo*
Herba Cistanchis	*Rou Cong Rong*
Radix Morindae Officinalis	*Ba Ji Tian*
Peni et Testes Callorhini	*Hai Gou Shen*
Hippocampus	*Hai Ma*

b. Herbs that tonify the Kidneys and strengthen tendons and bones

— These herbs are indicated for soreness and weakness of the lumbar region and knees due to Kidney Yang Deficiency and for osteoporosis, chronic Bi syndromes and hemiplegia. Commonly used herbs include:

Cortex Eucommiae	*Du Zhong*
Radix Dipsaci	*Xu Duan*
Rhizoma Cibotii	*Gou Ji*
Ramulus Loranthi	*Sang Ji Sheng*
Cortex Acanthopancis Radicis	*Wu Jia Pi*
Os Tigris	*Hu Gu*

c. Herbs that tonify the Kidneys and stimulate the reception of Qi

— These herbs are indicated for a weakness of the Kidneys' function of receiving the Qi, with symptoms of chronic cough or asthma. Commonly used herbs include:

Gecko	*Ge Jie*
Semen Juglandis	*Hu Tao Rou*
Umbilical cord	*Qi Dai*
Fructus Schisandrae	*Wu Wei Zi*
Fructus Psoraleae	*Bu Gu Zhi*
Cordyceps	*Dong Chong Xia Cao*
Lignum Aquilariae Resinatum	*Chen Xiang*

2. HERBS THAT TONIFY KIDNEY YIN

— These herbs are sweet, cold or slightly warm, nourishing and sticky in nature. They are indicated for Kidney Yin Deficiency with symptoms of soreness and weakness of the lumbar region and knees, tinnitus and tidal fever. Commonly used herbs include:

Radix Rehmanniae Praeparata	*Shu Di*
Radix Rehmanniae	*Sheng Di*
Radix Polygoni Multiflori	*He Shou Wu*
Fructus Corni	*Shan Zhu Yu*
Fructus Ligustri Lucidi	*Nu Zhen Zi*
Plastrum Testudinis	*Gui Ban*
Radix Scrophulariae	*Xuan Shen*

3. HERBS THAT STOP ENURESIS AND SPERMATORRHOEA

— These herbs are sour and astringent in nature and are indicated for patterns of Kidney Qi Not Firm, with symptoms of spermatorrhoea, enuresis and clear watery leucorrhoea. Commonly used herbs include:

Os Draconis	*Long Gu*
Concha Ostreae	*Mu Li*
Fructus Rosae Laevi	*Jin Ying Zi*
Semen Euryales	*Qian Shi*
Semen Nelumbinis	*Lian Zi*
Ootheca Mantidis	*Sang Piao Xiao*
Fructus Schisandrae	*Wu Wei Zi*
Fructus Corni	*Shan Zhu Yu*

4. HERBS THAT CLEAR EMPTY KIDNEY FIRE

— These herbs are bitter and cold in nature and are indicated for Empty Kidney Fire with sexual hyperfunction. Commonly used herbs include:

Rhizoma Anemarrhenae	*Zhi Mu*
Cortex Phellodendri	*Huang Bai*
Cortex Moutan Radicis	*Dan Pi*
Rhizoma Alismatis	*Ze Xie*

5. DIURETIC HERBS

— These herbs are sweet and bland in nature and are indicated for dysuria and oedema. Commonly used herbs include:

Poria	*Fu Ling*
Polyporus Umbellatus	*Zhu Ling*
Rhizoma Alismatis	*Ze Xie*
Semen Plantaginis	*Che Qian Zi*

6. HERBS THAT OPEN THE WATER PASSAGES

— These herbs are cold in nature and are indicated for urinary disturbance due to retention of Heat and for haematuria, urolithiasis or turbid urine. Commonly used herbs include:

Caulis Akebiae	*Mu Tong*

Herba Lysimachiae	*Jin Qian Cao*
Spora Lygodii	*Hai Jin Sha*
Folium Pyrrhosiae	*Shi Wei*
Herba Dianthi	*Qu Mai*

B. Interactions and combinations of herbs

1. HERBS THAT CLEAR KIDNEY FIRE AND HERBS THAT TONIFY KIDNEY YIN

— Herbs that clear Kidney Fire are indicated for Empty Heat due to Kidney Yin Deficiency. Herbs that clear Kidney Fire, such as Rhizoma Anemarrhenae and Cortex Phellodendri, are thus often combined with herbs that tonify Kidney Yin, such as Radix Rehmanniae and Fructus Corni.

2. HERBS THAT TONIFY KIDNEY YANG AND HERBS THAT TONIFY KIDNEY YIN

— Because Yin and Yang have the same root, Kidney Yang cannot flourish without the support of Kidney Yin. In the treatment of Kidney Yang Deficiency, herbs that tonify Kidney Yang are often combined with herbs that tonify Kidney Yin.

3. HERBS THAT STRENGTHEN TENDONS AND BONES, HERBS THAT STIMULATE THE RECEPTION OF QI AND HERBS THAT TONIFY KIDNEY YIN AND KIDNEY YANG

— Weakness of the tendons and bones due to Liver and Kidney Deficiency is rooted in

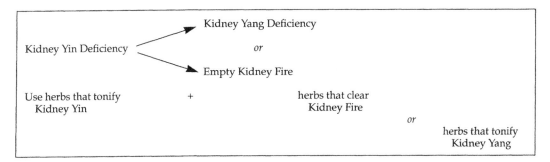

Fig. 26.1 Complications of Kidney Yin Deficiency.

deficiency of Kidney Yin and Kidney Yang. Dysfunction of the Kidneys' reception of Qi is also rooted in deficiency of Kidney Yin and Yang.

— Herbs that strengthen the tendons and bones, and herbs that stimulate the Kidney's reception of Qi, are therefore often combined with herbs that tonify Kidney Yin and Kidney Yang (Fig. 26.1)

4. HERBS THAT STOP SPERMATORRHOEA AND ENURESIS AND HERBS THAT TONIFY KIDNEY YIN AND KIDNEY YANG

— Nocturnal emission and spermatorrhoea are signs of a weakness of the Gate of Essence; enuresis is caused by failure of the Bladder to control urine; and clear watery leucorrhoea is due to weakness of the Dai channel in controlling vaginal discharge.

— All of these patterns are rooted in Kidney Deficiency. Herbs that stop spermatorrhoea, enuresis and leucorrhoea are therefore often combined with herbs that tonify the Kidneys.

5. HERBS THAT OPEN THE WATER PASSAGES AND PROMOTE DIURESIS AND HERBS THAT TONIFY KIDNEY YIN AND KIDNEY YANG

— When Kidney Yang is deficient, Qi does not transform Water, and this leads to retention of Water and Dampness with symptoms of oedema and dysuria. The treatment principle in such cases is to warm Yang and promote diuresis with herbs that open the water passages and warm Kidney Yang at the same time. For example, Polyporus Umbellatus, Poria and Rhizoma Alismatis are combined with Radix Aconiti Praeparata and Cortex Cinnamomi.

— On the other hand, when urinary disturbance is due to retention of Damp-Heat in the Bladder, the Heat will eventually damage Kidney Yin. Even if symptoms of Kidney Yin Deficiency are not apparent, diuretic herbs are themselves likely to deplete Fluids. Herbs that clear Heat and open the water passages are therefore combined with herbs that tonify Kidney Yin.

Questions

1. What is the clinical relationship between herbs that tonify Kidney Yin and Kidney Yang, herbs that promote diuresis and open the water passages and herbs that stop spermatorrhoea and enuresis?
2. What is the clinical relationship between herbs that tonify Kidney Yin and herbs that clear Empty Kidney Fire?

Part 4:
Combinations and comparisons of commonly used formulae

Formulae for Releasing the Exterior **27**

A. GUIDING PRINCIPLES FOR FORMULATING PRESCRIPTIONS TO RELEASE THE EXTERIOR

1. Formulae for Releasing the Exterior are indicated for invasion of the surface of the body (i.e. the skin, hair, muscles and channels) by any of the Six Pathogenic Factors. Symptoms of such a pattern include aversion to cold, fever, headache, nasal obstruction, a superficial pulse and a white tongue coating.
2. Formulae for Releasing the Exterior are prescribed when the treatment method consists of inducing diaphoresis to Release the Exterior and eliminate pathogenic factors.
3. The main ingredients of these formulae are herbs which are pungent in nature. The selection of formulae and herbs is based on the type of Exterior pattern, the method of treatment and the particular characteristics of individual herbs.

B. FORMULATING PRESCRIPTIONS FOR RELEASING THE EXTERIOR

1. Formulae for Releasing the Exterior with pungent and warm herbs

— Formulae for Releasing the Exterior with pungent and warm herbs disperse Wind-Cold and are thus indicated for patterns of Exterior Cold.
— Excess-type external patterns vary in severity. They may consist exclusively of Wind-Cold, or of Wind-Cold complicated with External Dampness, or the retention of Phlegm, or stagnation of Qi.
— Deficiency-type external patterns may be complicated with Yang Deficiency or Qi Deficiency.
— Mild patterns of the Excess type, with symptoms of mild aversion to cold, mild fever, nasal obstruction and runny nose, are treated with Bulbus Allii Fistulosi and Semen Sojae Praeparatum, which gently disperse pathogenic factors from the Defensive level.
— Severe exterior patterns of the Excess type, with symptoms of fever, aversion to cold, absence of sweating, dyspnoea and a tense superficial pulse, are treated with Herba Ephedrae and Ramulus Cinnamomi, which eliminate Wind-Cold more vigorously.
— If Wind-Cold is complicated with Dampness, with symptoms of fever, aversion to cold, headache, lethargy and general aching, herbs are chosen which not only Release the Exterior but also eliminate Dampness and relieve pain. Representative herbs include Rhizoma seu Radix Notopterygii, Radix Ledebouriellae and Radix Angelicae Dahuricae.
— Once the principal herbs have been selected according to these principles, combinations of secondary herbs are then prescribed according to the signs and symptoms of the particular case. For example:

  – for cough and dyspnoea add Semen Armeniacae Amarum and Fructus Perillae
  – for stagnation of Qi with fullness of the chest, add Rhizoma Cyperi and Pericarpium Citri Reticulatae
  – for Interior Heat with irritability, add Gypsum Fibrosum, Radix Rehmanniae and Radix Scutellariae
  – for Food Retention with abdominal distension, add Fructus Crataegi and Massa Fermentata Medicinalis
  – for retention of Phlegm-Fluid, add Rhizoma Pinelliae, Rhizoma Zingiberis and Herba Asari
  – to prevent warm and dry herbs from damaging Yin and consuming Lung Qi,

add Radix Paeoniae Alba and Fructus Schisandrae.

— Commonly used formulae include:

- *Cong Chi Tang*
  Spring Onion and Prepared Soybean Decoction
- *Cong Chi Jie Geng Tang*
  Spring Onion and Prepared Soybean Decoction with Platycodon
- *Ma Huang Tang*
  Ephedra Decoction
- *Jiu Wei Qiang Hu Tang*
- **Nine-Herb Decoction with Notopterygium**
- *Xiao Qing Long Tang*
- **Small Green Dragon Decoction**
- *Da Qing Long Tang*
  Major Blue-Green Dragon Decoction
- *Xiang Su San*
  Cyperus and Perilla Leaf Powder

— Deficient-type Exterior patterns manifest when there is a weak defensive response to pathogenic factors. Invasion of the Defensive level leads to disharmony between the Defensive (Wei) Qi and Nutritive (Ying) Qi with symptoms of aversion to Wind, spontaneous sweating and a superficial and slow or weak pulse. The method of treatment is to regulate Defensive Qi and Nutritive Qi with Ramulus Cinnamomi paired with Radix Paeoniae Alba, and Rhizoma Zingiberis Recens paired with Fructus Ziziphi Jujubae, to disperse the pathogenic factors and at the same time astringe the Nutrient Qi.
— Deficient-type Exterior patterns may be complicated with disorders of the Tai Yang channel, with symptoms of rigidity and stiffness of the neck and back. There may be impairment of the Lung functions of dispersing and descending, with symptoms of cough and wheeze. There may also be Yang Deficiency with cold limbs, or Qi Deficiency with a feeble pulse.
— For these complications, additional herbs are chosen such as:

- Radix Puerariae, to promote the smooth circulation of Qi in the muscles
- Cortex Magnoliae Officinalis and Semen Armeniacae Amarum to conduct Rebellious Lung Qi downward
- Radix Aconiti Praeparata to assist Yang
- Radix Ginseng to tonify Qi.

— Representative formulae include:

- *Gui Zhi Tang*
  Cinnamon Twig Decoction
- *Gui Zhi Jia Ge Gen Tang*
  Cinnamon Twig Decoction plus Kudzu
- *Gui Zhi Jia Hou Po Xing Zi Tang*
- **Cinnamon Twig Decoction plus Magnolia Bark and Apricot Kernel**
- *Gui Zhi Fu Zi Tang*
- **Cinnamon Twig Decoction plus Prepared Aconite**
- *Gui Zhi Jia Ren Shen Tang*
- **Cinnamon Twig Decoction plus Ginseng**

2. **Formulating prescriptions for Releasing the Exterior with pungent and cool herbs**

— Formulae for Releasing the Exterior with pungent and cool herbs disperse Wind-Heat and are indicated for Exterior Heat patterns. This type of pattern can present in several different ways and these require different methods of treatment.
— If the pattern is one of Wind-Heat at the Defensive level with pronounced signs of Heat, the method of treatment is to disperse Wind-Heat with pungent and cool herbs such as Flos Lonicerae and Fructus Forsythiae, assisted by herbs such as Semen Sojae Praeparata, Herba Menthae and Fructus Arctii.
— If the Heat enters the Lung channel and produces severe coughing, herbs are employed which not only disperse Wind-Heat but also promote the Lungs' functions of descending and dispersing, such as Folium Mori and Flos Chrysanthemi, assisted by Semen Armeniacae Amarum, Radix Platycodi and Radix Glycyrrhizae.
— Pathogenic Wind-Heat is Yang in nature and tends to consume Body Fluids and Yin; it can easily affect the throat and the Nutritive level. In this case, herbs such as Radix Adenophorae, Radix Ophiopogonis, Rhizoma Phragmitis, Radix Trichosanthis, Rhizoma Anemarrhenae and Gypsum Fibrosum should be added to the formula.
— Representative formulae are:

- *Yin Qiao San*
  Honeysuckle and Forsythia Powder
- *Sang Ju Yin*

Mulberry Leaf and Chrysanthemum Decoction

— Wind-Cold may turn to Heat, thus transforming an Exterior Cold pattern into an Exterior Heat pattern. Once this transformation takes place, the pathogenic factor will be transmitted inward to the Shao Yang and Yang Ming channels. The result will be that all three Yang channels will be affected, but primarily the Yang Ming channel. Signs and symptoms will then include high fever, mild aversion to cold, a bitter taste and dry mouth, headache, eye pain, dry nose, a yellow dry tongue coating and a slightly surging pulse.
— Alternatively, the heat produced may block the Lung channel, producing symptoms of cough and dyspnoea and a rapid pulse.
— To treat this pattern, a prescription must be formulated which addresses the mixed nature of the pathological pattern. Attention should be given to the relative proportion of pungent/warm and cold or cool herbs according to the presenting symptoms and signs.
— For example, when the three Yang channels are involved, the method of treatment is primarily to Release the Exterior with pungent and cool herbs and secondarily to clear internal Heat, using herbs such as Radix Bupleuri, Radix Puerariae, Rhizoma seu Radix Notopterygii, Radix Angelicae Dahuricae, Radix Scutellariae and Gypsum Fibrosum.
— In the treatment of Heat blocking the Lungs, the treatment method is to promote the function of the Lungs with pungent and cool herbs and to clear Lung Heat, using herbs such as Herba Ephedrae, Gypsum Fibrosum and Semen Armeniacae Amarum.
— If the Heat has consumed Yin, add Radix Paeoniae Alba and Radix Rehmanniae to nourish the Yin.
— Attention should be given to the relative proportions of pungent/warm herbs and cold or cool herbs.
— Representative formulae are:

  – *Chai Ge Jie Ji Tang*
    Bupleurum and Kudzu Decoction to Release the Muscle Layer
  – *Ma Xing Shi Gan Tang*
    Ephedra–Prunus–Gypsum–Glycyrrhiza Decoction

— Measles is caused by Yang toxins which rapidly turn to Heat. The onset of measles presents as an Exterior Heat pattern with symptoms of a mild rash, fever, aversion to cold, cough, runny nose and a superficial and rapid pulse. The correct method of treatment is Releasing the Exterior with pungent and cool herbs, with attention to promoting the expression of the rash and clearing toxins. Thus the prescription should consist primarily of herbs such as Rhizoma Cimicifugae, Radix Puerariae, Periostracum Cicadae, Fructus Arctii and Herba Menthae, plus one or two pungent and slightly warm herbs such as Herba Schizonepeta and Ramulus Tamarix Chinensis (Cheng Liu) which promote the expression of the rash.
— The toxic Qi of measles often invades the Spleen and Lung, damaging Yin and Blood and producing symptoms of fever, thirst, yellow urine, irritability, restlessness, cough, dyspnoea, poor appetite and a dark-red rash. In this event, combinations of herbs should be added to the formula such as:

  – Semen Armeniacae Amarum, Radix Platycodi and Radix Peucedani
  – Gypsum Fibrosum and Rhizoma Anemarrhenae
  – Radix Paeoniae Rubra and Radix Salviae Miltiorrhizae
  – Flos Lonicerae, Fructus Forsythiae and Herba Lophatheri.

— Representative formulae are:

  – *Sheng Ma Ge Gen Tang*
    Cimicifuga and Kudzu Decoction
  – *Zhu Ye Liu Bang Tang*
    Lophatheri–Tamarix–Arctii Decoction

3. Formulation of prescriptions to Release the Exterior and strengthen resistance to disease

— Formulae which both Release the Exterior and promote resistance to disease are indicated for Exterior patterns with Wei Qi Deficiency. External pathogens can be either Wind-Cold or Wind-Heat, and internal Deficiency may involve Qi, Blood, Yin or Yang, and these factors determine the selection of herbs.
— In most cases, Wind-Cold or Wind-Cold complicated with Dampness are likely to invade where there is Qi Deficiency or Yang Deficiency. The pattern thus produced is

cold in nature and the prescription will consist of:

a. pungent and warm herbs that Release the Exterior such as Herba Ephedrae, Ramulus Cinnamomi, Rhizoma seu Radix Notopterygii, Radix Ledebouriellae and Herba Asari

and

b. herbs that tonify Qi such as Radix Ginseng and Radix Astragali seu Hedysari

or

– herbs that tonify Yang such as Radix Aconiti Praeparata and Cortex Cinnamomi.

— The dosage of each herb depends upon the relative severity of symptoms.

— Commonly used formulae include:

– *Ma Huang Fu Zi Xi Xin Tang*
  Ephedra, Asarum and Prepared Aconite Decoction
– *Ren Shen Bai Du San*
  Ginseng Powder to Overcome Pathogenic Influences
– *Zai Zao San*
  Renewal Powder

— When there is an underlying pattern of Yin and Blood Deficiency, Wind-Heat is more likely to invade than Wind-Cold. In this case, the prescription consists of

a. pungent and cool herbs that Release the Exterior such as Radix Puerariae, Herba Menthae and Folium Mori

or

– pungent and slightly warm herbs that gently Release the Exterior such as Bulbus Allii Fistulosi and Semen Sojae Praeparata

and

b. herbs that nourish Yin such as Rhizoma Polygonati Odorati, Radix Ophiopogonis, Radix Adenophorae and Radix Glehniae

or

– herbs that tonify Blood such as Radix Angelicae Sinensis and Radix Rehmanniae Praeparata.

— Yin and Blood Deficiency can produce internal Heat which combines with External Wind-Heat to impair the Lungs' descending function. Symptoms may then include restlessness, five-palm heat, thirst, dry throat and cough. If this occurs, herbs such as Radix Ampelopsis, Rhizoma Anemarrhenae, Radix Trichosanthis, Gypsum Fibrosum,

Radix Platycodi, Radix Glycyrrhizae and Fructus Arctii should be added.

— Representative formulae include:

– *Jia Jian Wei Rui Tang*
  Modified Polygonatum Odoratum Decoction
– *Cong Bai Qi Wei Yin*
  Spring Onion Decoction with Seven Ingredients

C. POINTS TO REMEMBER IN FORMULATING PRESCRIPTIONS FOR RELEASING THE EXTERIOR

1. The actions of herbs that Release the Exterior are modified by dosage. For example, Radix Bupleuri in large doses Releases the Exterior and lowers fever; in moderate doses it harmonizes the Liver and relieves stagnation; and in small doses it raises the Yang.

— Folium Mori does not work in small doses, but only in large doses.

— Herba Asari in small doses stops cough but in large doses it may cause respiratory paralysis.

— Dosage will also be dictated by individual variations in sensitivity to herbs due to constitutional differences, and by the severity of the Exterior pattern itself.

2. Herbs that Release the Exterior are pungent and scattering in nature, and their active ingredients are volatile. It is therefore not advisable to decoct them for a long time over low heat, but rather to cook them quickly using strong heat.

— Such a decoction is taken warm, twice daily. To increase its diaphoretic action, the patient should eat hot porridge and be covered with thick bedclothes after taking the decoction.

— However, while absence of sweating does not allow the elimination of pathogenic factors, excessive sweating consumes Body Fluids and can lead to Collapse of Yang. It is best to induce moderate sweating only.

3. It is necessary to make an accurate diagnosis of the Exterior pattern before selecting a prescription. The book *Insight into Medicine* says:

To conclude, in case of deficiency of Yang, the treatment method of invigorating the Middle Burner and promoting diaphoresis is adopted. If signs of Heat are present, the method of clearing Heat and promoting diaphoresis is adopted. If signs of Cold are present, the method of warming the channels and promoting diaphoresis is adopted. In case of Retention of Food, the method of promoting digestion and promoting diaphoresis is adopted. If symptoms and signs are severe and the patient's constitution is strong, the method of producing vigorous sweating is adopted. If symptoms and signs are mild and the patient's constitution is weak, the method of causing mild sweating is adopted.

D. A COMPARISON OF COMMONLY USED FORMULAE FOR RELEASING THE EXTERIOR (TABLE 27.1)

1. – *Ma Huang Tang*
     Ephedra Decoction
   – *Gui Zhi Tang*
     Cinnamon Twig Decoction

— Both formulae contain Ramulus Cinnamomi and treated Radix Glycyrrhizae.
— Ephedra Decoction also contains Herba Ephedrae and Semen Armeniacae Amarum and thus strongly promotes diaphoresis and controls wheeze. This formula is indicated for Exterior patterns of the Excess type with symptoms of aversion to cold, fever, headache and general aching, with an absence of sweating and a superficial tense pulse.
— In Cinnamon Twig Decoction, Ramulus Cinnamomi and Radix Paeoniae Alba are combined with Rhizoma Zingiberis Recens and Fructus Ziziphi Jujubae. Its diaphoretic action is therefore weak, but it regulates Defensive and Nutritive Qi. This formula is indicated for Wind-Cold patterns of the Deficiency type with symptoms of sweating, and a superficial and weak pulse in addition to other symptoms of invasion of Wind-Cold.

2. – *Da Qing Long Tang*
     Major Blue-Green Dragon Decoction
   – *Xiao Qing Long Tang*
   – **Small Green Dragon Decoction**

— Both formulae contain Herba Ephedrae, Ramulus Cinnamomi and Radix Glycyrrhizae and are indicated for Exterior Cold patterns of the Excess type.
— **Major Blue-Green Dragon Decoction** also contains Semen Armeniacae Amarum, Rhizoma Zingiberis Recens and Fructus Ziziphi Jujubae to strengthen the effect of Releasing the Exterior, and Gypsum Fibrosum to clear Internal Heat. It is thus indicated for Exterior Cold complicated with Interior Heat, with symptoms of thirst, restlessness and irritability.
— **Small Green Dragon Decoction** also contains Radix Paeoniae Alba, Herba Asari, Rhizoma Zingiberis, Rhizoma Pinelliae and Fructus Schisandrae, to warm the Lungs and resolve Phlegm-Fluid. It is indicated for Exterior Cold patterns complicated with Interior Phlegm-Fluid, with symptoms of cough, dyspnoea and profuse clear sputum.

Table 27.1 Comparison of formulae for Releasing the Exterior

Formula	Actions	Indications
Ephedra Decoction	Strongly promotes diaphoresis Controls wheeze	Wind-Cold patterns of the Excess type
Cinnamon Twig Decoction	Regulates Defensive and Nutritive Qi	Wind-Cold patterns of the Deficiency type
Major Blue-Green Dragon Decoction	Releases the Exterior Clears Internal Heat	Wind-Cold complicated with Interior Heat
Small Green Dragon Decoction	Warms the Lungs Resolves Phlegm-Fluid	Wind-Cold complicated with Interior Phlegm-Fluid
Mulberry Leaf and Chrysanthemum Decoction	Disperses Wind-Heat Promotes the dispersing function of the Lungs	Mild patterns of Wind-Heat
Honeysuckle and Forsythia Powder	More strongly Releases the Exterior and clears Heat	More severe patterns of Wind-Heat

3. – *Sang Ju Yin*
      Mulberry Leaf and Chrysanthemum Decoction
   – *Yin Qiao San*
      Honeysuckle and Forsythia Powder

— Both formulae are pungent and cool in nature, and are indicated for the initial stages of Warm Disease. Both contain:

   – Herba Menthae to eliminate Wind and clear Heat
   – Fructus Forsythiae to clear Heat and Fire Poison
   – Radix Platycodi and Radix Glycyrrhizae to ease the throat and resolve Phlegm
   and
   – Rhizoma Phragmitis to clear Heat and promote Body Fluids.

— **Mulberry Leaf and Chrysanthemum Decoction** also contains Folium Mori, Flos Chrysanthemi and Armeniacae Amarum and is thus more effective in promoting the dispersing function of the Lungs to stop cough.
— **Honeysuckle and Forsythia Powder** also contains Herba Schizonepeta, Semen Sojae Praeparata, Fructus Arctii, Flos Lonicerae and Herba Lophatheri and is thus more effective in Releasing the Exterior and clearing Heat.
— The former is a mild formula and is indicated for mild Wind-Heat patterns, while the latter is a moderately strong formula and is indicated for more severe Wind-Heat patterns with symptoms of a sensation of heat, thirst and sore throat.

Questions

1. What principles should be observed in formulating prescriptions to Release the Exterior?
2. How would you formulate a prescription for the treatment of Deficient-type patterns of invasion by external pathogenic factors?

Purgative formulae 28

A. GUIDING PRINCIPLES FOR FORMULATING PURGATIVE PRESCRIPTIONS

1. Purgative formulae are prescribed when there is substantial accumulation due to pathogenic factors in the gastrointestinal tract with symptoms of abdominal pain, constipation and a forceful and full pulse.
2. These formulae are prescribed when the treatment method of choice is that of purging to remove obstruction in the Interior.
3. The formulae consist of purgative substances that relieve constipation and dispel substantial accumulation from the Interior. The selection of formulae depends upon the type of Excess pattern and the actions of individual herbs.

B. FORMULATING PURGATIVE PRESCRIPTIONS

1. Formulating cold purgative formulae

— Cold purgative formulae consist primarily of cold and cool purgatives. They remove obstruction from the Fu organs, clear Heat and dispel accumulation of Heat. They are thus indicated for patterns of accumulation of Heat in the Interior.
— The pathogenesis of such patterns is the retention of dry faeces in the intestinal tract due to Heat, which blocks the Qi of the Large Intestine. Clinical manifestations include constipation, distension, abdominal fullness and pain, tidal fever, a yellow tongue coating and a forceful full pulse.
— The main ingredients of such formulae are cold and bitter or salty substances such as Radix et Rhizoma Rhei and Natrii Sulfas.
— The accumulation of Full Heat tends to cause stagnation of Qi, or of both Qi and Blood. The pattern may be complicated with accumulation of Water or stagnation of Blood. The disorder is most often located in the Middle and Lower Burners but occasionally in the Middle and Upper Burners. If the accumulation of Heat blocks the circulation of Qi or Blood, herbs that regulate Qi or Blood and resolve Blood Stasis are added to promote bowel movement and relieve abdominal pain. Examples are Fructus Aurantii Immaturus and Cortex Magnoliae Officinalis in formulae such as *Da Cheng Qi Tang* (**Major Order the Qi Decoction**) and *Xiao Cheng Qi Tang* (**Minor Order the Qi Decoction**).

— Semen Persicae, Radix Paeoniae Rubra and Semen Raphani are similarly deployed in formulae such as *Fu Fang Cheng Qi Tang* (**Revised Major Order the Qi Decoction**).
— If Full Heat and stagnant Blood combine to block the intestinal tract and produce appendicitis with localized masses, herbs that activate the Blood, resolve Blood Stasis, relieve pain, disperse masses and relieve swelling are added.
— For Fire Poison with severe pain, herbs that activate the Blood, relieve pain and clear Heat and Fire Poison are even more important. Herbs such as Semen Persicae, Cortex Moutan Radicis and Semen Benincasae are used for this purpose in formulae such as *Da Huang Mu Dan Tang* (**Rhubarb and Moutan Decoction**), to which Flos Lonicerae and Herba Taraxaci can be added.
— If Water and Heat combine and are retained in the chest and abdomen with symptoms of constipation, dryness of the mouth and tongue, and epigastric and abdominal hardness, fullness and pain, strong purgatives that dispel retained Water should be added. An example of this type of combination is that of Radix et Rhizoma Rhei and Natrii Sulfas with Radix Euphorbiae Kansui

in *Da Xian Xiong Tang* (**Major Sinking into the Chest Decoction**).

2. Formulating warm purgative prescriptions

— These formulae are indicated for constipation with abdominal pain due to retention of Full Cold.
— The two factors of this pattern are the accumulation of faeces and pathogenic Cold. Pathogenic Cold is resolved by warming and the accumulation of faeces is relieved by purging. Warm purgative formulae therefore consist of herbs that warm the Interior and dispel Cold, and purgative herbs. Warm purgative herbs may be used, or a combination of warm and hot herbs with cold purgatives.
— For sudden distending and boring pain in the heart and abdomen, lockjaw and sudden syncope, powerful hot purgatives are combined with herbs that warm the Interior and dispel Cold, or with cold purgatives. An example is the combination of Fructus Crotonis (*Ba Dou*) with Radix et Rhizoma Rhei and dried Rhizoma Zingiberis in *San Wu Bei Ji Wan* (**Three-Substance Pill for Emergencies**).
— If the onset of the disorder is gradual, and pathological changes are not severe but consist of constipation, abdominal pain, a thick white tongue coating and a deep tense pulse, the correct method of treatment is warming the Interior, dispelling Cold and gently relieving constipation. In this case, herbs that warm the Interior are combined with cold purgatives, and Qi tonic herbs are added to the formula. Examples are the combination of Radix et Rhizoma Rhei with Radix Aconiti Praeparata and Herba Asari in *Da Huang Fu Zi Tang* (**Rhubarb and Prepared Aconite Decoction**) and the combination of Radix et Rhizoma Rhei with Radix Aconiti Praeparata, dried Rhizoma Zingiberis, Radix Ginseng and treated Radix Glycyrrhizae in *Wen Pi Tang* (**Warm the Spleen Decoction**).

3. Formulating moist purgative prescriptions

— Moist purgative formulae consist of moist and oily mild purgatives which relieve constipation by moistening the intestines. They are thus indicated for constipation due to intestinal dryness.
— The two factors in this pattern are the accumulation of dry faeces and the consumption of Body Fluids due to Full Heat, Empty Heat or damage to Essence and Blood following a prolonged illness or childbirth.
— In cases where Full Heat has consumed Body Fluids, resulting in dry constipation, the nature of the pattern is Excess complicated with Deficiency. Here, the method of moistening the intestines is combined with the method of purging by combining moist purgatives with herbs that nourish the Yin and harmonize the Interior and with herbs that clear Heat, regulate Qi and relieve constipation. An example is the combination of Fructus Cannabis, Semen Armeniacae Amarum, Radix Paeoniae Alba and Mel with Fructus Aurantii Immaturus, Cortex Magnoliae Officinalis and Radix et Rhizoma Rhei in *Ma Zi Ren Wan* (**Hemp Seed Pill**).
— If dry constipation is caused by a deficiency of Essence and Blood, the correct treatment method is to relieve constipation gently with warm and moist herbs, using herbs that warm the Kidneys, moisten the intestines and tonify Essence and Blood. However, moist herbs can produce stagnation, and purgatives may cause sinking of Qi in a weak person. Therefore, herbs that regulate Qi and herbs that raise Yang should be added.
— An example of such a formula is *Ji Chuan Jian* (**Benefit the River Decoction**) in which Herba Cistanchis tonifies Kidney Essence, moistens the intestines and relieves constipation; Radix Angelicae Sinensis tonifies Blood and moistens the intestines; Radix Achyranthis Bidentatae tonifies the Kidneys and strengthens the lumbar region; Fructus Aurantii relaxes the intestines and sends Qi downward; and Rhizoma Cimicifugae raises the clear Yang and conducts the turbid Yin downward

4. Formulae that drive out excess water

— Formulae for driving out water consist primarily of herbs that dispel water and relieve swelling. They are indicated for accumulated water in the chest and abdomen and for oedema with symptoms of distension and fullness.
— Herbs commonly used for this purpose include Radix Euphorbiae Kansui, Flos

Genkwa, Radix Euphorbiae Pekinensis, Semen Pharbitidis and Radix Phytolaccae, all of which dispel water via urine and stool.

— However, such herbs are powerful and somewhat toxic cathartics, and Fructus Ziziphi Jujubae or other Spleen tonics are generally added to these formulae to protect the Middle Burner, as in *Shi Zao Tang* (**Ten-Jujube Decoction**).

— If the pathological pattern includes oedema which blocks Qi circulation, as well as Full Heat with thirst, coarse breathing, a hard abdomen and constipation, herbs that regulate Qi should be added. An example of such a formula is *Zhou Che Wan* (**Vessel and Vehicle Pill**), in which Radix Euphorbiae Pekinensis, Radix Euphorbiae Kansui, Flos Genkwa and Semen Pharbitidis are combined with Pericarpium Citri Reticulatae Viride, Pericarpium Citri Reticulatae, Radix Aucklandiae, Semen Arecae and Radix et Rhizoma Rhei.

5. Formulating prescriptions to purge and tonify simultaneously

— These formulae consist of purgative herbs and tonic herbs in combination. They are indicated for an accumulation of pathogenic factors in the gastrointestinal tract complicated with a deficiency of the Upright (*Zheng*) Qi of the body. In such cases, purgative herbs alone will further damage the Upright Qi, while tonic herbs alone will strengthen the pathogenic factors.

— Interior patterns of Excess can consist either of accumulation of Heat or accumulation of Cold. Internal deficiency may involve Yin, Yang, Qi or Blood. The selection of formulae thus depends upon the individual case.

— If accumulation of Heat is severe, and Qi and Blood are deficient, the method of clearing Heat with powerful purgatives is combined with the method of tonifying Qi and Blood. An example of such a formula is *Huang Long Tang* (**Yellow Dragon Decoction**), in which **Major Order the Qi Decoction** is combined with Qi and Blood tonics such as Radix Ginseng and Radix Angelicae Sinensis.

— If there is an accumulation of Heat in Yang Ming which consumes Yin, producing dry constipation, the correct formula is *Zeng Ye Cheng Qi Tang* (**Increase the Fluids and Order the Qi Decoction**). In this formula, herbs such as Radix Scophulariae, Radix Rehmanniae and Radix Ophiopogonis, which nourish the Yin and promote Body Fluids, are combined with cold purgatives such as Radix et Rhizoma Rhei and Natrii Sulfas.

— If constipation is due to accumulation of Cold with Spleen Yang Deficiency, purgative herbs are combined with herbs that warm the Interior and tonify Qi. An example is *Wen Pi Tang* (**Warm the Spleen Decoction**), in which Radix et Rhizoma Rhei is combined with Radix Aconiti Praeparata, Rhizoma Zingiberis, Radix Ginseng and treated Radix Glycyrrhizae.

C. POINTS TO REMEMBER IN FORMULATING PURGATIVE PRESCRIPTIONS

1. Purgative formulae work in different ways, depending upon the dosage and the method of decoction and administration. For example, Major Order the Qi Decoction and Minor Order the Qi Decoction have different actions and indications despite having similar ingredients. If Fructus Aurantii Immaturus and Cortex Magnoliae Officinalis are prescribed in large dosages and Radix et Rhizoma Rhei is added toward the end of the cooking time, the purgative effect will be strong. If Fructus Aurantii Immaturus and Cortex Magnoliae Officinalis are used in small dosages and the three herbs are cooked together, the purgative effect will be weaker.

— Fructus Crotonis, an ingredient of **Three-Substance Pill for Emergencies**, is a powerful cathartic and should be administered in small doses, in the form of pills or powder with the oil removed in order to reduce its irritant effect on the stomach and intestines.

— Similarly, if Radix Euphorbiae Kansui is taken in large doses it will effectively drive out excess water but is likely to damage Stomach Qi. This side-effect is largely avoided if it is taken in small doses and combined with Jujube, as in **Ten-Jujube Decoction**, in order to minimize its toxicity.

2. Purgative formulae dispel accumulated pathogenic factors, but tend to damage Upright Qi. They are therefore contraindicated in cases of:

- extreme deficiency of Qi and Blood with a hesitant and feeble pulse
- Kidney Yang Deficiency with cold limbs
- Exterior patterns in which the pathogenic factors have not entered the Interior
- internal deficiency and Rebellious Qi with nausea, vomiting and hiccup
- dryness of the stool followed by loose stools.

— In his book *A Medical Text for Confucianists to Serve Family Members and Relatives*, Zhang Zihe says, 'Purgatives are prohibited in case of diarrhoea due to Cold, in case of Cold invasion with a superficial pulse, in case of deficiency of both the Exterior and the Interior and in case of cyanosis of the lips and cold limbs.'
— In his book *Insight into Medicine*, Cheng Zhongling points out, 'Constipation can be the result of dryness of Blood in old age, exhaustion of Blood following childbirth, consumption of Body Fluids and Blood due to prolonged illness.... Pathological conditions will deteriorate if purgatives are taken carelessly.'

D. A COMPARISON OF COMMONLY USED PURGATIVE FORMULAE (TABLE 28.1)

1. – *Da Cheng Qi Tang*
   Major Order the Qi Decoction

- *Xiao Cheng Qi Tang*
  Minor Order the Qi Decoction
- *Tiao Wei Cheng Qi Tang*
  Regulate the Stomach and Order the Qi Decoction

— These are known as **Three Purgative Decoctions**. All of them use Radix et Rhizoma Rhei to dispel accumulated Heat in the gastrointestinal tract and all are thus indicated for Yang Ming Fu patterns of Full Heat.
— In preparing **Major Order the Qi Decoction**, the herbs are cooked for a short time and Radix et Rhizoma Rhei and Natrii Sulfas are added toward the end of the cooking time. Fructus Aurantii Immaturus and Cortex Magnoliae Officinalis are used in large doses. These factors make this formula a powerful purgative and it is often prescribed in the treatment of severe Yang Ming Heat, characterized by distress, fullness and dryness.
— **Minor Order the Qi Decoction** does not contain Natrii Sulfas, and Radix et Rhizoma Rhei is cooked together with smaller doses of Fructus Aurantii Immaturus and Cortex Magnoliae Officinalis. The formula is thus milder in its action and is used in the treatment of less severe Yang Ming Heat, characterized by distress and fullness without dryness.
— **Regulate the Stomach and Order the Qi Decoction** does not contain Fructus Aurantii Immaturus and Cortex Magnoliae Officinalis. Radix et Rhizoma Rhei and Radix Glycyrrhizae are cooked together and

Table 28.1 Comparison of purgative formulae

Formula	Actions	Indications
Major Order the Qi Decoction	Purges strongly	Yang Ming Heat (severe) with distress, fullness, dryness
Minor Order the Qi Decoction	Purges less strongly	Yang Ming Heat (less severe) with distress and fullness only
Regulate the Stomach and Order the Qi Decoction	Purges mildly	Yang Ming Heat (mild) with no Qi stagnation
Yellow Dragon Decoction	Clears Heat Dispels accumulation Tonifies Qi and Blood	Interior Full Heat complicated with Qi and Blood Deficiency
Increase the Fluids and Order the Qi Decoction	Clears Heat Nourishes Yin and Fluids Relieves constipation	Acute febrile disease or Yang Ming Heat with Yin deficiency

Natrii Sulfas is added later. These factors make this formula even gentler in its action and it is often used in the treatment of mild cases of Yang Ming Heat with no signs of Qi Stagnation.

2. – *Huang Long Tang*
     Yellow Dragon Decoction
   – *Zeng Ye Cheng Qi Tang*
     Increase the Fluids and Order the Qi Decoction

— Both of these formulae combine purgation with tonification and contain Radix et Rhizoma Rhei and Natrii Sulfas. They are indicated for the accumulation of pathogenic factors in the Interior complicated with deficiency of Upright Qi.

— **Yellow Dragon Decoction** combines Natrii Sulfas and Radix et Rhizoma Rhei with Fructus Aurantii Immaturus and Cortex Magnoliae Officinalis in order to clear Heat, relieve constipation and dispel accumulation from the gastrointestinal tract. The formula also contains Radix Ginseng, Radix Glycyrrhizae and Radix Angelicae Sinensis to tonify Qi and Blood. It is thus indicated for Interior Full Heat patterns complicated with deficiency of Qi and Blood, with symptoms of constipation, abdominal distension, fullness and pain, a feverish sensation of the body, thirst, lassitude, a burnt yellow or dark tongue coating and a deficient pulse.

— **Increase the Fluids and Order the Qi Decoction** combines Natrii Sulfas and Radix et Rhizoma Rhei with Radix Scrophulariae, Radix Ophiopogonis and Radix Rehmanniae to nourish Yin, clear Heat, increase Body Fluids and relieve constipation. This formula is thus indicated for acute febrile diseases and Yang Ming Heat with Yin Deficiency, with symptoms of constipation, thirst, dry lips, a dry and burnt yellow tongue coating and a thready and rapid pulse.

Questions

1. What are the indications for purgative formulae?
2. How are cold purgative prescriptions formulated?

29 *Formulae for clearing Heat*

A. GUIDING PRINCIPLES FOR FORMULATING PRESCRIPTIONS TO CLEAR HEAT

1. Formulae for clearing Heat are indicated for Interior Heat patterns caused either by invasion of pathogenic Heat into the Interior or by Empty Heat in the Zang Fu. Symptoms include fever, restlessness, thirst with a preference for cold drinks, flushed face, a red tongue with yellow coating and a surging rapid pulse.
2. These formulae are prescribed when the treatment method consists of clearing Interior Heat.
3. The main ingredients of these formulae are herbs that clear Interior Heat.

B. FORMULATING PRESCRIPTIONS FOR CLEARING HEAT

1. Formulating prescriptions for clearing Qi level Heat

— Qi level Heat is caused by the invasion of pathogenic factors into the Interior, where they then transform to Heat, or by the retention of residual Heat after an illness. The Heat tends to involve the Lungs and Stomach.
— If the pattern is caused by the invasion of pathogenic factors, symptoms will include high fever, restlessness, profuse sweating and a surging and forceful pulse.
— If the pattern is caused by the retention of residual Heat after an illness, symptoms will include restlessness, dry mouth and lips, a red tongue with scanty coating and a deficient pulse.
— Commonly used herbs include Gypsum Fibrosum, Rhizoma Anemarrhenae, Fructus Gardeniae and Herba Lophatheri. Commonly used formulae include:

– *Bai Hu Tang*
White Tiger Decoction
– *Zhi Zi Dou Chi Tang*
Gardenia and Prepared Soybean Decoction

— Since Full Heat consumes Body Fluids, and residual Heat is often accompanied by deficiency of both Qi and Yin, herbs that tonify Qi and nourish Yin should be added. Examples are Radix Ginseng in *Bai Hu Jia Ren Shen Tang* (**White Tiger plus Ginseng Decoction**), and Radix Ginseng and Radix Ophiopogonis in *Zhu Ye Shi Gao Tang* (**Lophatherus and Gypsum Decoction**).
— If Qi level Heat is not resolved it may enter the Blood level, in which case herbs that clear Heat and cool Blood should be added. An example of such a formula is *Hua Ban Tang* (**Decoction for Relieving Feverish Rash**), which contains Cornu Rhinoceri Asiatici and Radix Scrophulariae. The Heat may stir up Liver Wind, in which case herbs should be added that calm the Wind and stop convulsion, as in *Ling Ma Bai Hu Tang* (**White Tiger Decoction with Antelopis and Gastrodia**), which contains Cornu Antelopis and Rhizoma Gastrodiae.
— Qi level Heat may also be complicated with pathogenic Dampness, in which case herbs that clear Heat and resolve Dampness should be added, as in *Bai Hu Jia Cang Zhu Tang* (**White Tiger Decoction with Atractylodis**), which contains Rhizoma Atractylodis. If Qi level Heat is complicated with Yang Ming Fu syndrome, herbs that purge Heat and relieve constipation should be added, as in *Bai Hu Cheng Qi Tang* (**White Tiger Decoction for Ordering the Qi**), which contains Radix et Rhizoma Rhei and Natrii Sulfas.

2. Formulating prescriptions for clearing Nutritive level Heat and cooling Blood

— These formulae consist primarily of herbs that clear Nutritive level Heat and cool Blood. They are indicated for invasion of the Nutritive and Blood levels by pathogenic Heat.

— Heat at the Nutritive level is a further development of Heat at the Qi level and is the beginning of the pattern of Heat at the Blood level. Nutritive Qi communicates with the Heart and pathological changes at the Nutritive level are characterized by consumption of Yin and disturbance of the Heart and Mind. The symptoms of Heat at the Nutritive level include a feverish sensation which is worse at night, delirium, indistinct skin eruptions, a deep-red dry tongue and a thready and rapid pulse. Once the pathogen has entered the Nutritive level, it may return to the Qi level or travel deeper to invade the Pericardium or stir up Liver Wind. Formulae for clearing Nutritive level Heat consist of:

  – salty and cold herbs that clear Nutritive level Heat and cool Blood, such as Cornu Rhinoceri Asiatici, Radix Scrophulariae and Radix Rehmanniae

  and

  – bitter and cold herbs that clear Heat, such as Radix Scutellariae, Rhizoma Coptidis and Fructus Gardeniae

  and

  – sweet and cold herbs that nourish Yin, such as Radix Ophiopogonis and Herba Dendrobii

  or

  – herbs that clear Nutritive level Heat through the Qi level, such as Flos Lonicerae, Fructus Forsythiae and Herba Lophatheri

  or

  – herbs that cool and activate Blood such as Radix Salviae Miltiorrhizae and Radix Paeoniae Rubra.

— The representative formula for this pattern is *Qing Ying Tang* (**Clear the Nutritive Level Decoction**).

— If pathogenic Heat at the Nutritive level goes deeper and results in delirium, or if it damages the Yin and stirs up Liver Wind, causing convulsions, the formula should be augmented with:

  – Rhizoma Acori Graminei and Radix Curcumae

  or

  – Cornu Antelopis and Ramulus Uncariae cum Uncis

  or

  – **Purple Snow Special Pill** (*Zi Xue Dan*) and **Calm the Palace Pill with Cattle Gallstone** (*An Gong Niu Huang Wan*).

3. Formulating prescriptions for clearing Heat and Fire Poison

— Formulae for clearing Heat and Fire Poison consist primarily of herbs that clear Heat and Fire Poison. They clear Heat and Fire Poison, purge Fire and treat skin ulcers and are thus indicated for severe deep-rooted Fire Poison such as infectious epidemic diseases, acute febrile diseases, and ulcers, boils and furuncles.

— Their main ingredients include Radix Scutellariae, Rhizoma Coptidis, Cortex Phellodendri, Fructus Gardeniae, Flos Lonicerae, Fructus Forsythiae, Radix Isatidis and Herba Andrographitis (*Chuan Xin Lian*).

— Other herbs should be added according to the areas affected by Fire Poison and other clinical manifestations.

— If the Fire Poison invades the Triple Burner, with symptoms of a feverish sensation of the body, restlessness, irritability, haemoptysis, epistaxis or skin eruptions, the method of clearing Heat and purging Fire should be followed by combining bitter and cold herbs such as Radix Scutellariae, Rhizoma Coptidis and Cortex Phellodendri with Fructus Gardeniae and Radix et Rhizoma Rhei. The representative formula is *Huang Lian Jie Du Tang* (**Coptis Decoction to Relieve Toxicity**).

— If Fire Poison is retained in the head and face, presenting with redness, swelling and a hot sensation of the head and face, red eyes, mouth ulcers and a painful swollen throat, the method of clearing is combined with the method of dispersing. This is done by prescribing:

  – herbs that purge Fire and clear Fire Poison in the Upper Burner, such as Radix Scutellariae, Rhizoma Coptidis, Radix Scrophulariae, Lasiosphaera seu Calvatia (*Ma Bo*), Fructus Forsythiae and Radix Isatidis *and*

- pungent and cool herbs that clear and disperse Heat, such as Fructus Arctii, Bombyx Batryticatus and Herba Menthae.

— The representative formula is *Pu Ji Xiao Du Yin* (**Universal Benefit Decoction to Eliminate Toxin**).

— If the Fire Poison moves to the pubic region or if Blood Stasis and Heat combine in the lower limbs, presenting with large carbuncles in the pubic region and gangrene of the toes, herbs that clear Heat are combined with:

- herbs that drain Dampness through the urine, such as Semen Plantaginis, Caulis Akebiae and Rhizoma Alismatis
and/or
- herbs that nourish and activate Blood such as Radix Angelicae Sinensis and Radix Salviae Miltiorrhizae.

— The representative formulae are *Long Dan Xie Gan Tang* (**Gentiana Draining the Liver Decoction**) for scrotal abscess and swelling of lymph nodes in the groin due to venereal disease and *Si Miao Yong An Tang* (**Four-Valiant Decoction for Well-being**) for gangrene of the toes.

— If Fire Poison is retained in the vessels and muscles, forming boils, ulcers and furuncles, herbs that clear Fire Poison and treat suppurating skin conditions, such as Flos Lonicerae, Fructus Forsythiae, Herba Taraxaci, Herba Violae and Flos Chrysanthemi are used. These are combined with herbs that activate Blood, relieve swelling and soften hard masses, such as the tail of Radix Angelicae Sinensis, Resina Olibani, Resina Myrrhae, Squama Manitis, Spina Gleditsiae and Bulbus Fritillariae.

— The representative formulae are *Wu Wei Xiao Du Yin* (**Five-Ingredient Decoction to Eliminate Toxin**) and *Xian Fang Huo Ming Yin* (**Sublime Formula for Sustaining Life**).

4. Formulating prescriptions for clearing Heat in the organs

— Each of the Zang Fu has its own physiological functions, channel and location and its own symptoms and signs of disease. Patterns of disease may involve a single organ or two or more organs simultaneously. Formulae for clearing Heat in the organs are prescribed according to the functions of the affected organs, their related channels, related organs and the actions of individual herbs.

— For example, before formulae for clearing Heat in the Heart are prescribed it must be known that the Heart houses the Mind, dominates the blood vessels, opens into the tongue, is externally – internally related to the Small Intestine and has a Fire–Water relationship to the Kidneys. It must also be known that Heart Fire can disturb the Mind, damage the Blood, cause Blood Stasis and move upward to affect the tongue or downward to affect the Small Intestine. Symptoms of Heart Fire can thus include a heat sensation in the heart and chest, restlessness, tongue ulcers, scanty deep-yellow urine, insomnia, haemorrhage and suppurating skin conditions.

— The herbs used to treat such a pattern include:

- bitter and cold herbs that enter the Heart channel and clear Heat, such as Rhizoma Coptidis and Fructus Gardeniae
- herbs that nourish Yin and Blood, such as Radix Rehmanniae, Radix Scrophulariae and Colla Corii Asini
- herbs that clear Heat through the urine, such as Herba Lophatheri, Caulis Akebiae and Semen Plantaginis
- herbs that clear Heat in the Heart and calm the Mind such as Cinnabaris and Succinum
- herbs that cool Blood and stop bleeding such as Rhizoma Imperatae and Herba Cephalanoploris.

— The representative formulae are *Dao Chi San* (**Eliminating Redness Powder**) and *Xie Xin Tang* (**Drain the Epigastrium Decoction**).

— Before prescribing formulae for clearing Liver Heat it must be understood that the Liver stores Blood, promotes the free flow of Qi, opens into the eyes, is externally – internally related to the Gall Bladder, has a Wood – Earth relationship with the Spleen and has a common origin with the Kidney; and that the Liver channel encircles the pubic region, passes through the hypochondrium, links with the eye system and reaches the vertex. It must also be understood that excessive Heat in the Liver channel can damage Liver Blood, impair the function of promoting the free flow of Qi, affect the Gall Bladder, disturb the head and eyes, invade the Spleen and Stomach and consume Kidney Yin, producing hypochondriac pain, acid regurgitation, a bitter taste in the mouth, poor appetite, headache, red eyes and turbid vaginal discharge.

— To clear Liver Heat, the primary herbs used are those which clear Heat in the Liver channel, such as Radix Gentianae, Radix Scutellariae, Rhizoma Coptidis, Indigo Naturalis, and Aloe. These are combined with:

 - herbs that nourish Liver Blood such as Radix Angelicae Sinensis, Radix Paeoniae Alba and Radix Rehmanniae

 or

 - herbs that clear Damp-Heat such as Caulis Akebiae, Rhizoma Alismatis and Semen Plantaginis

 or

 - herbs that harmonize the Liver and disperse Fire such as Radix Bupleuri and Radix Ledebouriellae.

— The representative formulae are *Long Dan Xie Gan Tang* (**Gentiana Draining the Liver Decoction**), *Zuo Jin Wan* (**Left Metal Pill**), and *Dang Gui Long Hui Wan* (**Dang Gui, Gentian and Aloe Pill**).

C. POINTS TO REMEMBER IN FORMULATING PRESCRIPTIONS FOR CLEARING HEAT

1. Interior Heat patterns may be patterns of Excess or Deficiency.
— Patterns of Excess are characterized by abrupt onset, short duration, severe symptoms and rapid pathological changes. They tend to consume Qi and Body Fluids and can cause the Blood to move recklessly. The main clinical manifestations include high fever, restlessness, flushed face, yellow urine, dry stool, a rapid and forceful pulse and a red tongue with yellow coating or thorns. In severe cases, there may be convulsions, mania and haemorrhage. The correct treatment method is clearing Heat.
— Patterns of Deficiency are characterized by slow onset, long duration, slow pathological changes, Yin Deficiency and excess of Yang. The primary treatment method is that of nourishing Yin with sweet and cold herbs;

the secondary treatment method is clearing Heat with cold and cool herbs.
— Patterns of Interior Heat may involve the Qi, Blood, Zang and/or Fu; clinical manifestations will vary according to the location of the disease and the method of treatment must be adapted accordingly.
— The severity of the pattern also determines which herbs are selected. Severe Interior Heat will not improve if only mild herbs are used. Conversely, if strong herbs are used to treat mild Interior Heat patterns, patterns of Cold will be created.
— The constitution of the patient is another relevant factor in the selection of herbs. Strong herbs should be used if the patient has a strong constitution and Interior Full Heat; even if the action of the herbs is too strong, it will not cause serious problems. However, if the patient has a weak constitution (e.g. women in the postpartum period), cold and cool herbs should not be prescribed in large doses even if there is high fever. In these cases, the Heat should be cleared gradually to avoid the situation wherein 'Heat is not cleared, but internal Cold is produced'.
2. Therapeutic results are also related to dosage and the method of decoction and administration. For example, Gypsum Fibrosum is a mineral and its active ingredients are not easily extracted by cooking. It is therefore often prescribed in large doses and decocted for a long time before adding other herbs.
— Flos Lonicerae and Herba Houttuyniae should not be decocted for a long time as this disperses their active ingredients.
— Extremely bitter and cold herbs such as Radix Scutellariae, Rhizoma Coptidis, Cortex Phellodendri and Radix Gentianae can easily damage the Stomach and Spleen. They should therefore not be prescribed in large doses, nor taken for a long time.
— Radix Rehmanniae is cold, nourishing and sticky in nature and when taken in large doses for a long time may impair the function of the Spleen and Stomach.
3. Formulae for clearing Heat are contraindicated in cases of persisting Exterior patterns, deficiency of the Spleen and Stomach with stagnation of Cold, Yang Deficiency with fever, and patterns of True Cold and False Heat.
— Patterns of Deficient Fire are treated by

tonification rather than clearing. For example, Empty Fire due to Kidney Yin Deficiency is treated by strengthening Water to control Fire. Floating Yang due to Kidney Yang Deficiency is treated by returning the Fire to its origin.

— In these cases, the method of clearing Heat would aggravate the pathological condition.

D. A COMPARISON OF FORMULAE FOR CLEARING HEAT (TABLE 29.1)

1. – *Bai Hu Tang*
   White Tiger Decoction
   – *Zhu Ye Shi Gao Tang*
   Lophatherus and Gypsum Decoction

— **Lophatherus and Gypsum Decoction** is **White Tiger Decoction** with Rhizoma Anemarrhenae removed and Radix Ginseng, Rhizoma Pinelliae, Radix Ophiopogonis and Herba Lophatherus added. Both formulae clear Heat and promote Body Fluids and are indicated for Qi level Heat.

— **White Tiger Decoction** is more powerful in clearing Heat and promoting Body Fluids and is thus indicated for Yang Ming Heat or patterns of Qi level Full Heat. Typical symptoms include high fever, profuse sweating, restlessness, severe thirst and a large and surging pulse.

— **Lophatherus and Gypsum Decoction** clears Heat more gently, but also nourishes Qi and Yin, harmonizes the Stomach and stops vomiting. It is thus indicated for the late stage of febrile disease marked by damage to Qi and Body Fluids and retention of residual Heat. Typical symptoms include a feverish sensation, profuse sweating, restlessness, thirst with desire to drink, a red tongue with scanty coating and a thready and rapid pulse.

— **White Tiger Decoction** is an extremely cold formula used in the treatment of severe Full Heat patterns. **Lophatherus and Gypsum Decoction** clears Heat but tonifies at the same time and is used in the aftermath of febrile disease to clear Heat from Deficiency.

2. – *Qing Ying Tang*
   Clear the Nutritive level Decoction
   – *Xi Jiao Di Huang Tang*
   Rhinoceros Horn and Rehmannia Decoction

Table 29.1 Comparison of Formulae for clearing heat

Formula	Actions	Indications
White Tiger Decoction	Strongly clears Heat Promotes Body Fluids	Yang Ming Heat Qi level Full Heat
Lophatherus and Gypsum Decoction	Clears Heat more gently Nourishes Qi and Yin Harmonizes the Stomach	Late stage febrile disease with residual Heat and damage to Fluids
Rhinoceros Horn and Rehmannia Decoction	Clears Heat from Nutritive and Blood levels Stops bleeding Resolves Stasis	Blood level Heat
Clear the Nutritive Level Decoction	Clears Heat from Nutritive and Blood levels Clears Qi level Heat Nourishes Yin	Nutritive level Heat
Clearing the Stomach Powder	Clears Stomach Fire Cools Blood	Stomach Fire
Jade Woman Decoction	Clears Stomach Heat Nourishes Yin	Stomach Heat complicated with Yin Deficiency
Expelling Whiteness Powder	Clears Lung Heat Nourishes the Stomach	Lung Heat which has damaged Yin, but Fire not severe
Reed Decoction	Clears Lung Heat Dispels Blood Stasis and pus	Lung abscess due to retention of stagnant Blood and Heat

— These are the representative formulae for clearing Nutritive level Heat and cooling Blood. Both contain Cornu Rhinoceri and Radix Rehmanniae to clear Heat from the Heart, clear Fire Poison, cool Blood and nourish Yin. Both are indicated for Heat at the Nutritive and Blood levels, with symptoms of fever which is more pronounced at night, mild thirst, restlessness, insomnia, delirium, a deep-red tongue and a rapid pulse.

— **Rhinoceros Horn and Rehmannia Decoction** consists of herbs that act only on the Blood level such as Cornu Rhinoceri, Radix Rehmanniae, Radix Paeoniae and Cortex Moutan Radicis. It is thus more effective in cooling Blood and stopping bleeding; it also resolves Blood Stasis. It is indicated for Blood level Heat with symptoms of haemoptysis, haematemesis, epistaxis, haematuria, bloody stools, dark-purple ecchymoses and petechiae and a deep-red or purple tongue.

— In addition to Cornu Rhinoceri and Radix Rehmanniae, **Clear the Nutritive Level Decoction** also contains Radix Salviae Miltiorrhizae, Radix Scrophulariae, Radix Ophiopogonis, Rhizoma Coptidis, Herba Lophatheri, Flos Lonicerae and Fructus Forsythiae. Because it contains herbs that clear Qi level Heat as well as herbs that clear Heat from the Nutritive and Blood levels, this formula is more effective in clearing Heat from the Nutritive level via the Qi level, and nourishing Yin. It is thus indicated for Heat at the Nutritive level, with symptoms of fever which is more pronounced at night, restlessness, insomnia, possible delirium and an indistinct skin rash, a deep-red dry tongue and a thready and rapid pulse.

3. – *Qing Wei San*
   Clearing the Stomach Powder
   – *Yu Nu Jian*
   Jade Woman Decoction

— **Clearing the Stomach Powder** consists of Radix Angelicae Sinensis, Rhizoma Coptidis, Radix Rehmanniae, Cortex Moutan Radicis and Rhizoma Cimicifugae. **Jade Women Decoction** consists of Gypsum Fibrosum, Radix Rehmanniae Praeparata, Radix Ophiopogonis, Rhizoma Anemarrhenae and Radix Achyranthis Bidentatae.

— Although the two formulae have different ingredients, both clear Stomach Heat. **Clearing the Stomach Powder** clears Stomach Fire and cools Blood and is thus indicated for toothache due to Stomach Fire and bleeding gums due to Heat damaging the blood vessels. **Jade Woman Decoction** clears Stomach Heat and nourishes Yin and is thus indicated for toothache, epistaxis, restlessness and thirst due to Stomach Heat complicated with Yin Deficiency.

4. – *Xie Bai San*
   Expelling Whiteness Powder
   – *Wei Jing Tang*
   Reed Decoction

— **Expelling Whiteness Powder** consists of Cortex Lycii Radicis, Cortex Mori Radicis, Radix Glycyrrhizae and non-glutinous rice. **Reed Decoction** consists of Rhizoma Phragmitis, Semen Coicis, Semen Benincasae and Semen Persicae. Both formulae clear Lung Heat and stop cough and are thus indicated for cough and dyspnoea due to Lung Heat.

— **Expelling Whiteness Powder** clears Heat as its primary function and nourishes the Stomach as a secondary function, in accordance with the concept of nourishing the Earth to strengthen Metal. It is indicated when Lung Heat has damaged the Yin, and when Qi fails to descend properly, but Upright Qi is not severely damaged and Fire is not severe.

— **Reed Decoction** not only clears Lung Heat but also dispels Blood Stasis and pus and is thus indicated for lung abscess formed by retention of stagnant Blood and Heat in the Lung, with symptoms of chest pain, foul sputum or spitting of purulent blood.

— Both formulae treat patterns involving pathogenic Heat, but **Expelling Whiteness Powder** is prescribed where there is a deficiency of Upright Qi, while **Reed Decoction** is prescribed when the patient's constitution is strong.

Questions

1. Compare and contrast formulae for clearing Heat at the Qi level and formulae for clearing Heat at the Blood level.
2. What are the guidelines for prescribing formulae for clearing Heat?

30 *Formulae for warming the Interior*

A. GUIDING PRINCIPLES FOR FORMULATING PRESCRIPTIONS TO WARM THE INTERIOR

1. Warming formulae are used to treat patterns of Interior Cold. Clinical manifestations of such patterns include absence of thirst or a preference for hot drinks, cold limbs, copious clear urine, loose stools, a deep and slow pulse and a pale tongue with a moist coating.
2. The treatment method is warming the Interior and dispersing Cold.
3. These formulae consist primarily of herbs that warm the Kidneys and Spleen and disperse internal Cold.

B. FORMULATING PRESCRIPTIONS TO WARM THE INTERIOR

1. Formulating prescriptions to warm the Middle Burner and disperse Cold

— These formulae warm and tonify the Spleen and Stomach and disperse Cold from the Middle Burner. They are indicated for deficiency of the Middle Burner with stagnation of Cold.
— If the Spleen and Stomach are constitutionally deficient and cold, or they are invaded by External Cold, or if the Yang of the Middle Burner is damaged by cold and raw food or incorrect herbal treatment, the Spleen's functions of transformation and transportation will be impaired and stagnation of Cold will occur. Clinical manifestations will include pain and a cold sensation in the epigastrium and abdomen, vomiting, diarrhoea, gustatory impairment, absence of thirst, cold limbs and a pale tongue with a moist white coating.
— To treat such patterns, the primary herbs are those that warm and invigorate the Middle Burner, such as Rhizoma Zingiberis, Rhizoma Alpiniae Officinalis, Fructus Evodiae, Pericarpium Zanthoxyli and Fructus Piperis Longi.
— However, Cold tends to damage Yang Qi, and deficiency of the Spleen and Stomach with stagnation of Cold may lead to Kidney Yang Deficiency, Blood Deficiency, Qi Stagnation and the production of internal Cold-Damp, and these complications must also be addressed.
— For Spleen and Stomach Qi Deficiency with symptoms of shortness of breath, lassitude, weak voice and a soft and weak pulse, Radix Ginseng, Radix Astragali seu Hedysari, Radix Codonopsis Pilosulae, Rhizoma Atractylodis Macrocephalae and treated Radix Glycyrrhizae are added to provide both warmth and tonification. Representative formulae include *Li Zhong Wan* (**Regulating the Middle Decoction**), *Wu Zhu Yu Tang* (**Evodia Decoction**) and *Da Jian Zhong Tang* (**Major Strengthening the Middle Decoction**).
— For Kidney Yang Deficiency with symptoms of aversion to cold, cold limbs and more severe diarrhoea, add Radix Aconiti Praeparata and Cortex Cinnamomi to invigorate the Spleen and Stomach. The representative formula is *Fu Zi Li Zhong Wan* (**Prepared Aconite Pill to Regulate the Middle**).
— For Blood Deficiency with symptoms of lingering abdominal pain, pale complexion, palpitations, restlessness and a thready and wiry pulse, add Saccharum Granorum, Radix Angelicae Sinensis, Radix Paeoniae Alba and Radix Rehmanniae Praeparata to warm the Middle Burner, harmonize Nutritive Qi and moderate acute pain. The representative formulae include *Xiao Jian Zhong Tang* (**Minor Strengthening the Middle Decoction**) and *Dang Gui Jian Zhong*

Tang (**Angelica Strengthening the Middle Decoction**).

— For obstruction of the Middle Burner by Cold Damp with symptoms of distension, fullness, epigastric and abdominal pain, loose stools or constipation and a white sticky tongue coating, add Cortex Magnoliae Officinalis, Pericarpium Citri Reticulatae, Semen Alpiniae Katsumadai, Fructus Tsaoko and Rhizoma Cyperi to warm the Middle Burner, disperse Cold, circulate Qi and resolve Dampness. The representative formula is *Hou Po Wen Zhong Tang* (**Magnolia Bark Decoction for Warming the Middle**).

2. Formulating prescriptions for restoring Collapsed Yang

— These formulae warm and tonify Heart, Spleen and Kidney Yang. They treat Collapse of Yang and thus deal with the decline of Yang Qi, retention of Cold in the Interior and patterns of False Heat above and True Cold below.

— Critical symptoms include cold limbs, aversion to cold, lying with the body curled up, diarrhoea with undigested food, feeble breathing, a pale tongue with white coating and a deep, feeble and fading pulse.

— This pattern may appear as the result of incorrect treatment, prolonged illness, or acute illness which damages Heart and Kidney Yang, producing Interior Cold. It is treated with strong pungent and hot herbs such as Radix Aconiti Praeparata, Rhizoma Zingiberis and Cortex Cinnamomi, to restore Collapsed Yang.

— However, Yang Deficiency rarely appears without complications and these must be addressed as well.

— Yang and Qi are closely related and deficiency of Yang inevitably involves Qi Deficiency. Severe Yang Deficiency also produces Internal Cold, or a pattern of True Cold and False Heat. Severe deficiency of Heart and Kidney Yang gives rise to related pathological patterns such as:

- leakage of Heart fluid, which causes profuse sweating
- stagnation of Blood with symptoms of painful limbs and cyanosis
- cold Water in the Interior with symptoms of oedema, palpitations, dizziness and vertigo

and
- inability of the Kidneys to receive Qi, with symptoms of dyspnoea and stuffiness of the chest.

— The core formula of Radix Aconiti Praeparata and Rhizoma Zingiberis must therefore be augmented with other herbs which address the actual combination of pathologies in the individual patient.

— For example, to restore Yang and at the same time benefit Qi, herbs such as Radix Ginseng, Radix Astragali seu Hedysari, Rhizoma Atractylodis and treated Radix Glycyrrhizae should be added. Representative formulae include *Si Ni Tang* (**Four-Rebellious Decoction**), *Si Ni Jia Ren Shen Tang* (**Four-Rebellious Decoction with Ginseng**) and *Shen Fu Tang* (**Panax–Aconitum Decoction**).

— For severe Internal Cold with exhaustion of Yang Qi, manifesting as Yin walling off Yang, or True Cold and False Heat, the three basic warming herbs should be prescribed in large doses and combined with Radix Ginseng, Rhizoma Atractylodis Macrocephalae, treated Radix Glycyrrhizae, Fructus Schisandrae and Moschus to restore Collapsed Yang, tonify Qi and restore the pulse. Representative formulae include *Tong Yang Si Ni Tang* (**Unblock the Yang Four-Rebellious Decoction**) and *Si Ni Jiu Ji Tang* (**Four-Rebellious Restore Collapsed Yang Decoction**).

— For Collapse of Yang with profuse sweating, add calcined Os Draconis, calcined Concha Ostreae, Fructus Corni, Radix Rehmanniae Praeparata and Radix Paeoniae Alba to stop the sweating, restore the Yang and benefit Yin. The representative formula is *Shen Fu Long Mu Tang* (**Panax–Aconitum Decoction with *Long Mu* and *Mu Li***).

— For stagnation of Blood, add Semen Persicae and Flos Carthami to warm the Yang and activate the Blood. The representative formula is *Hui Yang Jiu Ji Tang* (**Restore Collapsed Yang Decoction**).

— For retention of Internal Water and Dampness with symptoms of dysuria and oedema of the body and limbs, add Poria and Rhizoma Atractylodis Macrocephalae to warm the Yang and drain Water. Representative formulae include *Zhen Wu Tang* (**True Warrior Decoction**) and **Restore Collapsed Yang Decoction**.

3. Formulating prescriptions for warming the channels and dispersing Cold

— These formulae warm the channels, remove obstruction from the collaterals, disperse Cold and relieve stagnation. They are indicated for Yang Deficiency and invasion of the channels and collaterals by Cold.
— When Yang and Blood are deficient, Blood may stagnate and the channels and collaterals are vulnerable to invasion by pathogenic Cold. If this occurs, the Blood cannot circulate freely and Yang Qi cannot reach the four limbs. This produces symptoms such as cold limbs, painful joints and a purplish-blue skin tone.
— Retention of Cold-Phlegm in the muscles, tendons and bones produces generalized swelling with more soreness than pain and absence of discoloration.
— In either case, the treatment method is to warm the channels, disperse Cold, nourish the Blood and remove obstruction from the vessels with two main groups of herbs:

  – Ramulus Cinnamomi, Herba Asari, and Herba Ephedrae
  and
  – Radix Angelicae Sinensis, Radix Paeoniae Alba, Radix Rehmanniae Praeparata and Colla Cornus Cervi.

— Other herbs must then be added according to the pattern of the individual patient.
— For example, for severe blockage of channels and collaterals with symptoms of cold limbs, localized purplish-blue discoloration and numbness and pain in the lower back, hips and feet, add Medulla Tetrapanacis and Caulis Spatholobi to assist in removing obstruction from the vessels. The representative formula is *Dang Gui Si Ni Tang* (**Angelica Four-Rebellious Decoction**).
— For chronic Internal Cold complicated with upward Rebellion of Qi, add Fructus Evodiae and Rhizoma Zingiberis Recens to assist in warming the Middle Burner, dispersing Cold and conducting Rebellious Qi downward to stop vomiting. The representative formula is *Dang Gui Si Ni Jia Wu Zhu Yu Sheng Jiang Tang* (**Angelica Four-Rebellious Decoction with Evodia and Ginger**).
— For Cold-Phlegm in the muscles, tendons, bones and joints, add large doses of Radix Rehmanniae Praeparata and Colla Cornus

Cervi, plus smaller doses of baked Rhizoma Zingiberis, Cortex Cinnamomi, Herba Ephedrae and Semen Sinapsis Albae to warm the Yang, tonify Blood, disperse Cold and relieve stagnation. The representative formula is *Yang He Tang* (**Yang-Heartening Decoction**).

C. POINTS TO REMEMBER IN FORMULATING PRESCRIPTIONS FOR WARMING THE INTERIOR

1. Herbs for warming the Interior are all pungent, sweet and warm or extremely hot in nature. They warm the Interior and disperse pathogenic Cold but they also consume Yin and damage Body Fluids. Incorrect application of these formulae may cause side-effects and a correct diagnosis is vital.
— The book *Insight into Medicine* says:

  > For Cold invasion of the body surface in Winter, the method of providing warmth and dispersing Cold is adopted. For Wind invasion of the body in Winter, the method of providing warmth and dispersing Wind is adopted. For retention of Cold Phlegm, the method of providing warmth and resolving Phlegm is adopted. For injury to the Spleen and Stomach by cold food, the method of providing warmth and assisting digestion is adopted. For a weak constitution complicated with stagnation of Cold, the method of providing warmth and tonification is adopted.

— The method of providing warmth and dispersing is not adopted in cases of Yin Deficiency with hyperactive Yang or in Heat patterns with false Cold, as it may stir up Fire and damage Yin, thus aggravating the original condition.
2. Dosage and the method of decoction and administration can modify the therapeutic effects of formulae for warming the Interior. For example, Radix Aconiti Praeparata is toxic and correct dosage is important. To reduce its toxicity it must be decocted for a long time, often before other herbs are added. Overdose or improper preparation may cause poisoning or even death.
— On the other hand, Cortex Cinnamomi, Flos Caryophylli, Fructus Foeniculi and Fructus

Piperis Longi all contain volatile oils and their effects will be reduced if they are decocted at high temperatures or for a long time.

D. COMPARISON OF COMMON FORMULAE FOR WARMING THE INTERIOR (TABLE 30.1)

1. – *Li Zhong Wan*
   Regulating the Middle Pill
   – *Wu Zhu Yu Tang*
   Evodia Decoction
   – *Xiao Jian Zhong Tang*
   Minor Strengthening the Middle Decoction

— All three of these formulae consist of herbs that warm the Interior and tonify Qi. They warm the Middle Burner, eliminate Cold, tonify Qi and invigorate the Spleen and are thus indicated for deficiency of the Middle Burner with stagnation of Cold. Symptoms include abdominal pain, cold limbs, poor appetite, gustatory impairment, absence of thirst, a pale tongue with white coating and a deep and slow pulse.

— The main ingredient of **Regulating the Middle Pill** is Rhizoma Zingiberis, which is combined with Radix Ginseng, Rhizoma Atractylodis Macrocephalae and treated Radix Glycyrrhizae. This formula warms and invigorates Spleen Yang and dries Dampness, which makes it effective in warming the Spleen and stopping diarrhoea. It is indicated for deficiency of the Middle Burner with stagnation of Cold marked by abdominal pain, diarrhoea and poor appetite.

— The main ingredient of **Evodia Decoction** is Fructus Evodiae, which is combined with Radix Ginseng, Fructus Ziziphi Jujubae and a large dose of Rhizoma Zingiberis Recens. This formula disperses Cold, warms the Stomach and conducts Rebellious Qi downward to stop vomiting. It is indicated for deficiency of the Middle Burner with stagnation of Cold marked by vomiting, epigastric pain, acid regurgitation and an empty uncomfortable sensation in the stomach. It is also used to treat Jue Yin headache, retching and spitting of saliva, and for Shao Yin syndrome with vomiting, diarrhoea and cold limbs.

Table 30.1 Comparison of formulae for warming the interior

Formula	Actions	Indications
Regulating the Middle Pill	Warms and invigorates Spleen Yang Dries Damp	Deficiency of Middle Burner with Stagnation of Cold (abdominal pain and diarrhoea)
Evodia Decoction	Disperses Cold Warms the Stomach Regulates Rebellious Qi	Deficiency of Middle Burner with Stagnation of Cold (vomiting, epigastric pain) Jue Yin headache Shao Yin syndrome
Minor Strengthening the Middle Decoction	Harmonizes Yin and Yang Relieves abdominal pain	Deficiency of Middle Burner with Stagnation of Cold (intermittent abdominal pain) Fever due to disharmony of Yin and Yang Palpitations and restlessness due to Qi and Blood Deficiency
True Warrior Decoction	Warms the Interior to eliminate Water and Damp	Spleen and Kidney Yang Deficiency with retention of Water and Damp
Prepared Aconite Decoction	Strongly warms and tonifies to eliminate Cold Damp	Spleen and Kidney Yang Deficiency with retention of Cold Damp
Four-Rebellious Decoction	Restores Devastated Yang	Yang Deficiency (cold limbs)
Angelica Four-Rebellious Decoction	Warms the channels Disperses Cold Nourishes and invigorates Blood	Blood Deficiency and stagnation of Cold in channels and collaterals (cold extremities)

— The main ingredient of **Minor Strengthening the Middle Decoction** is Saccharum, which is combined with Ramulus Cinnamomi, Radix Paeoniae Alba and treated Radix Glycyrrhizae. The combination of Ramulus Cinnamomi and Radix Paeoniae treats disharmony of Yin and Yang while the combination of Radix Paeoniae and Radix Glycyrrhizae relieves abdominal pain. This formula is thus indicated for deficiency of the Middle Burner with stagnation of Cold marked by intermittent abdominal pain. It is also used to treat palpitations and restlessness due to deficiency of both Qi and Blood and for fever due to disharmony of Yin and Yang.

2. – *Zhen Wu Tang*
   True Warrior Decoction
   – *Fu Zi Tang*
   Prepared Aconite Decoction

— Both of these formulae consist of Radix Aconiti Praeparata, Rhizoma Atractylodis Macrocephalae, Poria and Radix Paeoniae Alba. They are effective in warming the Interior, relieving pain and eliminating Dampness and are indicated for Spleen and Kidney Yang Deficiency with retention of Water and Dampness in the Interior.
— **True Warrior Decoction** contains Rhizoma Zingiberis Recens but not Radix Ginseng. It is thus more effective in warming and dispersing to eliminate Water and Dampness and is indicated for Spleen and Kidney Yang Deficiency with retention of Water and Dampness marked by sluggishness and oedema.
— **Prepared Aconite Decoction** contains Radix Ginseng, but not Rhizoma Zingiberis Recens, and double the dosage of Radix Aconiti Praeparata and Rhizoma Atractylodis Macrocephalae. It is thus more effective in warming and tonifying to eliminate Cold Damp and is indicated for Spleen and Kidney Yang Deficiency with retention of Cold Damp marked by body and joint pain.

3. – *Si Ni Tang*
   Four-Rebellious decoction
   – *Dang Gui Si Ni Tang*
   Angelica Four-Rebellious Decoction

— Both of these formulae treat cold limbs, but from different causes.
— **Four-Rebellious Decoction** treats a pattern

in which the four limbs are not warmed and nourished due to the decline of Yang Qi. It uses powerful pungent and hot herbs to restore Collapsed Yang. It is indicated for coldness of the entire limb accompanied by systemic signs of deficiency and Cold.
— **Angelica Four-Rebellious Decoction** treats a pattern in which the limbs are not warmed and nourished due to a deficiency of Yang Qi and deficiency and stagnation of Blood. It uses the method of warming the channels, dispersing Cold, nourishing Blood and removing obstruction from the vessels. This formula is indicated for patterns of Blood Deficiency and stagnation of Cold in the channels and collaterals; the coldness of the limbs is relatively mild and is limited to the areas below the knees and elbows, with possible localized purplish-blue discoloration and a deep thready pulse.

Questions

1. Why do formulae for warming the Middle Burner and eliminating Cold contain Qi tonics such as Radix Ginseng and treated Radix Glycyrrhizae in addition to herbs that eliminate Cold? Give examples.
2. Explain the main principles for formulating prescriptions to restore Collapsed Yang.

Formulae that tonify 31

A. GUIDING PRINCIPLES FOR FORMULATING TONIC PRESCRIPTIONS

1. Tonic formulae are used for Deficiency patterns with symptoms of lassitude, palpitations, shortness of breath, dizziness, blurred vision, a sallow or pale complexion, malar flush, deficiency-type obesity or emaciation, cold limbs, five-palm heat, spontaneous sweating, night sweats, a swollen and delicate or pale tongue and a thready and weak pulse.
2. The treatment method is tonification.
3. These formulae consist primarily of herbs that are sweet and warm, neutral or cold in nature.

B. FORMULATING TONIC PRESCRIPTIONS

1. Formulating prescriptions to tonify Qi

— Formulae to tonify Qi consist mainly of sweet and warm herbs which tonify Qi and strengthen resistance to disease. They are indicated for Spleen and Lung Qi Deficiency.
— Qi Deficiency usually refers to Spleen and Lung Qi Deficiency.
— Spleen Qi Deficiency refers to a dysfunction of transportation and transformation which exhausts the source of Qi and Blood, produces Internal Dampness and causes a sinking of Central Qi.
— The Lungs dominate Qi. Lung Qi Deficiency refers to a dysfunction of dispersing and descending and a weak resistance to external pathogenic factors.
— In treating Dampness due to Spleen Deficiency, herbs that resolve or drain Dampness are included in the formula. Examples are Poria in *Si Jun Zi Tang* (**Four Gentlemen Decoction**) and Semen Coicis in

Shen Ling Bai Zhu San (**Panax–Poria–Atractylodis Powder**).
— For Damp-Phlegm, add herbs that dry Dampness and resolve Phlegm, such as Rhizoma Pinelliae in *Liu Jun Zi Tang* (**Six Gentlemen Decoction**). For Sinking of Central Qi, add herbs that lift the Qi such as Rhizoma Cimicifugae and Radix Bupleuri in *Bu Zhong Yi Qi Tang* (**Tonifying the Middle and Benefiting Qi Decoction**).
— Because Spleen Deficiency includes a weakness of transportation and transformation, herbs that regulate Qi are added to counter the tendency of tonic herbs to produce stagnation. Examples include Fructus Amomi in **Panax–Poria–Atractylodis Powder** and Pericarpium Citri Reticulatae in **Tonifying the Middle and Benefiting Qi Decoction.**
— Herbs that regulate Qi are also added where Qi Stagnation is already evident. An example is the use of Radix Aucklandiae, Fructus Amomi and Pericarpium Citri Reticulatae in *Xiang Sha Liu Jun Zi Tang* (**Six Gentlemen Decoction with Aucklandia and Amomum**).
— If Lung Deficiency is complicated with Yin Deficiency, herbs that nourish Yin and astringe the Lungs are added, such as Radix Ginseng combined with Radix Ophiopogonis and Fructus Schisandrae in *Sheng Mai San* (**Generating the Pulse Powder**), which clears and astringes while tonifying.
— For cough or dyspnoea, or in cases of disharmony between the Lungs and Kidneys, it is necessary to add herbs that tonify the Kidneys, stimulate the reception of Qi and stop cough and wheeze. Examples are Semen Armeniacae Amarum, Gecko, Bulbus Fritillariae and Cortex Mori Radicis in *Ren Shen Ge Jie San* (**Ginseng and Gecko Powder**).

2. Formulating prescriptions to tonify Blood

— Blood tonic formulae consist primarily of herbs that tonify and nourish Blood but must be adapted according to the actual condition of the patient.

— When there is a deficiency of Heart Blood, the Heart and Mind are deprived of nourishment, producing symptoms of palpitations, insomnia, poor memory and a thready and weak pulse. Herbs that nourish the Heart and calm the Mind must be included in the formula. An example is *Gui Pi Tang* (**Tonifying the Spleen Decoction**), which contains Radix Angelicae Sinensis and Arillus Longan to tonify Blood and nourish the Heart and Semen Ziziphi Spinosae, Poria cum Ligno Hospite and Radix Polygalae to soothe the Heart and calm the Mind.

— For deficiency of Heart Qi with symptoms of an intermittent pulse and palpitations, the method of treatment is primarily to tonify Blood and nourish the Heart and secondarily to tonify Qi and restore the pulse. The representative formula is *Zhi Gan Cao Tang* (**Glycyrrhiza Decoction**), which combines Radix Rehmanniae, Colla Corii Asini, Radix Ophiopogonis, treated Radix Glycyrrhizae, Radix Ginseng and Fructus Ziziphi Jujubae to tonify both Qi and Blood.

— When there is a deficiency of Liver Blood, the Liver's function of promoting the free flow of Qi and Blood is impaired and the eyes are deprived of nourishment. This produces symptoms of hypochondriac pain, blurred vision, dry eyes and a scanty and pale menstrual flow. Because the circulation of Blood is impaired, formulae to tonify Blood often include herbs that regulate Blood. The representative formula is *Si Wu Tang* (**Four-Substance Decoction**), which contains Radix Angelicae Sinensis, Radix Rehmanniae Praeparata and Radix Paeoniae Alba to tonify Blood and nourish the Liver, and Rhizoma Ligustici Chuanxiong to activate the Blood and resolve stagnation. Because this formula tonifies without causing stagnation, it is much used for tonifying Blood and regulating menstruation.

— If the Spleen is deficient, the source of Qi and Blood will be exhausted. Formulae for tonifying Blood therefore often include herbs that tonify Qi and these are sometimes used in large doses, as in *Dang Gui Bu Xue Tang* (**Angelica Decoction to Tonify the Blood**), which contains five times as much Radix Astragali seu Hedysari as Radix Angelicae Sinensis. When Qi flourishes, it produces sufficient Blood.

3. Formulating prescriptions to tonify Yin

— Yin Deficiency can refer either to deficiency of Liver and Kidney Yin or deficiency of Lung and Stomach Yin.

— Deficiency of Lung and Stomach Yin implies a deficiency of Body Fluids, manifesting as thirst and shortness of breath. Deficiency of Liver and Kidney Yin implies a deficiency of Blood, manifesting as dizziness, blurred vision and tinnitus.

— Lung Yin Deficiency can also produce dry cough and a dry sore throat. Stomach Yin Deficiency can manifest as spitting of white sticky foam. Liver Yin Deficiency often produces hypochondriac discomfort, restlessness and irritability. Kidney Yin Deficiency often results in sore and weak lower back and knees, nocturnal emissions and cloudy urine.

— All Yin tonics tonify Yin, but some are more effective in tonifying the Yin of the Lung and Stomach while others are more effective in tonifying the Yin of the Liver and Kidneys.

— Herbs that are more effective in tonifying Lung and Stomach Yin include Radix Adenophorae, Radix Glehniae, Radix Ophiopogonis, Bulbus Lilii, Herba Dendrobii and Rhizoma Polygonati Odorati. These are combined with other herbs according to the actual condition of the patient.

— For example, deficiency of Lung Yin may produce Empty Heat, which damages blood vessels and gives rise to cough, wheeze, blood-tinged sputum, a thready and rapid pulse and a red tongue with scanty coating. In this case, herbs that clear Lung Heat, stop bleeding, resolve Phlegm and stop cough are added to the formula, such as Colla Corii Asini combined with Fructus Aristolochiae, Fructus Arctii and Semen Armeniacae Amarum in *Bu Fei E Jiao Tang* (**Tonifying the Lung Decoction with Ass-Hide Gelatin**).

— In treating Kidney Yin Deficiency with symptoms of dry sore throat and tidal fever, it is necessary to tonify the Yin of both the Lungs and Kidneys. An example is *Bai He*

Gu Jin Tang (**Lily Bulb Decoction to Preserve the Metal**), which contains:

- Bulbus Lilii, Radix Ophiopogonis, Radix Rehmanniae, Radix Rehmanniae Praeparata and Radix Scrophulariae to tonify Lung and Kidney Yin
- Radix Angelicae and Radix Paeoniae Alba to nourish Blood

and

- Radix Platycodi and Bulbus Fritillariae Thunbergii to clear Lung Heat, resolve Phlegm and stop cough.

— If Lung and Kidney Yin Deficiency is complicated with Fire Poison, giving symptoms of a red, swollen sore throat or a white coating on the throat, herbs that clear Heat and Fire Poison are added. An example is *Yang Yin Qing Fei Tang* (**Nourish the Yin and Clear the Lungs Decoction**), which combines Radix Rehmanniae, Radix Scrophulariae and Radix Ophiopogonis with Herba Menthae, Cortex Moutan Radicis and Radix Glycyrrhizae. In severe cases, Radix Scutellariae and Fructus Forsythiae may be added.

— Simple deficiency of Stomach Yin may be treated either with *Yi Wei Tang* (**Benefiting the Stomach Decoction**), which consists of Radix Adenophorae, Radix Ophiopogonis, Rhizoma Polygonati Odorati, Radix Rehmanniae and crystalized brown sugar (*Bing Tang*), or with *Wu Zhi Yin* (**Five-Juice Decoction**), which consists of pear juice, lotus root, Radix Ophiopogonis, water-chestnut and Rhizoma Phragmitis.

— If deficiency of Stomach Yin is complicated with Qi Deficiency and Heat, herbs that tonify Qi and clear Heat are added. An example is the combination of Herba Dendrobii and Radix Ophiopogonis with Radix Panacis Qinquefolii, Rhizoma Coptidis, Herba Lophatheri, Rhizoma Anemarrhenae and watermelon peel in *Qing Shu Yi Qi Tang* (**Clear Summer Heat and Augment the Qi Decoction**).

— Herbs that are more effective in tonifying Liver and Kidney Yin include Radix Rehmanniae, Radix Rehmanniae Praeparata, Plastrum Testudinis, Carapax Trionycis, Fructus Ligustri Lucidi and Fructus Corni. These are combined with other herbs according to the condition of the patient.

— For Liver or Kidney Yin Deficiency complicated with Liver Qi Stagnation or Liver Yang Rising, with symptoms of pain in the chest, epigastrium and hypochondrium, acid regurgitation, a bitter taste in the mouth and a deficient wiry pulse, herbs that harmonize the Liver and regulate Qi should be added. An example is *Yi Guan Yin* (**Linking Decoction**), in which a large dose of Radix Rehmanniae is combined with Radix Glehniae, Radix Ophiopogonis, Radix Angelicae Sinensis, Fructus Lycii and Fructus Meliae Toosendan.

— For Yin Deficiency with hyperactive Yang, producing symptoms of dizziness and blurred vision, the method of nourishing Yin is combined with the method of suppressing Yang. An example is *Zhen Gan Xi Feng Tang* (**Pacifying the Liver and Subduing Wind Decoction**), which employs Plastrum Testudinis, Radix Scrophulariae, Radix Asparagi and Radix Paeoniae Alba to nourish Yin and clear Heat, and Radix Achyranthis Bidentatae, Haematitum, Os Draconis and Concha Ostreae to conduct Blood downward, suppress Yang and calm Liver Wind.

— Kidney Yin Deficiency is often complicated with Empty Fire, and herbs that tonify Yin are therefore often combined with herbs that clear Heat and Fire. For simple deficiency of Kidney Yin with symptoms of dizziness and blurred vision, sore and weak lumbar region and knees, nocturnal emissions, night sweats, a red tongue with scanty coating and a thready pulse, sweet herbs that nourish Yin are used to embrace the Yang, as in *Zuo Gui Yin* (**Restoring the Left Decoction**) and *Zuo Gui Wan* (**Restoring the Left Pill**).

— If Yin Deficiency is complicated with Flaring of Empty Fire with symptoms of five-palm heat, loose teeth, sore throat, a dry red tongue with scanty coating and a thready rapid pulse, herbs that clear Heat and Fire should be added. An example is *Liu Wei Di Huang Wan* (**Six-Flavour Rehmannia Pill**), in which Radix Rehmanniae Praeparata, Rhizoma Discoreae and Fructus Corni are combined with Cortex Moutan Radicis, Rhizoma Alismatis and Poria.

— If Liver and Kidney Yin Deficiency is complicated with more severe signs of Fire such as tidal fever, haemoptysis, irritability, restlessness and burning pain in the feet and knees, the dosage of herbs that clear Heat and Fire should be increased, as in *Da Bu Yin Wan* (**Great Tonify the Yin Pill**), in which

Radix Rehmanniae Praeparata and Plastrum Testudinis are combined with Rhizoma Anemarrhenae and Cortex Phellodendri.

4. Formulating prescriptions to tonify Yang

— Deficiency of Kidney Yang implies a lack of warmth. Symptoms may include soreness of the lumbar region and knees, aversion to cold, impotence, premature senility and copious clear urine. If the 'holding in' function of the Kidneys is impaired, there may be nocturnal emissions and enuresis; if the transformational function of the Kidneys is impaired, there may be dysuria and oedema.

— Yin and Yang share a common root and Yin tonics are often added to Yang tonic formulae both to support the Yang and to counter the warmth and dryness of Yang tonic herbs. Examples include *Shen Qi Wan* (**Kidney Qi Pill**) and *You Gui Wan* (**Restoring the Right Pill**), in which a large dose of Radix Rehmanniae Praeparata is combined with Rhizoma Dioscoreae and Fructus Corni.

— If Kidney Yang Deficiency leads to oedema, herbs that drain Dampness and open the Waterways are added, such as Poria and Rhizoma Alismatis in **Kidney Qi Pill** and Semen Plantaginis in *Ji Sheng Shen Qi Wan* (**Invigorate the Kidney Qi Pill**).

— For nocturnal or spontaneous emissions due to Kidney Deficiency and weakness of the seminal gate, astringent herbs that consolidate the Essence should be added, such as Semen Astragali Complanati, Semen Euryales, calcined Os Draconis and calcined Concha Ostreae in *Jin Suo Gu Jing Wan* (**Metal Lock Pill to Stabilize the Essence**).

C. POINTS TO REMEMBER IN FORMULATING TONIC PRESCRIPTIONS

1. Patterns of deficiency involve Qi, Blood, Yin or Yang and their related Zang Fu. For example, the Spleen and Lungs are involved in Qi Deficiency and it is treated with sweet and warm Qi tonic herbs which tonify the Spleen and Lungs.

— The Heart and Liver are involved in Blood Deficiency, which is treated either by tonifying Blood directly or, indirectly, by tonifying Qi in order to produce Blood. This is accomplished primarily via the Heart and Liver and secondarily via the Spleen and Stomach. The Spleen and Kidneys are involved in Yang Deficiency, which is treated by warming and tonifying these organs to benefit the source of Fire. The Liver, Kidneys, Lungs and Stomach are all involved in Yin Deficiency, which is treated with sweet and cold Yin tonics to benefit the Stomach, moisten the Lung, nourish the Kidneys and strengthen the Liver.

— For conditions of extreme deficiency, powerful tonics should be used in large doses and first aid should be administered for Collapse.

— For chronic conditions of deficiency, tonification should be achieved gradually, using mild herbs.

— For Yang Deficiency with Internal Cold, sweet and warm tonic herbs are used and herbs that clear Heat or moisten are contraindicated.

— For Yin Deficiency with Empty Heat, sweet and cool tonic herbs are used and pungent and dry herbs are contraindicated.

2. Qi, Blood, Yin and Yang are the four essential factors sustaining the vital activities of the human body.

— These factors are interrelated. For example, Qi and Blood share a common origin; Yin and Yang share a common root. Vigorous Qi produces Blood and abundant Yang produces Yin.

— When one of these factors is diseased, the others are affected. This produces complicated conditions, such as Qi Deficiency leading to Blood Deficiency, loss of Blood leading to Qi Deficiency, Yin Deficiency leading to hyperactivity of Yang and Yang Deficiency leading to weakness of Qi.

— Spleen Deficiency affects the Lungs, as Earth fails to produce Metal. Kidney Yang Deficiency causes Spleen Qi Deficiency, as Fire fails to warm Earth. Kidney Yin Deficiency produces Liver Fire, as Water fails to nourish Wood.

— These relationships are significant in the formulation of tonic prescriptions. For example, Yin tonics are added to Yang tonic formulae to support transformation; herbs that clear Heat are added to Yin tonic formulae to strengthen the Root and clear Empty Heat; Qi tonics are added to Blood tonic formulae to stimulate Qi to produce Blood.

— For Lung Deficiency with Spleen weakness, Earth should be strengthened to produce Metal. For Yang Deficiency with stagnation of Cold in the Spleen, Fire should be tonified to warm Earth. For Deficiency of Water with hyperactivity of Fire, Water should be nourished to produce Wood.

3. The Spleen and Stomach are the source of Qi and Blood. Tonic herbs tend to cause stagnation of Spleen and Stomach Qi, thus impairing the functions of transportation and transformation.
— If the Spleen and Stomach are weak, they cannot easily digest tonic herbs, and attention should therefore be given to invigoration of the Spleen in tonic formulae, using herbs that regulate Qi.
— It is also necessary to determine whether residual pathogens are present. When a weakness of Upright Qi is complicated with residual pathogens, tonification should be combined with the method of elimination of

pathogenic factors and both conditions should be treated at the same time.

4. The Spleen and Kidneys play an important role in the treatment of deficiency patterns, but medical scholars of all ages have held different views as to which should be tonified.
— Sun Simiao of the Tang Dynasty held, 'It is less effective to tonify the Kidneys than to tonify the Spleen', because the Spleen is the source of Qi and Blood and sufficient Spleen Qi makes it possible to transmit Essence to the various parts of the body.
— Xu Shuwei of the Song Dynasty held, 'It is less effective to tonify the Spleen than to tonify the Kidneys', because the Kidneys are the origin of the congenital constitution, the Yin and Yang of the Zang Fu all rely on the Kidneys and sufficiency of Kidney Qi ensures normal functioning of all the other organs.
— However, it is incorrect to overemphasize

Table 31.1 Comparison of tonic formulae

Formula	Actions	Indications
Four Gentlemen Decoction	Tonifies Qi Invigorates the Spleen	Spleen Qi Deficiency
Regulating the Middle Pill	Tonifies Qi Invigorates the Spleen Warms the Middle Burner and eliminates Cold	Deficiency of the Middle Burner with Stagnation of Cold
Panax–Poria–Atractylodis Powder	Tonifies Spleen and Lung Qi Eliminates Damp Harmonizes the Stomach	Spleen Deficiency complicated with Damp
Generating the Pulse Powder	Benefits Qi Promotes Body Fluids	Prostration due to Qi and Yin Deficiency (Yin Collapse)
Frigid Extremities Powder	Rescues Devastated Yang	Prostration due to Yang Deficiency (Yang Collapse)
Tonifying the Middle and Benefiting Qi Decoction	Tonifies Qi Raises sinking Qi Restores function of conducting the clear up and the turbid down	Spleen Deficiency Fever due to Deficiency Sinking of Central Qi
Tonifying the Spleen Decoction	Tonifies the Heart and Spleen Restores the function of producing and controlling Blood	Heart and Spleen Qi Deficiency Weakness of Spleen function of controlling Blood
Six-Flavour Rehmannia Pill	Tonifies Kidney, Spleen and Liver Yin	Kidney Yin Deficiency
Kidney Qi Pill	Tonifies Kidney Yin and Yang, but mainly Yang	Kidney Yang Deficiency

the importance of any one organ. *Insight into Medicine* says, 'It must be understood that if the Spleen is weak but the Kidneys are not deficient, the Spleen should be tonified; if the Kidneys are weak but the Spleen is not deficient, the Kidneys should be tonified; and if both the Spleen and Kidneys are deficient, they should both be tonified.'

D. A COMPARISON OF COMMON TONIC FORMULAE (TABLE 31.1)

1. – *Si Jun Zi Tang*
   Four Gentlemen Decoction
   – *Li Zhong Wan*
   Regulating the Middle Pill

— **Four Gentlemen Decoction** is a basic Qi tonic formula and only one ingredient differentiates it from **Regulating the Middle Pill**.

— Both formulae tonify Qi and invigorate the Spleen with Radix Ginseng, Rhizoma Atractylodis Macrocephalae and treated Radix Glycyrrhizae.

— Because **Four Gentlemen Decoction** uses Radix Ginseng as its Emperor (*Jun*) herb and combines it with Poria, it is more effective in tonifying Qi and invigorating the Spleen. It is thus indicated for Spleen and Stomach Qi Deficiency with impairment of transportation and transformation, manifesting as sallow complexion, reduced appetite, a pale tongue with white coating and a weak pulse.

— **Regulating the Middle Pill** uses Rhizoma Zingiberis as its Emperor herb. It is thus more effective in warming the Middle Burner and eliminating Cold and is indicated for deficiency of the Middle Burner with stagnation of Cold marked by aversion to cold, cold limbs, abdominal pain, loose stools, a pale tongue with white coating and a deep thready pulse.

2. – *Shen Ling Bai Zhu San*
   Panax–Poria–Atractylodis Powder
   – *Si Jun Zi Tang*
   Four Gentlemen Decoction

— **Panax–Poria–Atractylodis Powder** is made up of **Four Gentlemen Decoction** plus Rhizoma Dioscoreae, Semen Dolichoris Album, Semen Nelumbinis, Semen Coicis, Fructus Amomi and Radix Platycodi.

— Both formulae tonify Qi and invigorate the Spleen and are indicated for Spleen and Stomach Qi Deficiency with symptoms of

sallow complexion, lassitude, weak voice, poor digestion, loose stools, a pale tongue and a deficient pulse.

— **Four Gentlemen Decoction** is a basic formula for Spleen and Stomach Qi Deficiency with impairment of the functions of transportation and transformation. **Panax–Poria–Atractylodis Powder** has a stronger and more comprehensive action. It tonifies not only Spleen Qi but also Lung Qi; it also eliminates Dampness and harmonizes the Stomach. It is thus indicated for Spleen and Stomach Qi Deficiency complicated with Dampness.

3. – *Sheng Mai San*
   Generating the Pulse Powder
   – *Si Ni Tang*
   Frigid Extremities Decoction

— Both formulae are often used as first aid for prostration but from different causes.

— **Generating the Pulse Powder** is indicated for Yin Collapse, with symptoms of a hot sensation and profuse oily perspiration which is salty and sticky. The body and limbs are warm, or the body is warm but the limbs cold; the face is flushed and the tongue red and dry.

— **Frigid Extremities Decoction** is indicated for Yang Collapse, with symptoms of a cold sensation and profuse watery perspiration which is not salty or sticky. The body and limbs are cold, the complexion pale and the tongue pale and moist.

— **Generating the Pulse Powder** benefits Qi and promotes Body Fluids and is thus also indicated for deficiency of both Qi and Yin with symptoms of lassitude, shortness of breath, thirst, profuse sweating, dry mouth and throat and a rapid deficient pulse.

— **Frigid Extremities Decoction** rescues Devastated Yang and is thus indicated for extreme Yang Deficiency with cold limbs, abdominal pain, lassitude, somnolence, aversion to cold, lying with the body curled up, absence of thirst and a deep, thready and feeble pulse.

4. – *Bu Zhong Yi Qi Tang*
   Tonifying the Middle and Benefiting Qi Decoction
   – *Gui Pi Tang*
   Tonifying the Spleen Decoction

— Both formulae use Radix Ginseng, Radix Astragali seu Hedysari, Rhizoma

Atractylodis Macrocephalae and Radix Glycyrrhizae to benefit Qi and invigorate the Spleen and Radix Angelicae Sinensis to nourish Blood.

— **Tonifying the Middle and Benefiting Qi Decoction** is composed of herbs that tonify Qi and raise Yang, such as Rhizoma Cimicifugae and Radix Bupleuri, and is thus intended to tonify Qi, raise sinking Qi and restore the function of conducting the clear upward and the turbid downward.

— **Tonifying the Spleen Decoction** is composed of herbs that tonify Qi, plus herbs such as Arillus Longan, Semen Ziziphi Spinosae, Radix Polygalae and Poria cum Ligno Hospite, which nourish the Heart and calm the Mind. It is intended to tonify the Heart and Spleen and restore the function of producing and controlling Blood.

— The former is indicated for Spleen and Stomach Qi Deficiency with symptoms of lack of energy, dislike of speaking and fever from deficiency, or for Sinking of Central Qi with symptoms of prolapse or chronic diarrhoea.

— The latter is indicated for deficiency of Heart and Spleen Qi and Blood with symptoms of palpitations, poor memory and insomnia or for weakness of the Spleen's function of controlling Blood with symptoms of bloody stool or uterine bleeding.

5. – *Liu Wei Di Huang Wan*
     Six-Flavour Rehmannia Pill
    – *Shen Qi Wan*
     Kidney Qi Pill

— Both formulae consist of Radix Rehmanniae, Rhizoma Dioscoreae, Fructus Corni, Cortex Moutan Radicis, Rhizoma Alismatis and Poria. **Six-Flavour Rehmannia Pill** is **Kidney Qi Pill** minus Ramulus Cinnamomi (or Cortex Cinnamomi) and Radix Aconiti Praeparata. It tonifies Liver, Spleen and especially Kidney Yin and is thus indicated for Kidney Yin Deficiency with symptoms of sore and weak lower back and knees, dizziness, blurred vision, tinnitus, deafness, night sweats, nocturnal emissions, emaciation--thirst syndrome, a red tongue with scanty coating and a deep, thready and rapid pulse. It is also used to treat slow closure of fontanelles in infants.

— **Kidney Qi Pill** tonifies both Yin and Yang, but mainly warms and tonifies Kidney Yang. It is thus indicated for Kidney Yang Deficiency with symptoms of lumbago, weak legs, a cold sensation in the lower half of the body, dysuria or copious urination, a pale and swollen tongue and a weak pulse. It also treats beriberi and oedema.

Questions

1. Why do formulae for tonifying Spleen Qi often include herbs that eliminate Dampness and regulate Qi? Give examples.
2. Why are Qi tonic herbs often added to formulae for tonifying Blood? Give examples.
3. Why are herbs that clear Heat sometimes added to Yin tonic formulae? Give an illustrative example.

32 *Formulae that regulate Qi*

A. GUIDING PRINCIPLES FOR FORMULATING PRESCRIPTIONS TO REGULATE QI

— Formulae that regulate Qi treat patterns of Qi Stagnation or Rebellious Qi. These patterns may affect the upper or lower body, they may involve the Liver, Stomach or Lungs and they may be complicated with Cold, Heat, Phlegm-Dampness, Food Retention or Blood Stagnation.
— It is necessary at the outset to determine: 1) whether pathological changes are due to stagnation or rebellion of Qi; 2) where the disease is located; and 3) the nature and severity of any complications.

B. FORMULATING PRESCRIPTIONS TO REGULATE QI

1. Formulating prescriptions to invigorate the circulation of Qi

— Formulae that invigorate Qi circulation consist primarily of herbs that invigorate Qi circulation, relieve stagnation, harmonize the Liver and relieve depression. These formulae regulate Qi, relieve stagnation and remove obstruction from the channels and collaterals.
— Such formulae treat Qi Stagnation, which can be differentiated as either Liver Qi Stagnation or stagnation of Spleen and Stomach Qi.
— Liver Qi Stagnation manifests as distending pain in the costal and hypochondriac regions, irritability, restlessness, hernia and irregular menstruation or dysmenorrhoea. Herbs which treat this pattern include Radix Bupleuri, Fructus Meliae Toosendan, Radix Linderae, Rhizoma Cyperi, Radix Curcumae, Pericarpium Citri Reticulatae Viride and Semen Citri Reticulatae.

— Stagnation of Spleen and Stomach Qi is marked by distension and fullness of the epigastrium and abdomen, belching, acid regurgitation, nausea, vomiting and reduced appetite. Herbs which treat this pattern include Pericarpium Citri Reticulatae, Radix Aucklandiae, Fructus Aurantii, Cortex Magnoliae Officinalis, Fructus Amomi and Semen Amomi Cardamomi.
— Qi is the commander of Blood. Circulation of Qi leads to circulation of Blood and stagnation of Qi leads to stagnation of Blood. Prolonged stagnation of Qi is thus often complicated with stagnation of Blood, and in this event herbs that invigorate Blood and resolve Blood Stasis should be added to formulae which invigorate circulation of Qi. An example is *Chai Hu Shu Gan San* (**Bupleurum Soothing the Liver Decoction**), which uses Radix Bupleuri, Pericarpium Citri Reticulatae, Rhizoma Cyperi and Fructus Aurantii to harmonize the Liver, relieve stagnation, invigorate Qi and relieve pain, and Rhizoma Ligustici Chuanxiong and Radix Paeoniae to invigorate Blood and resolve Blood Stasis. This formula is commonly used in the treatment of stagnation of Liver Qi and Blood with symptoms of alternating chills and fever and pain in the costal and hypochondriac regions.
— *Yue Ju Wan* (**Gardenia–Ligusticum Pill**) is a representative formula for activating Qi circulation and relieving stagnation. It treats Qi Stagnation which is complicated with Phlegm, Fire, Dampness, Food Retention and Blood Stasis. This formula uses Rhizoma Cyperi as the Emperor herb and combines it with Rhizoma Ligustici Chuanxiong to activate Blood circulation and promote the smooth circulation of Qi.
— Another such formula is *Jin Ling Zi San* (**Melia Toosendan Powder**), which consists

of equal doses of Fructus Meliae Toosendan and Rhizoma Corydalis. Fructus Meliae Toosendan is the Emperor herb, acting to harmonize the Liver, clear Heat, activate Qi and relieve pain. Rhizoma Corydalis activates Blood circulation and promotes smooth circulation of Qi to reinforce the analgesic effect of the formula, which promotes the smooth circulation of both Qi and Blood.

— When Qi circulates smoothly, Dampness is resolved. Retardation of Qi circulation produces Dampness, which accumulates to form Phlegm. For patterns of Qi Stagnation complicated with Dampness and Phlegm, herbs that resolve Dampness and Phlegm should be added. An example is *Ban Xia Hou Po Tang* (**Pinellia and Magnolia Bark Decoction**), which is the main formula for treating Plum-stone Qi. This formula utilizes the combinations of Cortex Magnoliae Officinalis and Folium Perillae to activate Qi and relieve stagnation, and Rhizoma Pinelliae, Poria and Rhizoma Zingiberis Recens to resolve Phlegm and disperse masses. The entire formula relieves Plum-stone Qi by regulating Qi, relieving stagnation and resolving Phlegm.

— Another example is **Gardenia–Ligusticum Pill**, which uses Rhizoma Cyperi to activate Qi and relieve stagnation and Rhizoma Atractylodis (which is bitter and warm in nature) to resolve Dampness.

— Cold is characterized by contraction. When stagnation of Qi is complicated with Cold, it produces disorders such as hernia and cold epigastric pain. For this pattern, herbs that disperse Cold and warm the Interior should be added. An example is *Liang Gu Wan* (**Galangal and Cyperus Pill**), which treats epigastric pain, using one ingredient to activate Qi and the other to disperse Cold.

— Another example is *Nuan Gan Jian* (**Warm the Liver Decoction**), which treats hernia presenting as a cold sensation and pain in the lower abdomen. This formula combines Radix Linderae and Lignum Aquilariae Resinatum with Cortex Cinnamomi and Fructus Foeniculi.

— The Liver is a Yin organ and stores a Yin substance (Blood), but Liver Yang tends to rise. Severe stagnation of Liver Qi or transformation of stagnant Qi into Fire may damage Blood. In addition, herbs that activate Qi circulation are often aromatic and dry in nature and use of these herbs over a long time or in large doses will also damage Yin and Blood. Herbs that nourish Yin and Blood should therefore be added to formulae for harmonizing the Liver and regulating Qi. Examples include the use of Radix Angelicae Sinensis and Radix Paeoniae Alba in *Xiao Yao San* (**Free and Relaxed Powder**) and Radix Rehmanniae or Radix Rehmanniae Praeparata in *Hei Xiao Yao San* (**Black Free and Relaxed Powder**).

— Both Liver Qi Stagnation and stagnation of Spleen and Stomach Qi may impair the functions of transportation and transformation, producing a deficiency of Spleen Qi. In this case, herbs that tonify Qi and invigorate the Spleen should be added to the formula. Examples include the use of Rhizoma Atractylodis Macrocephalae and treated Radix Glycyrrhizae in **Free and Relaxed Powder** and the use of Radix Ginseng, Rhizoma Atractylodis Macrocephalae and treated Radix Glycyrrhizae in **Six Gentlemen Decoction with Aucklandia and Amomum**.

2. Formulating prescriptions to conduct Rebellious Qi downward

— Formulae that conduct Rebellious Qi downward consist primarily of herbs that conduct Qi downward and either soothe asthma or stop vomiting. Such formulae stop cough and wheeze, harmonize the Stomach and stop vomiting in patterns of Rebellious Qi of the Lung or Stomach, either of which may involve underlying Cold or Heat, Deficiency or Excess.

a. Formulae that conduct Rebellious Qi downward and soothe asthma

— Formulae that conduct Rebellious Qi downward and soothe asthma treat Rebellious Lung Qi. The Lungs' function of dispersing can be impaired either by invasion of the Lung by external pathogenic factors or by dysfunction of the Kidneys' reception of Qi, giving rise to symptoms of cough, dyspnoea, stuffiness of the chest and coarse breathing.

— These formulae often consist of herbs such as Fructus Perillae, Semen Armeniacae Amarum, Radix Asteris, Flos Farfarae, Cortex Mori Radicis and Lignum Aquilariae Resinatum, with the addition of other herbs according to the condition of the individual patient.

— For retention of Turbid Phlegm in the Lungs with impairment of dispersing and descending, herbs that dry Dampness and resolve Phlegm should be added. An example is *Su Zi Jiang Qi Tang* (**Perilla Seed Lowering Qi Decoction**), in which Fructus Perillae is the Emperor herb. This formula uses Cortex Magnoliae Officinalis to promote the Lungs' function of dispersing and descending in order to stop cough and wheeze, and Rhizoma Pinelliae and Radix Peucedani to dry Dampness and resolve Phlegm.

— For retention of Phlegm-Heat in the Interior which impairs the Lungs' descending function, herbs that clear Lung Heat and resolve Phlegm should be added. An example is *Ding Chuan Tang* (**Arrest Wheezing Decoction**), which uses Herba Ephedrae and Semen Ginkgo to soothe wheeze, Radix Scutellariae and Cortex Mori Radicis to clear Lung Heat and soothe wheeze and Rhizoma Pinelliae to resolve Phlegm.

— The Kidneys are responsible for reception of Qi. If retention of Turbid Phlegm in the Lungs is complicated with deficiency of the Kidneys' reception of Qi, there will be dyspnoea on exertion with more difficulty on inhalation than exhalation. In this case, herbs that warm the Kidneys and assist reception of Qi should be added, such as Lignum Aquilariae Resinatum, Cortex Cinnamomi and Gecko. An example is the use of Cortex Cinnamomi and Lignum Aquilariae Resinatum in **Perilla Seed Lowering Qi Decoction**, which is indicated for patterns in which the excess in the upper body (i.e. retention of Turbid Phlegm and Rebellious Qi) is more pronounced than the deficiency in the lower body (Kidney Yang Deficiency with failure to receive Qi).

— If asthma is caused simply by deficiency of the Lungs and Kidneys, the treatment method should be primarily tonification.Representative formulae include *Ren Shen Hu Tao Tang* (**Ginseng and Walnut Decoction**) and *Ren Shen Ge Jie San* (**Ginseng and Gecko Powder**).

b. Formulae that conduct Rebellious Qi downward and stop vomiting

— Formulae which conduct Rebellious Qi downward and stop vomiting treat Rebellious Stomach Qi. When the Stomach functions properly, Stomach Qi descends. Improper diet or retention of pathogenic factors impair the descending function of the Stomach and gives rise to symptoms of vomiting, hiccup, belching and retching.

— These formulae consist primarily of herbs such as Flos Inulae, Haematitum, Rhizoma Pinelliae, Rhizoma Zingiberis Recens, Caulis Bambusae in Taeniam and Calyx Kaki. Because the causes of Rebellious Stomach Qi differ, other herbs are added according to the condition of the individual patient.

— In cases of pathogenic Cold, the correct treatment method is to warm the Middle Burner and conduct Rebellious Qi downward. An example is *Ding Xiang Shi Di Tang* (**Clove and Persimmon Calyx Decoction**), which uses Flos Caryophylli to warm the Stomach, disperse Cold and conduct Rebellious Qi downward and Calyx Kaki to conduct Rebellious Qi downward and stop hiccup.

— If Rebellious Qi is due to retention of Empty Heat in the Stomach, herbs that clear Heat should be added, such as Pericarpium Citri Reticulatae, Rhizoma Zingiberis Recens and Caulis Bambusae in Taeniam in *Ju Pi Zhu Ru Tang* (**Tangerine Peel and Bamboo Shaving Decoction**).

— If Rebellious Qi is due to Stomach Qi Deficiency and is complicated with retention of Turbid Phlegm, herbs that resolve Phlegm should be added. An example is *Xuan Fu Dai Zhe Tang* (**Inula and Haematite Decoction**), in which Flos Inulae and Haematitum are combined with Rhizoma PInelliae and Rhizoma Zingiberis to conduct Rebellious Qi downward, resolve Phlegm and stop vomiting.

— Failure of Stomach Qi to descend is closely related to deficiency of Stomach Qi. The foregoing formulae therefore often include herbs that tonify Qi, invigorate the Spleen, harmonize the Stomach and produce Body Fluids, such as Radix Ginseng, treated Radix Glycyrrhizae or Fructus Ziziphi Jujubae.

C. POINTS TO REMEMBER IN FORMULATING PRESCRIPTIONS TO REGULATE QI

1. Disorders of Qi can arise from either deficiency or excess. Formulae for regulating

Qi are indicated for Qi disorders of the excess type. If tonification is used to treat Qi Stagnation of the excess type, the condition will be aggravated. On the other hand, if distension and fullness due to deficiency are treated by invigorating the circulation of Qi rather than tonifying, Qi will be further damaged and deficiency will be aggravated.

— In the treatment of patterns of combined excess and deficiency, a small dose of Qi tonic herbs is added to formulae that activate the circulation of Qi in order to treat both Ben and Biao.

2. Formulae to regulate Qi consist primarily of herbs that are pungent, warm, aromatic and dry in nature. These herbs tend to consume Qi and Yin and must be prescribed in the correct dosage.

— Such herbs are contraindicated in cases of Qi Deficiency and Empty Fire due to Yin Deficiency. They should be used with caution in the treatment of Qi Stagnation complicated with Yin Deficiency, and in pregnant women, and should be balanced by herbs that are sweet and cold in nature and promote Body Fluids or nourish Blood.

3. Because most herbs that regulate Qi are aromatic and pungent in nature, their active ingredients will evaporate and be lost if they are decocted for a long time or if the lid of the cooking pot is removed from time to time during cooking. Aromatic herbs such as Radix Aucklandiae and Lignum Aquilariae Resinatum should be added in the last 4 or 5 minutes of cooking.

D. A COMPARISON OF COMMONLY USED FORMULAE TO REGULATE QI (TABLE 32.1)

1. – *Yue Ju Wan*
     Gardenia–Ligusticum Pill
   – *Chai Hu Shu Gan San*
     Bupleurum Soothing the Liver Decoction

— Both formulae activate Qi circulation, relieve stagnation and stop pain.

— **Gardenia-Ligusticum Pill** consists of Rhizoma Cyperi, Rhizoma Ligustici Chuanxiong, Rhizoma Atractylodis, Fructus Gardeniae and Massa Fermentata Medicinalis. It activates Qi circulation and relieves stagnation as its primary action and activates Blood circulation, clears Heat, resolves Dampness and assists digestion as secondary actions. It is thus indicated for Six Stagnations (i.e. stagnation of Qi, Blood, Phlegm, Fire, Dampness and Food), with symptoms of distress and stuffiness in the chest and diaphragm, epigastric and abdominal pain, acid regurgitation, vomiting and poor digestion. It is necessary to determine which of the six stagnations is the most pronounced before additional ingredients of the formula can be selected.

— **Bupleurum Soothing the Liver Decoction** consists of Radix Bupleuri, Rhizoma Cyperi, Pericarpium Citri Reticulatae, Fructus Aurantii, Rhizoma Ligustici Chuanxiong, Radix Paeoniae and treated Radix Glycyrrhizae. It is indicated for Liver Qi Stagnation and stagnation of Blood with symptoms of alternating chills and fever, hypochondriac pain, a pale purplish tongue with white coating and a wiry pulse.

2. – *Tian Tai Wu Yao San*
     Top-Quality Lindera Powder
   – *Nuan Gan Jian*
     Warm the Liver Decoction

— Both formulae contain Radix Linderae and Fructus Foeniculi, and both formulae activate Qi circulation and disperse Cold. They are otherwise quite different.

— **In Top-Quality Lindera Powder**, Radix Linderae is combined with herbs that strongly relieve Qi Stagnation, such as Radix Aucklandiae, Pericarpium Citri Reticulatae Viride and Semen Arecae, and the action of invigorating Qi circulation is therefore more pronounced. Fructus Meliae Toosendan, though bitter and cold in nature, is prepared with Fructus Crotonis (which is removed from the formula after preparation), thus intensifying its action of warming and dispersing; Rhizoma Alpiniae Officinalis and Fructus Foeniculi combine to treat long-standing accumulated Cold.

— This formula is commonly used in the treatment of Cold-type hernia with symptoms of hardness and swelling of the scrotum and violent pain radiating to the lower abdomen. Because all the ingredients of this formula eliminate pathogenic factors, this formula treats excess-type patterns only.

— In addition to Radix Linderae and Fructus Foeniculi, **Warm the Liver Decoction** contains Lignum Aquilariae Resinatum, Cortex Cinnamomi, Radix Angelicae

Table 32.1 Comparison of formulae that regulate Qi

Formula	Actions	Indications
Gardenia–Ligusticum Pill	Activates Qi circulation and relieves stagnation Activates Blood circulation Clears Heat Resolves Damp Assists digestion	Six Stagnations
Bupleurum Soothing the Liver Decoction	Activates Qi circulation and relieves stagnation	Liver Qi Stagnation Blood Stagnation
Top-Quality Lindera Powder	Activates Qi Circulation Strongly warms and disperses pathogenic Cold	Excess-type patterns of Cold accumulation (especially hernia)
Warm the Liver Decoction	Activates Qi circulation Disperses Cold Tonifies Liver and Kidneys	Liver and Kidney Deficiency complicated with invasion of Cold
Perilla Seed Lowering Qi Decoction	Conducts Rebellious Qi downward Warms and resolves Cold Phlegm Assists Kidney reception of Qi	'Excess above and Deficiency below', i.e. cough and wheeze due to Kidney Deficiency and Phlegm
Arrest Wheezing Decoction	Stimulates Lung functions of descending and dispersing Resolves Phlegm	Recurrent asthma, due to Wind-Cold with underlying Internal Phlegm-Heat
Inula and Haematite Decoction	Conducts Stomach Qi downward Tonifies Qi Resolves Phlegm	Rebellious Stomach Qi due to Stomach Qi Deficiency and retention of Turbid Phlegm
Tangerine Peel and Bamboo Shaving Decoction	Clears Heat Conducts Stomach Qi downward Tonifies Qi Nourishes the Stomach	Rebellious Stomach Qi due to Empty Stomach Heat
Clove and Persimmon Calyx Decoction	Warms the Stomach Conducts Stomach Qi downward Activates Qi circulation	Hiccup or vomiting due to Stomach Deficiency with Stagnation of Cold

Sinensis, Fructus Lycii, Poria and Rhizoma Zingiberis Recens. This formula is indicated for Liver and Kidney Deficiency and Blood Deficiency complicated with invasion of Cold, as seen in Cold-type hernia marked by deficiency complicated with excess. Symptoms include a cold sensation and pain in the scrotum, inability to attain an erection, pale complexion, cold feet, a white tongue coating and a deep pulse.

3. – *Su Zi Jiang Qi Tang*
   Perilla Seed Lowering Qi Decoction
   – *Ding Chuan Tang*
   Arrest Wheezing Decoction

— Both formulae are indicated for asthma but their use requires a differentiation of the underlying pattern.

— **Perilla Seed Lowering Qi Decoction** consists of Fructus Perillae, Rhizoma Pinelliae, Cortex Magnoliae Officinalis, Radix Peucedani, Cortex Cinnamomi, Radix Angelicae Sinensis and Radix Glycyrrhizae. It conducts Rebellious Qi downward, soothes wheeze and warms and resolves Cold Phlegm as its primary actions and warms the Kidneys to assist reception of Qi as its secondary action. It is indicated for cough and wheeze due to retention of profuse Phlegm marked by excess in the upper body (i.e. the Lungs) and deficiency of the lower body (i.e. the Kidneys).

— **Arrest Wheezing Decoction** consists of Semen Ginkgo, Herba Ephedrae, Fructus Perillae, Rhizoma Pinelliae, Flos Farfarae, Semen Armeniacae Amarum, Cortex Mori

Radicis, Radix Scutellariae and Radix Glycyrrhizae. This formula is a collection of many different types of herbs that treat wheeze, including cold herbs, warm herbs, herbs which stimulate the dispersing function of the Lungs and herbs which astringe the Lungs. It stimulates the functions of dispersing and descending, soothes wheeze and resolves Phlegm and is thus indicated for recurrent asthma due to exposure to external Wind-Cold with Internal Phlegm-Heat. Symptoms include profuse sticky yellow sputum, a sticky yellow tongue coating and a rolling and rapid pulse. There may also be fever and aversion to cold.

4. – *Xuan Fu Dai Zhe Tang*
   Inula and Haematite Decoction
   – *Ju Pi Zhu Ru Tang*
   Tangerine Peel and Bamboo Shaving Decoction
   – *Ding Xiang Shi Di Tang*
   Clove and Persimmon Calyx Decoction

— All three formulae conduct Stomach Qi downward, stop belching and hiccup, tonify Qi and harmonize the Stomach. All are indicated for Stomach Deficiency with symptoms of hiccup and belching but have important differences.
— **Inula and Haematite Decoction** consists of Flos Inulae, Haematitum, Rhizoma Pinelliae, Rhizoma Zingiberis Recens, Radix Ginseng, Radix Glycyrrhizae and Fructus Ziziphi Jujubae. Using Flos Inulae and Haematitum as the Emperor herbs, this formula eliminates Phlegm and conducts Rebellious Qi downward.
— This formula is indicated for Rebellious Stomach Qi due to Stomach Qi Deficiency and retention of Turbid Phlegm with symptoms of epigastric distress, frequent belching, vomiting, a white slippery and sticky tongue coating and a deficient wiry pulse. It is very effective in relieving epigastric distress and nausea.
— **Tangerine Peel and Bamboo Shaving Decoction** consists of Pericarpium Citri Reticulatae, Caulis Bambusae in Taeniam, Rhizoma Zingiberis Recens, Radix Ginseng, Fructus Ziziphi Jujubae and Radix Glycyrrhizae. Using Pericarpium Citri Reticulatae and Caulis Bambusae in Taeniam as the Emperor herbs, this formula clears Heat, conducts Rebellious Qi downward,

tonifies Qi and nourishes the Stomach. It is indicated for Rebellious Stomach Qi due to Empty Heat in the Stomach, with symptoms of hiccup, vomiting, a tender red tongue and a rapid deficient pulse.
— **Clove and Persimmon Calyx Decoction** consists of Flos Caryophylli, Calyx Kaki, Radix Ginseng and Rhizoma Zingiberis Recens. Using Flos Caryophylli and Calyx Kaki as the Emperor herbs, this formula warms the Stomach and conduct Rebellious Qi downward. It is effective in warming the Middle Burner, activating Qi circulation and stopping hiccup.
— This formula is indicated for hiccup due to Stomach Deficiency with stagnation of Cold and Rebellious Stomach Qi. It also treats vomiting due to stagnation of Cold in the Stomach. In either case, symptoms include hiccup, vomiting, clear and dilute sputum, epigastric distress, a pale tongue with white coating and a slow pulse.

Questions

1. Why are herbs that activate Blood circulation added to formulae that activate Qi circulation? Illustrate this with a prescription.
2. For which pattern are herbs that warm the Kidneys and assist reception of Qi added to formulae for conducting Rebellious Qi downward and soothing wheeze?

33 *Formulae that regulate Blood*

A. GUIDING PRINCIPLES FOR FORMULATING PRESCRIPTIONS THAT REGULATE BLOOD

— Formulae that regulate Blood treat Blood Stagnation and haemorrhage.
— The formulation of prescriptions that regulate Blood is based on the constitution of the patient, the location of the disease, the duration and severity of pathological conditions and the actions and characteristics of the herbs. The primary treatment method is activating Blood circulation and resolving Stasis.
— When the aetiology, pathogenesis and complications have been determined, secondary treatment methods such as clearing Heat, warming, tonifying or purging may be selected.
— Haemorrhage is treated primarily by the method of stopping bleeding, but haemorrhagic patterns vary in nature, location and severity. Herbs that stop bleeding should therefore be combined with herbs that clear Fire, invigorate the Spleen, warm the Yang or resolve Stasis, as appropriate to the patient's condition.

B. TYPES OF FORMULA THAT REGULATE BLOOD

1. Formulae that activate Blood circulation and resolve Blood Stasis

— Formulae that activate the Blood and resolve Stasis smooth the circulation of Qi and Blood in the channels and collaterals and disperse stagnant Blood.
— Qi and Blood are intimately related. Circulation of Qi leads to circulation of Blood, stagnation of Qi leads to stagnation of Blood and stagnation of Blood can retard the circulation of Qi.

— To assist in resolving Blood Stasis, herbs that activate Qi are often added to formulae that activate Blood and resolve Blood Stasis. One example is the use of Radix Bupleuri and Fructus Aurantii in *Xue Fu Zhu Yu Tang* (**Blood Mansion Eliminating Stasis Decoction**). Another is *Dan Shen Yin* (**Salvia Decoction**), in which Radix Salviae Miltiorrhizae is the Emperor herb and Lignum Santalum and Fructus Amomi are included to activate Qi and relieve pain. This formula is indicated for pain in the heart and stomach due to stagnation of Blood and Qi.
— If Blood Stagnation is caused by Cold, herbs that warm the channels and disperse Cold should be added. An example is *Wen Jing Tang* (**Warm the Menses Decoction**), in which Radix Angelicae Sinensis, Radix Paeoniae and Rhizoma Ligustici Chuanxiong are the Emperor herbs, acting to activate Blood circulation and resolve Stasis, while Fructus Evodiae and Ramulus Cinnamomi assist by warming the channels and dispersing Cold. This formula is indicated for stagnation of Blood with deficiency and coldness of the Chong and Ren channels; symptoms include irregular menstruation, dysmenorrhoea, uterine bleeding and infertility.
— Chronic Blood Stagnation prevents the production of new Blood, thus leading to deficiency of Qi and Blood. Conversely, Qi and Blood Deficiency can lead to stagnation of Blood. When stagnation is complicated with deficiency, herbs that nourish Blood and tonify Qi should be added as appropriate. For example, **Blood Mansion Eliminating Stasis Decoction** includes Radix Rehmanniae and Radix Angelicae Sinensis to nourish Blood; *Bu Yang Huan Wu Tang* (**Tonify the Yang to Restore Five-Tenths Decoction**), which is indicated for hemiplegia due to Qi

Deficiency and Blood Stasis, includes a large dose of Radix Astragali seu Hedysari.

— If Blood Stagnation is complicated with pathogenic Heat which gives rise to disorders in the lower body, bitter and cold purgative herbs should be added, such as Radix et Rhizoma Rhei and Natrii Sulfas. *Tao Ren Cheng Qi Tang* (**Peach Pit Decoction to Order the Qi**), which is indicated for a combination of Blood Stagnation and Heat in the Lower Burner, is made up of *Tiao Wei Cheng Qi Tang* (**Regulate the Stomach and Order the Qi Decoction**) plus Semen Persicae and Ramulus Cinnamomi.

— If stagnant Blood forms palpable abdominal masses, herbs that activate the Blood generally will not be effective and substances that break stagnation and resolve masses will be needed. Such substances include Hirudo, Tabanus, Eupolyphaga seu Steleophaga, Rhizoma Sparganii and Rhizoma Zedoariae. The representative formula is *Bie Jia Jian Wan* (**Turtle Shell Pill**).

2. Formulae that stop bleeding

— Formulae that stop bleeding treat both internal and external bleeding. Haemorrhagic patterns can arise from excess or deficiency and may involve different Zang Fu, and these factors will determine the selection of herbs.

— The most common cause of haemorrhagic patterns is Fire, which damages blood vessels and causes the Blood to leave the vessels. Symptoms include haemoptysis, epistaxis, haematemesis, uterine bleeding and bloody stool. The treatment method is to clear Heat, cool Blood and stop bleeding.

— *Shi Hui San* (**Ten Partially-Charred Substance Powder**) is a commonly used formula which cools Blood and stops bleeding with Herba seu Radix Cirsii Japonici, Herba Cephalanoploris, Folium Nelumbinis, Cacumen Biotae, Radix Rubiae, Rhizoma Imperatae and Cortex Trachycarpi. It also includes Fructus Gardeniae, Cortex Moutan Radicis and Radix et Rhizoma Rhei to clear Heat and Fire and conduct Heat downward. The haemostatic effect of the formula is enhanced by charring the ingredients to ash. It is indicated for haemoptysis, haematemesis, bloody stool and haematuria caused by reckless movement of Blood due to Heat.

— For fresh blood in the stool, the correct treatment method is to clear Heat from the intestines and stop bleeding with *Huai Hua San* (**Sophora Japonica Flower Powder**). This formula uses Flos Sophorae to clear Damp-Heat from the intestines and stop bleeding and includes Cacumen Biotae and charred Herba Schizonepetae to enhance its haemostatic effect.

— For urinary disturbance with haematuria, the method of treatment is to cool Blood, stop bleeding, promote urination and open the Waterways. The representative formula is *Xiao Ji Yin Zi* (**Cephalanoplos Decoction**), in which Herba Cephalanoploris and Radix Rehmanniae are combined with Nodus Nelumbinis Rhizomatis and Pollen Typhae to cool Blood, stop bleeding and resolve Blood Stasis.

— In Cold deficient patterns, haemorrhage is caused by Spleen deficiency with impairment of the Spleen's function of controlling Blood, and deficiency of the Chong and Ren channels. The treatment method is to warm and tonify to stop bleeding. *Huang Tu Tang* (**Yellow Earth Decoction**) is a formula commonly used in the treatment of bloody stool, haemoptysis and epistaxis due to deficiency of the Middle Burner with stagnation of Cold. This formula contains Terra Flava Usta or Halloysitum Rubrum which warm the Yang to stop bleeding, and Rhizoma Atractylodis Macrocephalae, Radix Aconiti Praeparata and Radix Glycyrrhizae which warm the Yang and invigorate the Spleen to restore the Spleen's function of controlling Blood.

— *Jiao Ai Tang* (**Ass-Hide Gelatin and Mugwort Decoction**) is indicated for uterine bleeding. It contains Colla Corii Asini and Folium Artemisiae Argyi to stop bleeding and nourish Blood, and Radix Rehmanniae Praeparata, Radix Paeoniae Alba, Radix Angelicae Sinensis and Rhizoma Ligustici Chuanxiong to nourish Blood and regulate menstruation. It treats both the Biao and the Ben of bleeding due to deficiency of the Chong and Ren channels.

— Blood coagulates on exposure to Cold; warmth causes it to circulate. Large doses of herbs that cool Blood and stop bleeding tend to cause stagnation of Blood and herbs that activate the Blood and resolve Stasis should be added to formulae that stop bleeding to counter this effect. An example is the inclusion of Radix Rubiae and Cortex Moutan Radicis in **Ten Partially-Charred Substance Powder**.

C. POINTS TO REMEMBER IN FORMULATING PRESCRIPTIONS TO REGULATE BLOOD

1. In using formulae to regulate Blood, it is necessary to identify the cause, location and duration of the disease. In an acute case, the Biao is treated; in a chronic case, both the Biao and Ben are treated. Simply treating the symptoms of Stasis or bleeding is not therapeutically effective.

2. Formulae that activate Blood circulation or resolve Stasis tend to consume Blood and Qi; formulae that stop bleeding may produce stagnation of Blood. Herbs that benefit Qi and nourish Blood are therefore often added to formulae that activate Blood and resolve Stasis in order to avoid damage to the Upright Qi, and herbs that activate Blood and resolve Stasis are often added to formulae that stop bleeding in order to avoid producing Stasis. Formulae that activate Blood and resolve Stasis should be used with caution on pregnant women and patients with profuse menstrual bleeding.

D. A COMPARISON OF COMMONLY USED FORMULAE THAT REGULATE BLOOD (TABLE 33.1)

1. – *Xue Fu Zhu Yu Tang*
       Blood Mansion Eliminating Stasis Decoction
     – *Fu Yuan Huo Xue Tang*
       Revive Health by Invigorating the Blood Decoction

— In both formulae, herbs that activate the Blood and resolve Stasis are combined with herbs that harmonize the Liver and activate Qi, such as Semen Persicae, Flos Carthami, Radix Angelicae Sinensis, Radix Bupleuri and Radix Glycyrrhizae.

— **Blood Mansion Eliminating Stasis Decoction** also contains Rhizoma Ligustici Chuanxiong, Radix Paeoniae Rubra, Radix Achyranthis Bidentatae, Radix Rehmanniae, Radix Platycodi and Fructus Aurantii to enhance the effect of activating Qi and Blood and resolving Stasis.

— **Revive Health by Invigorating the Blood Decoction** also contains Squama Manitis, Radix et Rhizoma Rhei and Radix Trichosanthis, making it even more effective in activating Blood and resolving Stasis.

— Although both formulae are indicated for stagnation of Blood, the former is more effec-

Table 33.1 Comparison of formulae that regulate Blood

Formula	Actions	Indications
Blood Mansion Eliminating Stasis Decoction	Activates Qi and Blood Resolves Stasis	Stagnation of Blood in the chest
Revive Health by Invigorating the Blood Decoction	More strongly activates Blood and resolves Stasis	Stagnation of Blood in the hypochondrium due to traumatic injury
Cephalanoplos Decoction	Clears Heat Cools Blood Promotes urination	Haematuria due to stagnation of Blood and Heat in the Lower Burner
Eliminating Redness Decoction	Clears Heart Heat Promotes urination	Urinary disturbance due to Heart Heat
Sophora Japonica Flower Decoction	Cools Blood and stops bleeding	Bloody stool due to Wind and Fire Poison or Damp-Heat at the Blood level of the Spleen and Stomach
Yellow Earth Decoction	Warm Yang Invigorates the Spleen and promotes the control of Blood	Bloody stool due to Spleen Yang Deficiency

tive in treating stagnation of Blood in the chest with symptoms of chest pain, palpitations, insomnia, dream-disturbed sleep, irritability and afternoon fever; the latter is more effective in treating stagnation of Blood in the hypochondrium due to traumatic injury, with the symptom of intolerable hypochondriac pain.

2. – *Xiao Ji Yin Zi*
   Cephalanoplos Decoction
   – *Dao Chi San*
   Eliminating Redness Powder

— Both formulae clear Heat and promote urination and are thus indicated for urinary disturbances.
— Cephalanoplos Decoction is made up of **Eliminating Redness Powder** plus Herba Cephalanoploris, Pollen Typhae, Nodus Nelumbinis Rhizomatis and Radix Angelicae Sinensis to cool Blood and stop bleeding, and Fructus Gardeniae and Talcum to clear Heat and Fire and promote urination. It is thus more effective in clearing Heat and cooling Blood and is indicated for urinary disturbance with haematuria due to stagnation of Blood and Heat in the Lower Burner, with symptoms of haematuria, hesitant burning and painful urination, a red tongue and a rapid pulse.
— **Eliminating Redness Powder** clears Heart Heat and promotes urination and is thus indicated for urinary disturbance due to Heart Heat moving down to the Small Intestine, with symptoms of painful and hesitant passage of dark urine with mild haematuria.

3. – *Huai Hua San*
   Sophora Japonica Flower Powder
   – *Huang Tu Tang*
   Yellow Earth Decoction

— Both formulae are indicated for bloody stool, but one treats a Full Heat pattern while the other treats a Cold deficient pattern.
— The main ingredients of **Sophora Japonica Flower Powder** are Flos Sophorae and Cacumen Biotae. The formula cools Blood and stops bleeding; it treats bloody stool resulting from an invasion of pathogenic Wind and Fire Poison or Damp-Heat into the Blood level of the Spleen and Stomach, with the key symptom of an explosive discharge of bright red blood before or after stools.
— **Yellow Earth Decoction** consists of Terra Flava Usta, Rhizoma Atractylodis Macrocephalae, Radix Aconiti Praeparata and Colla Corii Asini. The formula warms Yang, invigorates the Spleen and stimulates the control of Blood. It treats bloody stool due to Spleen Yang Deficiency with an impairment of the Spleen's function of controlling the Blood; the key symptom is a dribbling discharge of dark or pale blood following the stool. Accompanying symptoms include a sallow complexion, pale tongue with white coating and a deep, thready and weak pulse.

Questions

1. Give examples to illustrate why herbs that activate Qi circulation are often added to formulae that activate Blood and resolve Blood Stasis.
2. What are the functions of Fructus Gardeniae and Radix et Rhizoma Rhei in **Ten Partially-charred Substance Powder**?

34 *Formulae that expel Dampness*

A. GUIDING PRINCIPLES FOR FORMULATING PRESCRIPTIONS THAT EXPEL DAMPNESS

— The formulation of prescriptions that expel Dampness is based on the nature and location of the disease, the particular Zang Fu involved and whether there are other pathogenic factors complicating the condition.

— As a general rule, if pathogenic Dampness affects the upper or exterior parts of the body, herbs that induce diaphoresis are primarily used to eliminate the pathogen by mild sweating. If pathogenic Dampness affects the lower or interior parts of the body, diuretic herbs are primarily used to drain Dampness through urination.

— In the treatment of interior Dampness, especially Damp-Heat, the location of the pathology within the Triple Burner must be determined. For example, if Dampness affects the Upper Burner and the Lung channel, pungent herbs are used to promote the Lungs' dispersing function so that Dampness can be resolved.

— If Dampness affects the Middle Burner, aromatic herbs are used to resolve Dampness and regulate the Spleen, or bitter and dry herbs are used to dry Dampness and invigorate the Spleen's function of transportation and transformation.

— If Dampness affects the Lower Burner and involves the Kidneys and Bladder, diuretic herbs that relieve oedema or open the Waterways are used to eliminate Water and Dampness.

— If Dampness transforms to Cold, one must also adopt the method of warming; if Dampness transforms to Heat, then the Heat must be cleared.

— If a patient with a strong constitution has an excess of Water or Dampness, harsh purgatives may be used. If the patient has a weak constitution, the treatment method must be combined with strengthening Upright Qi.

— If pathogenic Dampness is complicated with pathogenic Wind, herbs that eliminate Wind-Damp must be included.

B. TYPES OF FORMULA THAT EXPEL DAMPNESS

1. Formulae that dry Dampness and harmonize the Stomach

— Formulae that dry Dampness and harmonize the Stomach consist primarily of bitter and warm herbs that dry Dampness and aromatics that resolve turbidity. These formulae not only dry Dampness and resolve turbidity but also invigorate the Spleen's function of transportation and transformation. They are indicated for retention of Turbid Dampness and disharmony between the Spleen and Stomach.

— The Spleen and Stomach receive food, and transport and transform Water and Dampness. They like dryness and the aromatic smell, and dislike Dampness. These formulae therefore consist largely of aromatics that dry Dampness, such as Herba Agastachis, Herba Eupatorii and Rhizoma Atractylodis.

— Dampness is a Yin pathogen and tends to consume Yang Qi; it obstructs Qi circulation, prevents Stomach Qi from descending and may be complicated with external pathogens that invade the surface of the body. These factors determine the auxiliary herbs to be used in formulae to expel Dampness.

— When retention of Dampness in the Spleen and Stomach obstructs the circulation of Qi and gives rise to epigastric and abdominal distension and fullness, poor appetite and a sticky white tongue coating, herbs that activate Qi circulation should be included in the formula, as in *Ping Wei San* (**Balancing the Stomach Powder**), where Cortex Magnoliae Officinalis and Pericarpium Citri Reticulatae assist the Emperor herb Rhizoma Atractylodis in activating Qi and resolving Dampness.

— If Stomach Qi fails to descend, producing symptoms of nausea and vomiting, one must harmonize the Stomach and conduct Rebellious Qi downward as well. An example is *Bu Huan Jin Zheng Qi San* (**Rectify the Qi Powder Worth More Than Gold**), in which Rhizoma Atractylodis and Herba Agastachis are combined with Rhizoma Pinelliae and Rhizoma Zingiberis Recens.

— If internal Turbid Dampness is complicated with invasion of External Cold-Wind, the method of resolving Dampness must be combined with the method of Releasing the Exterior. An example is *Huo Xiang Zheng Qi San* (**Agastache Upright Qi Powder**), in which the Emperor herb, Herba Agastachis, is combined with Radix Angelicae Dahuricae to disperse Wind-Cold and with Cortex Magnoliae Officinalis, Pericarpium Citri Reticulatae, Pericarpium Arecae, Rhizoma Pinelliae and Poria to resolve Dampness and regulate Qi.

2. Formulae that clear Damp-Heat

— Formulae that clear Damp-Heat are made up of herbs that clear Heat and either resolve Dampness or drain Dampness through urination. They are indicated for patterns of Dampness turning to Heat, or combined patterns of Dampness and Heat.

— The combination of pathogenic Dampness and Heat is characterized by slow onset and long duration and the resulting pathological changes are difficult to treat. Simply clearing Heat will not eliminate Dampness and simply eliminating Dampness will not clear Heat. Dampness is a Yin pathogen and cannot be resolved without using warm herbs; Heat is a Yang pathogen and cannot be cleared without using cool herbs. Formulae that clear Damp-Heat are thus complex and can be classified into four categories:

a. **Herbs that clear Heat and Dampness**, such as Radix Scutellariae, Rhizoma Coptidis, Cortex Phellodendri, Fructus Gardeniae and Herba Artemisiae Scopariae

b. **Herbs that drain Dampness through urination**, such as Poria, Polyporus Umbellatus, Rhizoma Alismatis, Semen Coicis and Medulla Tetrapanacis, and diuretic herbs that open the Waterways, such as Talcum, Semen Plantaginis, Herba Dianthi, Herba Polygoni Avicularis, Folium Pyrrosiae and Herba Lysimachiae

c. **Aromatics that resolve Dampness**, such as Herba Agastachis, Herba Eupatorii, Fructus Amomi Cardamomi and Rhizoma Acori Graminei

d. **Bitter and warm herbs that dry Dampness**, such as Rhizoma Atractylodis, Rhizoma Pinelliae and Cortex Magnoliae Officinalis.

— The way in which these herbs are combined depends upon the relative severity of Dampness and Heat and the location of the disease. As a general rule, if Dampness is more severe than Heat, the primary treatment method is to expel Dampness and the secondary method is to clear Heat. An example is *San Ren Tang* (**Three-Nut Decoction**), which employs Semen Armeniacae Amarum, Fructus Amomi Cardamomi, Semen Coicis, Rhizoma Pinelliae and Cortex Magnoliae Officinalis to resolve Dampness and regulate Qi, and Herba Lophatheri, Medulla Tetrapanacis and Talcum to clear Heat and drain Dampness. This formula treats Damp-Heat in all three Burners at the same time.

— If Heat is more severe than Dampness, the primary treatment method is to clear Heat and the secondary method is to expel Dampness. An example is *Bai Hu Jia Cang Zhu Tang* (**White Tiger plus Atractylodis Decoction**), which employs Gypsum Fibrosum and Rhizoma Anemarrhenae to clear Heat and Fire, and Rhizoma Atractylodis to dry Dampness.

— If Dampness and Heat are of equal severity, the methods of clearing Heat and expelling Dampness are given equal emphasis. An example is *Gan Lu Xiao Du Dan* (**Sweet Dew Special Pill to Eliminate Toxin**), in which the main herbs, Talcum, Herba Artemisiae Scopariae and Radix Scutellariae, are combined with Fructus Forsythiae, Caulis Akebiae, Rhizoma Acori Graminei,

Herba Agastachis and Fructus Amomi Cardamomi.

— If the pathological changes are most apparent in the Middle Burner, with symptoms of epigastric distress and poor appetite, the treatment method is to resolve Dampness and harmonize the Middle Burner. An example is **Three-Nut Decoction**, which contains Fructus Amomi Cardamomi, Cortex Magnoliae Officinalis and Rhizoma PInelliae.

— If the disease is located in the Upper Burner, with symptoms of dizziness, sore throat, fever and aversion to cold, herbs that promote the Lungs' dispersing function should be added, for example Semen Armeniacae Amarum in **Three-Nut Decoction**.

— If the Damp-Heat moves downward to the Lower Burner, giving rise to symptoms of urinary disturbance and leucorrhoea, the treatment method is to clear Damp-Heat in the Lower Burner. Examples include the use of Talcum, Semen Plantaginis, Herba Dianthi and Herba Polygoni Avicularis in *Ba Zheng San* (**Eight-Herb Powder for Rectification**), and the use of Cortex Phellodendri and Rhizoma Atractylodis in *Er Miao San* (**Two-Marvel Powder**).

3. Diuretic formulae that drain Dampness

— Formulae that expel Dampness through the urine consist primarily of herbs that are sweet and bland in nature. They are indicated for retention of excess Water and Dampness with symptoms of oedema and retention of urine.

— Oedema and urinary retention due to excess Water and Dampness are treated with the method of draining Water and Dampness through urination. There is a saying, 'If urination is not promoted in the treatment of Damp syndromes, the method is wrong.'

— These formulae consist primarily of herbs such as Polyporus Umbellatus, Poria, Rhizoma Alismatis and Semen Coicis. Complications such as overflow of Water to the muscles, obstruction of Qi circulation in the Interior or impairment of the Bladder's function of controlling urine require the addition of other herbs.

— If Water and Dampness are retained in the muscles due to invasion of external pathogenic Wind and deficiency of Defensive Qi, the correct treatment method consists of benefiting Qi and promoting diuresis. The representative formula is *Fang Ji Huang Qi Tang* (**Stephania and Astragalus Decoction**), in which Radix Stephaniae Tetrandrae is combined with Radix Astragali seu Hedysari, Rhizoma Atractylodis Macrocephalae and Radix Glycyrrhizae to promote diuresis without damaging the Upright Qi.

— When Dampness obstructs Qi, giving rise to symptoms of oedema with distension and fullness in the epigastrium and abdomen, the correct treatment method consists of activating Qi circulation and promoting diuresis. The representative formula is *Wu Pi San* (**Five-Peel Powder**), which combines Poria peel, Cortex Mori Radicis and ginger peel with Pericarpium Arecae and Pericarpium Citri Reticulatae to activate Qi in order to activate fluid circulation.

— When the Bladder's function of controlling urine is impaired, causing retention of Water in the Lower Burner with symptoms of oedema and dysuria, the correct treatment method consists of strengthening Qi and promoting diuresis. The representative formula is *Wu Ling San* (**Five 'Ling' Powder**), which combines Rhizoma Alismatis, Polyporus Umbellatus, Poria and Rhizoma Atractylodis Macrocephalae with Ramulus Cinnamomi or Cortex Cinnamomi to strengthen the Bladder's function of controlling urine.

— If Water and Dampness turn to Heat which damages Yin, giving rise to symptoms of dysuria, fever and thirst, the correct treatment method consists of clearing Heat, nourishing Yin and promoting diuresis. The representative formula is *Zhu Ling Tang* (**Polyporus Decoction**), which combines Polyporus Umbellatus, Poria and Rhizoma Alismatis with Colla Corii Asini and Talcum to drain Dampness, clear Heat and nourish Yin simultaneously.

4. Formulae that warm and expel Water and Dampness

— Formulae that warm and expel Water and Dampness act to warm Yang, disperse Cold and drain Dampness through urination. They are indicated for patterns of transformation of Dampness into Cold and patterns of Spleen and Kidney Yang Deficiency with

impairment of transportation and transformation of fluids. Symptoms include oedema, urinary disturbance and turbid urine.
— Patterns of Cold Damp are characterized by Internal Cold, retention of Water and Dampness in the Interior, and Spleen and Kidney Yang Deficiency. Pathogenic Cold cannot be eliminated without warming; Water and Dampness cannot be eliminated without diuresis; and Spleen and Kidney Yang Deficiency cannot be rectified without tonification.
— Patterns of Cold Damp are therefore treated by combining the methods of warming and invigorating the Spleen and Kidneys with the methods of dispelling Cold and activating fluid circulation. Formulae include:

  - herbs that warm Yang and disperse Cold, such as Ramulus Cinnamomi, Radix Aconiti Praeparata and Rhizoma Zingiberis
  - herbs that drain Dampness, such as Polyporus Umbellatus, Poria and Rhizoma Alismatis
  - herbs that invigorate the Spleen and benefit Qi, such as Radix Codonopsis Pilosulae, Rhizoma Atractylodis Macrocephalae and Radix Glycyrrhizae.

— The representative formulae include *Ling Gui Zhu Gan Tang* (**Poria–Ramulus Cinnamomi–Atractylodes–Glycyrrhiza Decoction**) and *Zhen Wu Tang* (**True Warrior Decoction**). The former is more effective in warming Yang and resolving retained fluid; it is thus indicated for retention of Phlegm and fluid with symptoms of palpitations, dizziness and vertigo, cough and dyspnoea. The latter is more effective in warming the Kidneys and promoting diuresis; it is thus indicated for oedema due to Kidney Yang Deficiency.
— Retention of Cold-Damp in the Interior obstructs the circulation of Qi, giving rise to abdominal distension. Invasion of the lower body by Dampness affects the channels and collaterals, causing the ankles to swell. Urinary disturbance with turbid urine is related to Kidney Deficiency. When there is Qi stagnation, one should activate the Qi; when there is Kidney Deficiency, one should astringe in order to tonify the Kidneys; when the channels and collaterals are invaded by Dampness, one should relax the tendons and

remove obstruction from the collaterals. Herbs that activate Qi, eliminate Dampness and relax the tendons, or tonify and astringe the Kidneys, are therefore added to formulae for these patterns. The representative formulae are:
  - *Shi Pi San* (**Strengthening the Spleen Decoction**), which uses Radix Aucklandiae, Cortex Magnoliae Officinalis, Semen Arecae and Fructus Tsaoko
  - *Ji Ming San* (**Powder to Take at Cock's Crow**), which uses Fructus Chaenomelis and Semen Arecae

and
  - *Bei Xie Fen Qing Yin* (**Dioscorea Hypoglauca Decoction to Separate the Clear**), which uses Fructus Alpiniae Oxyphyllae and Radix Linderae.

5. Formulae that expel Wind-Damp

— Formulae that expel Wind-Damp treat Bi syndromes and relieve pain. They are indicated for invasion of the muscles, channels and collaterals, tendons, bones and joints by Wind-Damp; symptoms include aversion to cold, fever, a heavy sensation and pain in the head and body, lumbago, pain in the knees and numbness.
— Disorders of Wind-Damp vary in location and complications and the selection of herbs will vary accordingly.
— If the upper body (i.e. the head, face and muscles) are affected, giving rise to pain in the head, shoulders and back, or if there is fever and aversion to cold, herbs such as Rhizoma seu Radix Notopterygii, Radix Ledebouriellae, Rhizoma Ligustici Chuanxiong and Radix Angelicae Dahuricae are selected.
— If the lower body (i.e. the lower back, knees and ankles) are affected, with symptoms of lumbago, pain in the knees and reduced mobility of joints, herbs such as Radix Angelicae Pubescentis, Radix Stephaniae Tetrandrae and Fructus Chaenomelis are chosen.
— *Qiang Huo Sheng Shi Tang* (**Notopterygium Dispelling Dampness Decoction**) is a commonly used formula for the treatment of invasion by external Wind-Damp. In this formula, Rhizoma seu Radix Notopterygii and Radix Angelicae Pubescentis are the Emperor herbs, to disperse Wind-Damp from all parts of the body. Radix

Ledebouriellae and Rhizoma Ligustici are the Minister, to relieve headache by expelling Wind-Damp; Rhizoma Ligustici Chuanxiong and Fructus Viticis are the Assistant, to eliminate Wind and relieve pain; and Radix Glycyrrhizae is the Messenger, to harmonize the ingredients of the formula. The overall formula promotes diaphoresis, expels Dampness and relieves pain.

— Chronic painful joints due to invasion by Wind-Damp often affect the Liver and Kidneys, giving rise to Qi and Blood Deficiency. Herbs that nourish Blood, activate Blood circulation, tonify Qi, invigorate the Spleen and tonify the Liver and Kidneys are therefore added. The representative formula is *Du Huo Ji Sheng Tang* (**Angelica Pubescens–Loranthus Decoction**).

C. POINTS TO REMEMBER IN FORMULATING PRESCRIPTIONS TO EXPEL DAMPNESS

1. Patterns of Dampness vary in location and according to the Zang Fu affected and treatment must be adapted to the actual condition of the patient. Pathological conditions will be aggravated if Dampness affects the Exterior but the Interior is treated, or if Dampness affects the upper body but the lower body is treated, or if the Spleen is affected but the Kidney is treated.
2. Pathogenic Dampness in the body may turn to Cold or Heat; it may combine with other pathogenic factors to form Cold-Damp, Damp-Heat, Summer Heat-Damp or Wind-Damp.
— If Dampness turns to Cold, the correct treatment method consists of warming and resolving Dampness. If Dampness turns to Heat, the correct treatment method consists of clearing Heat and expelling Dampness. If pathogenic Dampness combines with pathogenic Wind, the treatment method consists of eliminating Wind-Damp. If pathogenic Dampness combines with Summer Heat, the treatment method consists of clearing Summer Heat and eliminating Dampness. If exterior symptoms are present, they must be addressed as well.
3. Dampness is a Yin pathogen and tends to damage Yang Qi. Excessive use of bitter, dry

and warm herbs also damages Body Fluids and consumes Yin.

— Excessive use of bitter and cold herbs to clear Damp-Heat damages not only Yin but also Yang Qi. If Yang Qi is damaged, pathogenic Dampness will persist. If Yin is consumed, Dampness will turn to Heat.
— The method of clearing Damp-Heat will further damage Yin; the method of nourishing Yin will then aggravate Dampness.
— Attention should therefore be given to protecting Qi and Yin when using formulae that expel Dampness.

D. A COMPARISON OF COMMONLY USED FORMULAE THAT EXPEL DAMPNESS (TABLE 34.1)

1. – *Huo Xiang Zheng Qi San*
   Agastache Upright Qi Powder
   – *Ping Wei San*
   Balancing the Stomach Powder

— Both formulae dry Dampness, activate Qi and harmonize the Stomach; they are thus indicated for retention of Dampness in the Middle Burner with symptoms of distension and fullness in the epigastrium and abdomen, and abdominal pain.
— **Agastache Upright Qi Powder** is more effective in activating Qi and resolving Dampness as it combines Herba Agastachis with Rhizoma Pinelliae, Cortex Magnoliae Officinalis, Pericarpium Citri Reticulatae, Pericarpium Arecae and Poria. It also Releases the Exterior and disperses Cold with Folium Perillae and Radix Angelicae Dahuricae.
— **Balancing the Stomach Powder** is more effective in drying Dampness and invigorating the Spleen as it combines a large dose of Rhizoma Atractylodis with Cortex Magnoliae Officinalis and Pericarpium Citri Reticulatae. It does not Release the Exterior.
— The first formula is thus indicated for invasion of external Wind-Cold complicated with retention of interior Dampness; the second is indicated for Dampness invading the Spleen and Stomach with stagnation of Qi.

2. – *Gan Lu Xiao Du Dan*
   Sweet Dew Special Pill to Eliminate Toxin

Table 34.1 Comparison of formulae that expel Dampness

Formula	Actions	Indications
Agastache Upright Qi Powder	Activates Qi Resolves Damp Releases the Exterior and disperses Cold	Invasion of Wind-Cold complicated with Interior Damp
Balancing the Stomach Powder	Dries Damp Invigorates the Spleen	Damp invading the Spleen and Stomach with stagnation of Qi
Sweet Dew Special Pill to Eliminate Toxin	Clears Heat and Fire Poison Expels Damp	Febrile disease due to invasion of Damp and Heat in equal degrees
Three-Nut Decoction	Regulates Qi Resolves Damp Heat	Invasion of Damp-Heat, with more Damp than Heat
Five 'Ling' Powder	Invigorates Qi and Yang Invigorates the Spleen Promotes diuresis	Dysuria due to impairment of the Bladder's control of urine
Polyporus Decoction	Clears Heat Promotes diuresis Nourishes Yin	Dysuria due to combination of Water and Heat, complicated with Yin Deficiency

- *San Ren Tang*
  Three-Nut Decoction

— Both formulae clear Heat and expel Dampness with Talcum and Fructus Amomi Cardamomi and are indicated for pathogenic Damp-Heat at the Qi level.
— **Sweet Dew Special Pill to Eliminate Toxin** contains more bitter and cold herbs that eliminate Heat, Dampness and Fire Poison, e.g. large doses of Herba Artemisiae Scopariae and Radix Scutellariae combined with Fructus Forsythiae and Herba Menthae.
— **Three-Nut Decoction** contains more pungent and dry herbs that resolve Dampness and regulate Qi. In this formula, Semen Armeniacae Amarum and Semen Coicis are combined with Rhizoma Pinelliae, Cortex Magnoliae Officinalis, Herba Lophatheri and Medulla Tetrapanacis to regulate Qi and drain Dampness through urination.
— The first formula effectively clears Heat and Fire Poison, expels Dampness and resolves turbidity. The second promotes the smooth circulation of Qi and clears Damp-Heat; it is more effective in resolving Dampness and regulating Qi.
— **Sweet Dew Special Pill to Eliminate Toxin** is indicated for febrile disease due to invasion of seasonal pathogenic Damp-Heat; in this pattern, Dampness and Heat are of equal severity. **Three-Nut Decoction** is indicated for the early stages of patterns of Damp-Heat, when Dampness is more pronounced than Heat. The key to their differentiation is the relative severity of Dampness and Heat.

3. — *Wu Ling San*
  Five 'Ling' Powder
  - *Zhu Ling Tang*
  Polyporus Decoction

— Both formulae promote diuresis to drain Dampness and are indicated for Internal Water and Dampness with dysuria.
— **Five 'Ling' Powder** treats dysuria due to impairment of the Bladder's function of controlling urine, with retention of Water in the Lower Burner. In this formula, Rhizoma Alismatis, Polyporus Umbellatus and Poria are combined with Ramulus Cinnamomi to invigorate Yang and produce Qi, and Rhizoma Atractylodis is added to invigorate the Spleen and promote diuresis.
— **Polyporus Decoction** treats dysuria due to combined Water and Heat, complicated with Yin Deficiency. In this formula, Poria, Polyporus Umbellatus and Rhizoma Alismatis are combined with Talcum to clear Heat and relieve urinary disturbance, and Colla Corii Asini is added to nourish Yin and moisten dryness.
— The first formula is indicated for dysuria with clear urine, fullness in the lower

abdomen but no pain on urination, and a pale tongue with white coating. The second formula is indicated for dysuria with deep-yellow urine, burning pain on urination, restlessness, insomnia and a red tongue with scanty coating.

Questions

1. Why are herbs that activate Qi circulation added to formulae that dry Dampness and harmonize the Stomach?
2. How do **Three-Nut Decoction** and **Sweet Dew Special Pill to Eliminate Toxin** differ in their actions and indications?

Formulae that eliminate Phlegm **35**

A. GUIDING PRINCIPLES IN FORMULATING PRESCRIPTIONS TO ELIMINATE PHLEGM

— Phlegm is a pathological product of the body, arising from a dysfunction of the Zang Fu, particularly the Spleen and the Lungs. There is a saying, 'The Spleen produces Phlegm and the Lungs store it.'
— Before deciding upon a treatment method and selecting a formula to treat a Phlegm pattern, it is important to clarify the nature of the pattern.
— Phlegm is Biao, i.e. a symptom, not the Ben of disease. The book *Complete Collection of Jin Yue's Treatises* says, 'Good doctors treat the source of Phlegm.' One must not only eliminate Phlegm but also treat the source of Phlegm.
— Phlegm tends to move with Qi, affecting various parts of the body including the chest, diaphragm, intestines, stomach, channels and collaterals, and the four limbs. Stagnation of Qi causes accumulation of Phlegm and smooth circulation of Qi is necessary in order to eliminate Phlegm. Herbs that regulate Qi must therefore be included in formulae that eliminate Phlegm.
— In addition, the organs involved in Phlegm patterns must be treated, e.g. the Spleen must be invigorated, the Lungs regulated and the Kidneys tonified.

B. TYPES OF FORMULA THAT ELIMINATE PHLEGM

1. Formulae that dry Dampness and resolve Phlegm

— Formulae that dry Dampness and resolve Phlegm consist primarily of bitter, warm and dry herbs that eliminate Phlegm. Such formulae dry Dampness, invigorate the Spleen, resolve Phlegm and regulate Qi. They are indicated for Phlegm-Damp patterns.
— Patterns of Phlegm-Damp are caused by impairment of the Spleen's function of transportation and transformation, leading to retention of Turbid Damp. They are characterized by cough with profuse white sputum which is easy to expectorate, stuffiness of the chest, poor appetite and a slippery or sticky white tongue coating.
— Rhizoma Pinelliae and Rhizoma Arisaematis are often used as the main herbs in these formulae; they are combined with herbs that expel Dampness and invigorate the Spleen, such as Poria and Rhizoma Atractylodis Macrocephalae, to treat the source of Phlegm.
— Because retention of Phlegm leads to stagnation of Qi, herbs that activate Qi, such as Pericarpium Citri Reticulatae, Fructus Aurantii and Fructus Aurantii Immaturus, are often added. Examples include the use of Pericarpium Citri Reticulatae in *Er Chen Tang* (**Two Old Decoction**) and the use of Pericarpium Citri Reticulatae and Fructus Aurantii Immaturus in *Wen Dan Tang* (**Warming the Gall Bladder Decoction**).
— If Phlegm production is due to Spleen Deficiency, herbs that tonify Qi and invigorate the Spleen should be added, e.g. Radix Codonopsis Pilosulae, Rhizoma Atractylodis Macrocephalae and treated Radix Glycyrrhizae in *Liu Jun Zi Tang* (**Six Gentlemen Decoction**).

2. Formulae that clear Heat and resolve Phlegm

— These formulae consist primarily of herbs that clear Heat and herbs that resolve Phlegm. They eliminate Turbid Phlegm and clear Internal Heat, and are indicated for Phlegm-Heat patterns.

— Patterns of Phlegm-Heat are caused by Internal Heat acting on the Lungs to condense Body Fluids into Phlegm. Symptoms include cough with thick sticky yellow sputum which is difficult to expectorate, a red tongue with sticky yellow coating and a rolling rapid pulse.

— These formulae consist of a combination of:

  – herbs that clear Heat and resolve Phlegm, such as Fructus Trichosanthis, Radix Platycodi, Arisaemae cum Felle Bovis, Bulbus Fritillariae and Chlorite-schist
  and
  – herbs that clear Heat, such as Radix Scutellariae, Rhizoma Coptidis, Fructus Gardeniae and Flos Lonicerae.

— The representative formula is *Qing Qi Hua Tan Wan* (**Clearing Heat–Resolving Phlegm Decoction**), in which herbs that activate Qi circulation (Fructus Aurantii Immaturus and Pericarpium Citri Reticulatae) are combined with Poria, which drains Dampness and invigorates the Spleen.

— Phlegm-Heat patterns tend to be complicated. In addition to cough with sticky yellow sputum, they may present with other symptoms, such as an accumulation of pathogens in the chest. In this event the treatment method consists of using pungent herbs to open the chest, combined with bitter herbs to send Rebellious Qi downward, resolve Phlegm and disperse masses. The representative formula is *Xiao Xian Xiong Tang* (**Small Sinking Chest Decoction**), in which Rhizoma Pinelliae is combined with Herba Trichosanthis and Rhizoma Coptidis.

— If Phlegm and Heat cloud the Mind they may produce manic-depressive disorders; if they disturb the Heart they may produce palpitations and insomnia. The representative formula for this pattern is *Meng Shi Gun Tan Wan* (**Chlorite–Schist Pill for Chronic Phlegm Syndromes**), in which Chlorite-schist and Nitrum are combined with Radix et Rhizoma Rhei, Radix Scutellariae and Lignum Aquilariae Resinatum.

3. Formulae that warm and resolve Phlegm-Fluid

— These formulae consist primarily of herbs that eliminate Phlegm and herbs that warm the Interior. They resolve Phlegm and retained Fluid, warm the Interior and disperse Cold, and are indicated for patterns of Cold-Phlegm with retained Fluid.

— Patterns of Phlegm-Fluid are marked by cough with clear watery sputum, dyspnoea, recurrent acute episodes provoked by exposure to cold, a pale tongue with a slippery white coating and a deep slow pulse. Such patterns affect the Spleen and Stomach primarily and the Kidneys secondarily.

— The pathogenesis is Spleen Yang Deficiency with retention of Internal Cold and Fluid, or retention of Cold and Fluid in the Lung; it is sometimes also related to Kidney Yang Deficiency. In any event, the Lungs are always involved.

— The book *Synopsis of the Golden Cabinet* says, 'In the treatment of retention of Phlegm and Fluid, warm herbs are used to mediate the condition.' Formulae that treat Phlegm-Fluid consist of:

  – herbs that warm the Lungs and Spleen, such as Rhizoma Zingiberis, Herba Asari, and Ramulus Cinnamomi
  – herbs that dry Dampness and resolve Phlegm, such as Rhizoma Pinelliae and Semen Sinapis Albae
  and
  – herbs that invigorate the Spleen and resolve Dampness, such as Poria and Rhizoma Atractylodis Macrocephalae.

— The representative formulae are *Ling Gui Zhu Gan Tang* (**Poria–Ramulus Cinnamomi–Atractylodes–Glycyrrhiza Decoction**) and *Ling Gan Wu Wei Jiang Xin Tang* (**Poria-Glycyrrhiza–Schisandra–Zingiber–Asarum Decoction**).

— If Food Retention, or impairment of transportation and transformation, give rise to poor appetite and abdominal distension, herbs that promote digestion and invigorate the Stomach should be added. An example is *San Zi Yang Qin Tang* (**Three-Seed Nourishing Parents Decoction**), which employs Fructus Perillae and Semen Sinapis Albae to resolve Phlegm and soothe asthma and Semen Raphani to promote digestion and relieve stagnation. When Qi circulates smoothly, Phlegm and Retained Food are resolved and cough and asthma will disappear spontaneously.

4. Formulae that moisten dryness and resolve Phlegm

— Formulae that moisten dryness and resolve Phlegm consist of herbs that clear Heat and resolve Phlegm, and herbs that nourish Yin and moisten the Lungs. Such formulae moisten the Lungs, resolve Phlegm, nourish Yin and promote Body Fluids. They are indicated for patterns of Dry-Phlegm.

— Patterns of Dry-Phlegm primarily involve the Lungs. The pathogenesis is invasion of the Lungs by Dryness and Heat, which cause Body Fluids to condense into Phlegm. Symptoms include thick sticky sputum which is difficult to expectorate, and Lung Yin Deficiency with dry throat, choking cough and hoarse voice. To treat such patterns, Lung Dryness should be moistened, Phlegm should be resolved and pathogenic Heat should be cleared. Formulae that treat Dry-Phlegm therefore consist of:

  – herbs that nourish Yin and moisten the Lungs, such as Radix Adenophorae, Radix Ophiopogonis, Radix Asparagi and Bulbus Lilii

  and

  – herbs that clear Heat and resolve Phlegm, such as Bulbus Fritillariae, Fructus Trichosanthis, Radix Platycodi and Succus Bambusae.

— The representative formula is *Bei Mu Gua Lou San* (**Fritillaria–Trichosanthes Powder**), which uses Bulbus Fritillariae, Fructus Trichosanthis, Radix Platycodi and Radix Trichosanthis to moisten dryness and resolve Phlegm, and Exocarpium Citri Grandis and Poria to regulate Qi and resolve Phlegm. When the Lungs' function of descending is restored, dry cough and sputum will be relieved.

— However, patterns of Dry Phlegm can also be caused by invasion of External Heat and Dryness damaging Lung Yin, or by Empty Fire due to Lung and Kidney Yin Deficiency which condenses Body Fluids into Phlegm.

— If Phlegm is due to damage by External Heat and Dryness, herbs that promote the Lungs' dispersing function and eliminate pathogenic Dryness should be added. The representative formula is *Sang Xing Tang* (**Mulberry Leaf and Apricot Kernel Decoction**), which includes Folium Mori and Semen Sojae Praeparata to promote the Lungs' function of dispersing and eliminate pathogenic Dryness; Semen Armeniacae Amarum and Bulbus Fritillariae Thunbergii to stop cough and resolve Phlegm; Radix Adenophorae and pear peel to promote Body Fluids and moisten dryness; and Fructus Gardeniae to clear Lung Heat.

— If Phlegm is due to Empty Fire arising from Lung and Kidney Yin Deficiency, herbs that nourish Yin and clear Fire should be added. The representative formula is *Bai He Gu Jin Tang* (**Lily Bulb Decoction to Preserve the Metal**), which includes Radix Rehmanniae, Radix Rehmanniae Praeparata, Radix Ophiopogonis, Bulbus Lilii, Radix Scrophulariae, Radix Paeoniae Alba and Radix Angelicae Sinensis to nourish Yin and clear Heat; and Radix Platycodi and Bulbus Fritillariae to clear Heat and resolve Phlegm.

— When the Lungs and Kidneys are nourished, Empty Fire is reduced and Phlegm-Heat is resolved, patterns of Dry Phlegm will resolve spontaneously.

5. Formulae to expel Wind and resolve Phlegm

— Formulae that expel Wind and resolve Phlegm consist primarily of herbs that expel Phlegm and herbs that subdue Wind. They are indicated for patterns of Wind-Phlegm.

— Because Phlegm follows the movement of Qi and the smooth circulation of Qi resolves Phlegm, herbs that regulate Qi must be included in such formulae.

— Wind-Phlegm patterns are related not only to the Liver but also to the Spleen. If Wind-Phlegm disturbs the clear Yang, giving rise to dizziness, vertigo and headache, further additions must be made:

  – herbs that dry Dampness and resolve Phlegm, such as Rhizoma Pinelliae
  – herbs that invigorate the Spleen and eliminate Dampness, such as Rhizoma Atractylodis Macrocephalae and Poria

  and

  – herbs that subdue Wind, such as Rhizoma Gastrodiae.

— The representative formula is *Ban Xia Bai Zhu Tian Ma Tang* (**Pinellia–Atractylodes–Gastrodia Decoction**).

— If Internal Phlegm-Heat stirs up Liver Wind

and clouds the Mind, producing symptoms of epilepsy, the formula must include:

- herbs that clear Heat and resolve Phlegm, such as Bulbus Fritillariae, Arisaemae cum Felle Bovis and Succus Bambusae
- herbs that subdue Wind, such as Rhizoma Gastrodiae, Scorpio and Bombyx Batryticatus
- herbs that clear Heat such as Rhizoma Coptidis and Radix Ophiopogonis

and

- herbs that open the orifices and calm the Mind, such as Rhizoma Acori Graminei, Radix Curcumae, Radix Polygalae, Cinnabaris and Succinum.

— The representative formula is *Ding Xian Wan* (**Arrest Seizures Pill**).

C. POINTS TO REMEMBER IN FORMULATING PRESCRIPTIONS TO EXPEL PHLEGM

1. Phlegm is the result of an accumulation of Body Fluids. Qi is the motive force in the circulation of Body Fluids. The formation of Phlegm is thus often related to disorders of Qi, and Qi must be regulated in order to treat Phlegm patterns.
   — The production of Phlegm is also related to the Lungs, Spleen and Kidneys. Dysfunction of the Lungs in dispersing, descending and regulating the Waterways, dysfunction of the Spleen in transportation and transformation of Water and Dampness, and dysfunction of the Kidneys in dominating water metabolism can all lead to retarded circulation of Water and Dampness and Phlegm will be produced as a consequence.
   — In formulating prescriptions to eliminate Phlegm, attention must therefore be given to regulating Qi and to the functions of the Lungs, Spleen and Kidneys.
2. Phlegm easily combines with Cold, Heat, Dampness, Dryness and Wind. As a rule, Phlegm is the Biao of the disease, while the cause of Phlegm is the Ben. Formulae that eliminate Phlegm often treat Biao and Ben simultaneously, with emphasis on the Ben.
   — When the causes of Phlegm are resolved, the Phlegm itself will resolve. Focusing on the Phlegm itself in the treatment yields poor results.

— However, herbs that expel Phlegm differ in nature; they may be warm, dry, cool or moist. It is essential to identify the nature of the Phlegm in formulating prescriptions to expel Phlegm.

D. A COMPARISON OF COMMONLY-USED FORMULAE THAT ELIMINATE PHLEGM (TABLE 35.1)

1. – *Er Chen Tang*
   Two Old Decoction
   – *Bei Mu Gua Lou Tang*
   Fritillaria–Trichosanthes Powder

— Both formulae contain Pericarpium Citri Reticulatae and Poria to regulate Qi, expel Dampness and resolve Phlegm; both are indicated for Phlegm patterns.
— **Two Old Decoction** is a representative formula for patterns of Phlegm-Damp. In addition to Pericarpium Citri Reticulatae and Poria, it features Rhizoma Pinelliae as the Emperor herb to dry Dampness, resolve Phlegm and conduct Rebellious Qi downward to stop vomiting; Radix Glycyrrhizae is included as the Messenger herb, and to invigorate the Spleen and harmonize the Middle Burner. The whole formula dries Dampness, resolves Phlegm, regulates Qi and harmonizes the Middle Burner. It is indicated for patterns of Phlegm-Damp with symptoms of cough with profuse thin sputum, distension and fullness of the chest and diaphragm, nausea, vomiting, dizziness, palpitations and a pale tongue with a slippery white coating.
— **Fritillaria–Trichosanthes Powder** is a representative formula for patterns of Dry Phlegm. In addition to Pericarpium Citri Reticulatae and Poria, it features Bulbus Fritillariae as the Emperor herb. It also contains Fructus Trichosanthis and Radix Platycodi to clear Heat, resolve Phlegm, moisten the Lungs and stop cough, and Radix Trichosanthis to promote Body Fluids and moisten dryness.
— The whole formula moistens dryness, resolves Phlegm, regulates Qi and stops cough. It is indicated for Phlegm patterns due to Lung Dryness with symptoms of a choking cough with difficult expectoration, a dry sore throat, thirst, dry lips and a thin, dry, white tongue coating.

Table 35.1 Comparison of formulae that eliminate Phlegm

Formula	Actions	Indications
Two-Old Decoction	Dries Damp Resolves Phlegm Regulates Qi and harmonizes the Middle Burner	Patterns of Phlegm-Damp
Fritillaria–Trichosanthes Powder	Moistens dryness Resolves Phlegm Regulates Qi and stops cough	Phlegm patterns due to Lung Dryness
Poria–Glycyrrhiza–Schisandra–Zingiber–Asarum Decoction	Warms the Lungs to resolve retained Fluid Invigorates the Spleen and drains Damp	Patterns of Phlegm-Fluid
Small Green Dragon Decoction	Releases the Exterior and disperses Cold Dries Damp and resolves Phlegm Harmonizes Nutritive and Defensive Qi	Invasion of Wind-Cold complicated with retention of fluid
Chlorite–Schist Pill for Chronic Phlegm Patterns	Clears Fire Expels long-standing Phlegm	Phlegm-Heat patterns, especially affecting the Mind
Clearing Qi – Resolving Phlegm Decoction	Clears Heat Resolves Phlegm Regulates Lung Qi	Internal Heat and Phlegm (cough with thick yellow sputum)

2. – *Ling Gan Wu Wei Jiang Xin Tang*
   Poria–Glycyrrhiza–Schisandra-Zingiber –Asarum Decoction
   – *Xiao Qing Long Tang*
   Small Green Dragon Decoction

— Both formulae use Rhizoma Zingiberis, Herba Asari, Fructus Schisandrae and Radix Glycyrrhizae to warm the Lungs and resolve retained Fluids. Both are indicated for retention of Cold in the Lungs with symptoms of cough, profuse sputum and dyspnoea.

— **Poria–Glycyrrhiza–Schisandra–Zingiber –Asarum Decoction** is more effective in warming the Lungs and resolving retained Fluids; it is thus indicated for patterns of Phlegm-Fluid with symptoms of cough with occasional expectoration of thin sputum, fullness in the chest, dyspnoea, a slippery white tongue coating and a deep slow pulse. Poria is used in this formula to invigorate the Spleen and drain Dampness.

— **Small Green Dragon Decoction** is also effective in Releasing the Exterior and dispersing Cold and is thus indicated for invasion by External Wind-Cold compli-cated with retention of fluid. Symptoms include aversion to cold, fever, absence of sweating, cough, dyspnoea, profuse thin sputum, a moist and slippery tongue coating and a tense superficial pulse. This formula also contains Herba Ephedrae and Ramulus Cinnamomi, to Release the Exterior and promote the Lungs' dispersing function; Rhizoma Pinelliae to dry Dampness and resolve Phlegm; and Radix Paeoniae Alba to nourish Blood and astringe Yin; in combination with Ramulus Cinnamomi it harmonizes Nutritive and Defensive Qi.

3. – *Mang Shi Gun Tan Wan*
   Chlorite-Schist Pill for Chronic Phlegm Patterns
   – *Qing Qi Hua Tan Wan*
   Clearing Qi–Resolving Phlegm Decoction

— Both formulae contain Radix Scutellariae to clear Fire in the Upper Burner; both are indicated for Phlegm-Heat patterns.

— **Chlorite–Schist Pill for Chronic Phlegm Patterns** is aimed at treating Internal Heat and long-standing retained Phlegm. In this formula, Chlorite-schist and Natrium are calcined to expel long-standing Phlegm; Radix et Rhizoma Rhei relieves substantial stagnation and, together with Radix Scutellariae, treats the source of Phlegm; Lignum Aquilariae Resinatum regulates Qi to assist in resolving Phlegm.

— The whole formula clears Fire and expels Phlegm and is thus indicated for patterns of Heat and Phlegm with symptoms of manic and depressive mental disorders, palpitations, coma, cough with profuse thin sputum, dyspnoea, stuffiness of the chest, dizziness and vertigo.

— **Clearing Qi–Resolving Phlegm Decoction** is a representative formula for Phlegm-Heat patterns. This formula contains Radix Scutellariae, Arisaemae cum Felle Bovis and Fructus Trichosanthis to clear Heat and resolve Phlegm; Fructus Aurantii Immaturus and Pericarpium Citri Reticulatae to circulate Qi in order to resolve Phlegm; Poria to drain Dampness and invigorate the Spleen; Semen Armeniacae Amarum to send Qi downward and stop cough; and Rhizoma Pinelliae to resolve Phlegm and conduct Rebellious Qi downward.

— The whole formula clears Heat, resolves Phlegm, regulates Qi and stops cough. It is indicated for Internal Heat and Phlegm with symptoms of cough with thick sticky yellow sputum, distress and fullness in the chest and epigastrium, dyspnoea, nausea, deep-yellow urine, a sticky yellow tongue coating and a rolling rapid pulse.

Questions

1. Why are herbs that regulate Qi added to formulae that expel Phlegm? Give an illustrative example.
2. Compare and contrast formulae for clearing Heat and resolving Phlegm, and formulae for moistening Dryness and resolving Phlegm.

Formulae that expel Wind 36

A. GUIDING PRINCIPLES FOR FORMULATING PRESCRIPTIONS TO EXPEL WIND

— In treating patterns involving Wind, it is necessary at the outset to determine whether Wind is external or internal, whether it is complicated with Cold or Heat and whether it is due to Excess or Deficiency.

— In cases of External Wind, the treatment method consists of dispersing it with pungent herbs; in cases of Internal Wind, the treatment method consists of subduing it.

— If pathogenic Wind is complicated with Cold, Dampness, Heat, Phlegm or Stagnant Blood, the treatment method must include eliminating these additional pathogenic factors.

— In cases of mixed Excess and Deficiency, the method of promoting Upright Qi is combined with the method of eliminating pathogenic factors in order to treat both Biao and Ben.

— External and Internal Wind may influence each other. External Wind may induce Internal Wind; Internal Wind may be complicated with External Wind. In the treatment of such complicated conditions, first priority is given to the predominating pattern, while still considering the secondary pattern in the formulation of a prescription.

B. TYPES OF FORMULA THAT EXPEL WIND

1. Formulae that disperse External Wind

— Formulae that disperse External Wind consist primarily of herbs that expel Wind, relieve itching and pain and expel Dampness.

— Patterns of External Wind are caused by a weakness of Defensive Qi complicated with invasion of pathogenic Wind. These patterns differ from Wind patterns such as the common cold, which are the result of invasion of the skin and hair by pathogenic Wind and present with mainly exterior symptoms; such patterns can be relieved by herbs that Release the Exterior.

— In the External Wind patterns discussed here, Defensive Qi is weak and pathogenic Wind invades deeper layers of the body such as the head, face, muscles, channels and collaterals, joints, tendons and bones, giving rise to more severe pathological conditions. Commonly used herbs that eliminate External Wind include Rhizoma Ligustici Chuanxiong, Rhizoma seu Radix Notopterygii, Radix Ledebouriellae, Radix Angelicae Dahuricae, Herba Schizonepetae, Rhizoma Typhonii and Radix Gentianae Macrophyllae.

— Wind tends to combine with other pathogenic factors. For invasion of External Wind-Cold with symptoms of headache, *Chuan Xiong Cha Tiao San* (**Ligusticum–Green Tea Regulating Powder**) is a representative formula. Rhizoma Ligustici Chuanxiong, Radix Angelicae Dahuricae and Rhizoma seu Radix Notopterygii are jointly the Emperor herbs; these are combined with Herba Schizonepeta and Radix Ledebouriellae to expel Wind and relieve pain; Herba Asari to disperse Cold and relieve pain; Herba Menthae to clear Heat from the head and eyes; and treated Radix Glycyrrhizae to harmonize all the ingredients of the formula.

— If External Wind is complicated with Damp-Heat, herbs that expel Dampness and clear Heat should be added. An example is *Xiao Feng San* (**Eliminate Wind Powder**), in which Herba Schizonepeta, Radix

Ledebouriellae, Fructus Arctii and Periostracum Cicadae are jointly the Emperor herbs, to expel Wind and Release the Exterior; these are combined with Rhizoma Atractylodis, to expel Wind and dry Dampness; Radix Sophorae Flavescentis, to clear Heat and dry Dampness; Caulis Akebiae to drain Damp-Heat through the urine; and Rhizoma Anemarrhenae and Gypsum Fibrosum to clear Heat and Fire. This formula is commonly used in the treatment of rubella and eczema.

— Invasion of the channels and collaterals by pathogenic Wind retards the circulation of Qi, Blood and Body Fluids, resulting in stagnation of Blood and the formation of Phlegm-Damp. When this occurs it is even more difficult to expel Wind, and herbs that activate Blood and relieve pain must be added. There is a saying, 'To treat Wind, treat Blood first. Smooth circulation of Blood extinguishes Wind.'

— The representative formula for this pattern is *Xiao Huo Luo Dan* (**Minor Invigorate the Collaterals Special Pill**), which contains Resina Olibani and Resina Myrrhae.

— If pathogenic Wind combines with Phlegm-Damp to obstruct the channels and collaterals, it may produce deviation of the mouth and eye. In this event, herbs that expel Wind and resolve Phlegm such as Rhizoma Arisaematis and Rhizoma Typhonii should be added. The representative formula is *Qian Zheng San* (**Lead to Symmetry Powder**).

2. Formulae that subdue Internal Wind

— Formulae that subdue Internal Wind consist primarily of herbs that pacify Liver Wind; they may also contain herbs that nourish Yin and Blood. Such formulae subdue Wind and stop convulsions.

— Patterns of Internal Wind are caused by Liver Wind, which may originate from Liver Yang Rising, extreme Heat producing Wind, or Blood Deficiency giving rise to Wind. Symptoms include dizziness, vertigo, tremor, slurred speech, motor impairment, fits, loss of consciousness, deviation of the mouth and eye, and hemiplegia. The methods of treatment vary according to the cause of the condition.

a. Formulae that suppress Liver Yang and subdue Wind

— These formulae are indicated for patterns of Liver Yang Rising with stirring of Liver Wind. They consist primarily of herbs that suppress Liver Yang, such as Concha Haliotidis, Os Draconis, Concha Ostreae and Haematitum.

— Because Liver Yang Rising is closely associated with Liver and Kidney Yin Deficiency, herbs that nourish Yin are added. An example is *Zhen Gan Xi Feng Tang* (**Pacifying the Liver and Subduing Wind Decoction**), which contains Haematitum, Os Draconis and Concha Ostreae to conduct Rebellious Qi downward, suppress hyperactive Yang and calm Liver Wind, and Plastrum Testudinis, Radix Paeoniae Alba, Radix Scrophulariae and Radix Asparagi to nourish Yin and Blood.

— If Liver Yang Rising is complicated with pronounced Internal Heat, herbs that clear Heat and quell Fire should be added to clear Heat from the Liver Channel. An example is *Tian Ma Gou Teng Yin* (**Gastrodia–Uncaria Decoction**), which contains Fructus Gardeniae and Radix Scutellariae.

b. Formulae that cool the Liver and subdue Wind

— These formulae are indicated when extreme pathogenic Heat in the Liver Channel gives rise to Wind. They consist primarily of herbs that cool the Liver and subdue Wind, such as Cornu Antelopis, Ramulus Uncariae cum Uncis, Folium Mori and Flos Chrysanthemi.

— Wind and Fire combine to consume Body Fluids; the tendons are deprived of Blood and nourishment, and this is the cause of convulsions. This condition requires the use of herbs that nourish Yin and relax the tendons, such as Radix Rehmanniae, Radix Paeoniae Alba, Radix Scrophulariae and Radix Ophiopogonis.

— *Ling Jiao Gou Teng Tang* (**Antelope Horn and Uncaria Decoction**) is a formula commonly used in the treatment of extreme Heat producing Wind. In this formula, Cornu Antelopis and Ramulus Uncariae are jointly the Emperor herbs; they are combined with Folium Mori and Flos Chrysanthemi, to cool the Liver, subdue Wind, clear Heat and stop convulsions; and Radix Rehmanniae and Radix Paeoniae Alba to nourish Yin, promote Body Fluids and relax the tendons.

— Excess Heat tends to condense Body Fluids

into Phlegm; Wind and Phlegm may then combine and move upward to worsen the condition. In this case, herbs that clear Heat and resolve Phlegm are added, such as Bulbus Fritillariae Cirrhosae and (fresh) Caulis Bambusae in Taeniam, as in Antelope Horn and Uncaria Decoction.

c. Formulae that nourish Yin and subdue Wind

— These formulae are indicated for consumption of Yin, Blood and Body Fluids in the late stage of febrile disease, with stirring of Liver Wind of the Deficient type. They consist primarily of herbs that nourish Yin and Blood and promote Body Fluids, such as Radix Rehmanniae, Radix Paeoniae Alba, Radix Ophiopogonis, Plastrum Testudinis, Colla Corii Asini and egg yolk.

— To strengthen their effect in stopping convulsion, herbs that suppress the Liver and subdue Wind are added. Examples include *E Jiao Ji Zi Huang Tang* (**Ass-Hide Gelatin and Egg Yolk Decoction**) and *Da Ding Feng Zhu* (**Major Arrest Wind Pearl**), both of which contain Colla Corii Asini, egg yolk, Radix Rehmanniae and Radix Paeoniae Alba to nourish Yin and Blood, and Concha Ostreae and Concha Haliotidis to suppress hyperactive Yang.

C. POINTS TO REMEMBER IN FORMULATING PRESCRIPTIONS THAT EXPEL WIND

1. Wind patterns tend to be complicated and to change quickly. It is essential to determine whether the Wind is external or internal, whether it is complicated with Cold, Heat, Dampness, Phlegm or Stagnant Blood and whether it is of the Deficiency or Excess type. Herbs must be selected according to the nature of the pattern.

2. In the treatment of External Wind, the treatment method consists of dispersing. In the treatment of Internal Wind, the treatment method consists of pacifying, and pungent dispersing herbs should be avoided. Pungent herbs that disperse Wind are usually warm and dry in nature and can consume Body Fluids and produce Fire. They should be used with caution where there is deficiency of Body Fluids, or Yin Deficiency with Empty Heat or hyperactive Yang.

D. A COMPARISON OF COMMONLY USED FORMULAE THAT EXPEL WIND (TABLE 36.1)

1. – *Ling Jiao Gou Teng Tang*
     Antelope Horn and Uncaria Decoction
   – *Zhen Gan Xi Feng Tang*
     Pacifying the Liver and Subduing Wind Decoction
   – *Da Ding Feng Zhu*
     Major Arrest Wind Pearl

— All three formulae pacify Internal Wind.
— Antelope Horn and Uncaria Decoction is more effective in clearing Heat, cooling the Liver and stopping convulsion. It features Cornu Antelopis and Ramulus Uncariae cum Uncis as the Emperor herbs, to clear Heat, cool the Liver, pacify Wind and stop convulsions. These are combined with Folium Mori and Flos Chrysanthemi to assist in clearing Heat and pacifying Wind.
— This formula is indicated for Wind due to excess Heat in the Liver channel, with

Table 36.1 Comparison of formulae that subdue Liver Wind

Formula	Actions	Indications
Antelope Horn and Uncaria Decoction	Clears Heat Cools the Liver Stops convulsion	Liver Wind due to extreme Heat
Pacifying the Liver and Subduing Wind Decoction	Suppresses hyperactive Yang Conducts Qi and Blood downward Pacifies Wind	Wind-Stroke due to Liver Yang Rising with Liver Wind
Major Arrest Wind Pearl	Nourishes Yin and Blood Suppresses hyperactive Yang Pacifies Wind	Deficiency-type Liver Wind due to consumption of Yin

symptoms of high fever, irritability, restlessness and convulsions.

— **Pacifying the Liver and Subduing Wind Decoction** combines Radix Achyranthis Bidentatae, which conducts Blood downward and tonifies the Liver and Kidneys, with Haematitum, Os Draconis and Concha Ostreae, which suppress Liver Yang and pacify Liver Wind. This formula is thus more effective in suppressing hyperactive Yang, conducting Rebellious Qi downward and pacifying Wind and is indicated for Wind-Stroke due to Liver Yang Rising with Liver Wind.

— **Major Arrest Wind Pearl** has as its main ingredients herbs that nourish Yin and Blood, in combination with herbs that suppress Liver Yang. It includes (among other ingredients) Colla Corii Asini, egg yolk, Radix Rehmanniae, Radix Paeoniae Alba, Radix Ophiopogonis, Plastrum Testudinis and Carapax Trionycis. This formula is thus more effective in nourishing Yin, suppressing hyperactive Yang and pacifying Wind of the deficiency type. It is indicated for stirring of Wind in the late stage of febrile disease due to extreme consumption of Yin.

Questions

1. Why do formulae that pacify Internal Wind contain herbs that nourish Yin?
2. What is the difference between formulae that cool the Liver and pacify Wind and formulae that nourish Yin and pacify Wind? Give illustrative examples.

Formulae that calm the Mind   **37**

A. GUIDING PRINCIPLES FOR FORMULATING PRESCRIPTIONS TO CALM THE MIND

— Formulae that calm the Mind are indicated for restlessness, which may be caused by fear, shock, emotional stress, pensiveness or deficiency of Qi and Blood. The Heart, Liver and Kidneys are affected, producing symptoms of palpitations, insomnia, dream-disturbed sleep, anxiety and irritability.

— Restlessness may be due to patterns of Excess or Deficiency. The Excess type is treated by the method of soothing the Heart and calming the Mind. The Deficiency type is treated by the method of nourishing the Heart and calming the Mind. In complicated cases of both Excess and Deficiency involving Heat and Phlegm, the treatment method consists of nourishing and soothing the Heart as the primary action and clearing Heat and resolving Phlegm as a secondary action. Both Biao and Ben must be treated.

B. TYPES OF FORMULA THAT CALM THE MIND

1. Formulae that soothe the Heart and calm the Mind

— These formulae consist of herbs that soothe the Heart and calm the Mind. They are indicated for restlessness of the Excess type caused by fear, shock or other emotional factors.

— If there is Empty Fire in the Heart or Liver, with signs of hyperactive Yang, herbs that clear Heat and quell Fire are added, such as Rhizoma Coptidis, Radix Rehmanniae and Cornu Antelopis. The representative formula for clearing Heat and calming the Mind is *Zhu Sha An Shen Wan* (**Cinnabar Pill to Calm the Spirit**), which contains Cinnabaris and Rhizoma Coptidis.

— If Empty Fire in the Heart and Liver consumes Yin and Blood, herbs that clear Heat are combined with herbs that nourish Yin and Blood, such as Radix Angelicae Sinensis, Radix Rehmanniae Praeparata and Radix Ophiopogonis. An example is the use of Radix Angelicae Sinensis and Radix Rehmanniae Praeparata in **Cinnabar Pill to Calm the Spirit**.

— Empty Fire in the Heart and Liver may condense Body Fluids and produce Phlegm-Fire which moves upward to cause manic and depressive mental disorders. In this case, herbs that clear Heat and resolve Phlegm are added, such as Arisaemae cum Felle Bovis, Bulbus Fritillariae Cirrhosae and bamboo fungus. The representative formula is *Sheng Tie Luo Yin* (**Iron Filings Decoction**).

2. Formulae that nourish the Heart and calm the Mind

— These formulae consist primarily of herbs that nourish the Heart and calm the Mind. They are indicated for restlessness due to deficiency of Yin, Blood and Heart Qi. The Heart dominates Blood and the Liver stores it, and deficiency of Yin and Blood deprive the Heart and Liver of nourishment. This is the most common cause of restlessness.

— For this pattern, herbs that nourish Yin and Blood are used. An example is *Tian Wang Bu Xin Dan* (**Heavenly Emperor Tonifying the Heart Pill**), which combines herbs that nourish the Heart and calm the Mind, such as Semen Ziziphi Spinosae, Semen Biotae, Poria, Radix Polygalae and Fructus Schisandrae, with herbs that nourish Yin and Blood, such as Radix Angelicae Sinensis, Radix Rehmanniae, Radix Asparagi and Radix Ophiopogonis.

— Yin and Blood Deficiency tends to produce Empty Heat, and some herbs that clear Heat should therefore be included in such prescriptions. Examples include the use of Radix Scrophulariae in **Heavenly Emperor Tonifying the Heart Pill**, and the use of Rhizoma Anemarrhenae in *Suan Zao Ren Tang* (**Sour Jujube Decoction**).

C. POINTS TO REMEMBER IN FORMULATING PRESCRIPTIONS THAT CALM THE MIND

1. Formulae that soothe the Heart and calm the Mind contain substances that are heavy and descending in their action and difficult to digest. They can only be administered for a short time.
— Some of these substances are also toxic, and should be administered with caution, especially to patients with abnormal liver and kidney function. For example, a large dosage of Cinnabaris may cause mercury poisoning.
— These substances are also hard, and it is thus more difficult to extract their active ingredients. They should be broken into pieces and cooked for some time before adding other ingredients of the formula.
2. Restlessness is often linked to emotional problems and herbal treatment should be combined with psychotherapy to achieve better therapeutic results.

D. A COMPARISON OF COMMONLY USED FORMULAE THAT CALM THE MIND (TABLE 37.1)

1. – *Zhu Sha An Shen Wan*
   Cinnabar Pill to Calm the Spirit
   – *Ci Zhu Wan*
   Magnetite and Cinnabar Pill

— In both formulae, Cinnabaris is used to soothe the Heart and calm the Mind.
— In **Cinnabar Pill to Calm the Spirit**, Cinnabaris is combined with Rhizoma Coptidis, Radix Angelicae Sinensis, Radix Rehmanniae and treated Radix Glycyrrhizae. This formula clears Heart Heat, nourishes Yin and Blood and calms the Mind. It is indicated for Heart Fire consuming Yin and Blood, with symptoms of restlessness, palpitations, insomnia, dream-disturbed sleep, a sensation of heat in the chest, a red tongue with yellow coating and a thready and rapid pulse.
— In **Magnetite and Cinnabar Pill**, Cinnabaris is combined with Magnetitum and Massa Fermentata Medicinalis. This formula harmonizes the Heart and Kidneys, improves vision and calms the Mind. It is indicated for disharmony between the Heart and Kidneys with symptoms of palpitations, insomnia, blurred vision, tinnitus and deafness.

2. – *Suan Zao Ren Tang*
   Sour Jujube Decoction

Table 37.1 Comparison of formulae that calm the Mind

Formula	Actions	Indications
Cinnabar Pill to Calm the Spirit	Clears Heart Heat Nourishes Yin and Blood Calms the Mind	Heart Fire consuming Yin and Blood
Magnetite and Cinnabar Pill	Harmonizes the Heart and Kidney Improves vision Calms the Mind	Disharmony between the Heart and Kidneys
Sour Jujube Decoction	Nourishes Liver Blood Clears Heat Calms the Mind	Liver Blood Deficiency and hyperactive Liver Yang
Heavenly Emperor Tonifying the Heart Pill	Nourishes the Heart and Kidneys Tonifies Yin and Blood Clears Heat Calms the Mind	Yin and Blood Deficiency

- *Tian Wang Bu Xin Dan*
  Heavenly Emperor Tonifying the Heart Pill

— Both formulae nourish the Heart, calm the Mind and clear Heat.

— Sour Jujube Decoction is more effective in nourishing Liver Blood. It is indicated for Liver Blood Deficiency and hyperactive Liver Yang with symptoms of insomnia, dizziness, vertigo, blurred vision, dry mouth and throat and a thready and wiry pulse.

— **Heavenly Emperor Tonifying the Heart Pill** is more effective in nourishing the Heart and Kidneys and tonifying Yin. It is indicated for Yin and Blood Deficiency with symptoms of palpitations, insomnia, poor memory, dream-disturbed sleep, dry stool, mouth ulcers, a red tongue with scanty coating and a thready and rapid pulse.

Questions

1. Both **Cinnabar Pill to Calm the Spirit** and **Magnetite and Cinnabar Pill** are formulae that soothe the Heart and calm the Mind. Why do both contain treated Radix Glycyrrhizae and Massa Fermentata Medicinalis?

2. Why do formulae that nourish the Heart and calm the Mind contain herbs that nourish Yin and Blood, and herbs that clear Heat? Give illustrative examples.

38 *Formulae that reduce Food Stagnation and dissipate masses*

A. GUIDING PRINCIPLES FOR FORMULATING PRESCRIPTIONS THAT REDUCE FOOD STAGNATION AND DISSIPATE MASSES

— These formulae are indicated for Retention of Food and palpable abdominal masses. These conditions may be complicated with Phlegm, Dampness, parasites, Qi Stagnation or Blood Stagnation, and other methods of treatment may be required in addition to the formulae given here.
— For cases of deficiency of Upright Qi due to a constitutional Spleen and Stomach Deficiency, or in cases of long-term stagnation, herbs that invigorate the Spleen should be added to the formula in order to resolve stagnation without further damaging the Upright Qi. For cases of severe stagnation, purgatives may be required as well in order to remove substantial pathogens.

B. TYPES OF FORMULAE THAT REDUCE FOOD STAGNATION AND DISSIPATE MASSES

1. Formulae that reduce Food Stagnation and promote digestion

— These formulae consist primarily of herbs that promote digestion; they are indicated for patterns of Food Stagnation. The Spleen and Stomach form a pivot regulating the ascent and descent of Qi. Retention of food in the Middle Burner obstructs the circulation of Qi, causing distension, fullness and pain in the epigastrium and abdomen. Herbs that activate Qi and resolve Stagnation are therefore added to formulae in order to assist in promoting digestion; such herbs include Pericarpium Citri Reticulatae, Radix Aucklandiae, Fructus Amomi, Cortex Magnoliae Officinalis and Fructus Aurantii Immaturus.
— A representative formula is *Bao He Wan* (**Preserving and Harmonizing Pill**), which contains Fructus Crataegi, Massa Fermentata Medicinalis and Semen Raphani to promote digestion and resolve stagnation, and Pericarpium Citri Reticulatae to activate Qi circulation.
— Long-term stagnation may turn to Heat, producing symptoms of deep-yellow urine, constipation and a red tongue with a thick sticky yellow coating. In this case, herbs that clear Damp-Heat should be used, such as Radix Scutellariae, Rhizoma Coptidis, Fructus Forsythiae, Rhizoma Pinelliae and Poria. Examples include the use of Fructus Forsythiae, Rhizoma Pinelliae and Poria in *Bao He Wan* (**Preserving and Harmonizing Pill**), and the use of Radix Scutellariae, Rhizoma Coptidis, Poria and Rhizoma Alismatis in *Zhi Shi Dao Zhi Wan* (**Citrus aurantius Eliminating Stagnation Pill**).
— Improper diet and overeating tend to damage the Spleen and Stomach. Old people, or those with constitutional deficiency of the Spleen and Stomach, easily develop Food Stagnation with symptoms of reduced appetite, poor digestion, distension and fullness in the epigastrium and abdomen, lassitude, sallow complexion, loose stools and a weak deficient pulse. In treating such cases of complicated Deficiency and Excess, herbs that tonify Qi and invigorate the Spleen should be added, such as Radix Codonopsis Pilosulae, Rhizoma Atractylodis Macrocephalae, Rhizoma Discoreae and Radix Glycyrrhizae. It is necessary to determine the relative severity of the Food Stagnation and the Spleen Deficiency and to adjust the treatment accordingly.
— *Da An Wan* (**Great Tranquillity Pill**) consists

of **Preserving and Harmonizing Pill** with the addition of Rhizoma Atractylodis Macrocephalae and is thus more effective in promoting digestion. *Jian Pi Wan* (**Strengthen the Spleen Pill**) combines Qi tonics such as Radix Ginseng, Rhizoma Atractylodis Macrocephalae, Rhizoma Dioscoreae and Radix Glycyrrhizae with digestives such as Fructus Crataegi, Massa Fermentata Medicinalis and Fructus Hordei Germinatus; it also contains Semen Myristicae. This formula promotes digestion and invigorates the Spleen, with greater emphasis on tonification.

2. Formulae that dissipate masses and resolve stagnation

— Formulae that dissipate masses and resolve stagnation consist of:

  – herbs that soften hardness and disperse masses, such as Carapax Trionycis
  – herbs that break Blood Stasis, such as Semen Persicae, Eupolyphaga seu Steleophaga, Rhizoma Sparganii and Rhizoma Zedoariae

  and

  – herbs that activate Qi circulation, such as Fructus Aurantii Immaturus, Cortex Magnoliae Officinalis, Pericarpium Citri Reticulatae Viride and Rhizoma Cyperi.

— Palpable abdominal masses can present with distension or pain. Examples include enlargement of the liver and spleen, and tumours. These conditions are the result of the combination of Cold, Heat, Phlegm or Dampness with Stagnant Qi and Blood. They therefore often require the addition of herbs that resolve Phlegm and eliminate Dampness, such as Rhizoma Pinelliae, Poria, Folium Pyrrosiae, Herba Dianthi and Semen Lepidii seu Descurainiae.

— In cases of combined Cold and Heat, herbs that warm the Interior and disperse Cold are often combined with herbs that clear Heat. For chronic cases with deficiency of Qi and Blood, herbs that tonify Qi and nourish Blood should be added, such as Radix Ginseng, Rhizoma Atractylodis Macrocephalae, Radix Angelicae Sinensis, Radix Paeoniae Alba, Radix Rehmanniae and Colla Corii Asini. *Zhi Shi Xiao Pi Wan* (**Immature Bitter Orange Pill to Reduce Focal Distension**) is a representative

formula for distress in the chest; *Bie Jia Jian Wan* (**Decocted Turtle Shell Pill**) is a commonly used formula for palpable masses in the hypochondrium.

C. POINTS TO REMEMBER IN FORMULATING PRESCRIPTIONS TO REDUCE FOOD STAGNATION AND DISSIPATE MASSES

1. Food Stagnation and palpable masses should be treated gradually in order to achieve good therapeutic results. It is not advisable to prescribe large doses of herbs; formulae are often administered in the form of pills, which have a gradual but consistent action.
— For Excess patterns of severe stagnation, powerful purgatives are required, and formulae that reduce Food Stagnation and dissipate masses are inappropriate as they would delay a resolution of the condition.
2. Food Stagnation, and especially palpable masses, have a complicated pathogenesis which may involve Qi Stagnation, Blood Stagnation, Phlegm-Damp, Cold, Heat and combinations of Deficiency and Excess. The various treatment methods of activating Qi and Blood, resolving Phlegm, eliminating Dampness, dispersing Cold, clearing Heat and tonifying are often used in combination.

D. A COMPARISON OF COMMONLY USED FORMULAE THAT REDUCE FOOD STAGNATION AND DISSIPATE MASSES (TABLE 38.1)

1. – *Bao He Wan*
     Preserving and Harmonizing Pill
   – *Zhi Shi Dao Zhi Wan*
     Citrus aurantius Eliminating Stagnation Pill

— Both formulae promote digestion, harmonize the Stomach, clear Heat and eliminate Dampness. They are indicated for Food Stagnation with symptoms of distension, fullness and pain in the epigastrium and abdomen, foul belching, acid regurgitation and a thick, sticky, yellow tongue coating.
— **Preserving and Harmonizing Pill** is more effective in promoting digestion and is

Table 38.1 Comparison of formulas that reduce Food Stagnation and dissipate masses

Formula	Actions	Indications
Preserving and Harmonizing Pill	Promotes digestion Harmonizes the Stomach (Clears Damp-Heat)	Food Stagnation with stagnation of Qi and mild Damp-Heat
Citrus Aurantius Eliminating Stagnation Pill	Clears Damp-Heat Harmonizes the Stomach (Promotes digestion)	Combined Damp-Heat and retained food
Strengthen the Spleen Pill	Invigorates the Spleen and tonifies Qi Promotes digestion Activates Qi Clears Damp-Heat	Spleen and Stomach Deficiency with impaired digestion and pronounced signs of Damp-Heat and Qi Stagnation

indicated for Food Stagnation with symptoms of Qi Stagnation and mild Damp-Heat.

— **Citrus aurantius Eliminating Stagnation Pill** is more effective in clearing Damp-Heat. It is indicated for patterns of combined Damp-Heat and retained food with symptoms of distension, abdominal fullness and pain, and diarrhoea.

2. – *Bao He Wan*
   Preserving and Harmonizing Pill
   – *Jian Pi Wan*
   Strengthen the Spleen Pill

— Both formulae contain Fructus Crataegi, Massa Fermentata Medicinalis, Pericarpium Citri Reticulatae and Poria. Both promote digestion and harmonize the Stomach and are indicated for Food Stagnation with symptoms of distension and fullness in the epigastrium and abdomen and a thick, sticky tongue coating.

— The difference between the two formulae lies in the fact that **Preserving and Harmonizing Pill** is indicated for the initial stage of Food Stagnation, with only mild symptoms of Spleen and Stomach Deficiency, Damp-Heat and Qi Stagnation. It does not contain herbs that invigorate the Spleen and tonify Qi.

— **Strengthen the Spleen Pill** is indicated for Spleen and Stomach Deficiency with impaired digestion and more pronounced signs of Damp-Heat and Qi Stagnation. Its primary action is to invigorate the Spleen and tonify Qi and secondarily to promote digestion, activate Qi, resolve Dampness and clear Heat.

Questions

1. Why do formulae that reduce Food Stagnation and promote digestion contain herbs that activate Qi and resolve Dampness?

2. What is the difference between **Preserving and Harmonizing Pill** and **Strengthen the Spleen Pill**?

Astringent formulae

39

A. GUIDING PRINCIPLES FOR THE FORMULATION OF ASTRINGENT FORMULAE

— Astringent formulae are indicated for patterns of consumption and loss of Qi, Blood, Essence and Body Fluids with symptoms of spontaneous sweating, night sweats, spermatorrhoea, urinary incontinence, chronic diarrhoea and dysentery, uterine bleeding and leucorrhoea.

— Their main ingredients are astringent herbs, combined with other herbs according to the causes and severity of the condition, so that both Biao and Ben are treated.

— If external pathogenic factors are involved, they should be eliminated first. If the external pathogens are mild, the treatment methods of astringing and Releasing the Exterior are combined in order to astringe without retaining the pathogens.

— In the treatment of extreme Deficiency or Collapse, the use of astringent herbs alone will not be effective; it is necessary to act promptly to tonify the Upright Qi strongly.

B. TYPES OF ASTRINGENT FORMULA

1. Formulae that consolidate the Exterior and stop sweating

— These formulae consist primarily of astringent herbs that stop sweating. They are indicated for spontaneous sweating and night sweats.

— Spontaneous sweating is due to Qi Deficiency, and particularly a weakness of the Defensive Qi and the body surface. Symptoms include spontaneous sweating, pallor, palpitations, dyspnoea, a pale and swollen tongue and a weak, deficient pulse. The main herbs used are those which are sour, astringent, warm and mild in nature and which tonify Qi, consolidate the Exterior and stop sweating. Examples include calcined Concha Ostreae, Radix Ephedrae, Fructus Tritici Levis, Fructus Corni, Fructus Schisandrae, Radix Astragali seu Hedysari and Rhizoma Atractylodis Macrocephalae. The representative formula is *Mu Li San* (**Oyster Shell Powder**), in which Concha Ostreae is the Emperor, to astringe and stop sweating, assisted by Radix Ephedrae, Fructus Tritici Levis and Radix Astragali seu Hedysari.

— Another such formula is *Yu Ping Feng San* (**Jade Wind-Screen Powder**), in which a large dose of Radix Astragali seu Hedysari is used as the Emperor herb to tonify Qi and consolidate the Exterior, assisted by Rhizoma Atractylodis Macrocephalae to strengthen the effect of tonification. When the body surface is deficient, pathogenic Wind can invade easily, and a small dose of Radix Ledebouriellae is therefore added to expel Wind. This combination of Radix Astragali seu Hedysari and Radix Ledebouriellae consolidates the Exterior without retaining pathogens and eliminates pathogens without damaging the Upright Qi.

— Sweat and Blood have the same origin, and prolonged sweating will inevitably damage Blood. In the same way, Qi Deficiency can develop into Yang Deficiency. Herbs should therefore be added to formulae according to the actual pathological condition.

— Night sweating results from Yin Deficiency with Empty Heat. It is often accompanied by restlessness, five-palm Heat, a red tongue with scanty coating and a thready, rapid pulse. Prescriptions should include:

  – herbs that astringe and stop sweating, such as Fructus Corni, Fructus Tritici, Concha Ostreae, and Radix Oryzae Glutinosae

- herbs that nourish Yin and Blood, such as Radix Rehmanniae, Radix Rehmanniae Praeparata, Radix Angelicae Sinensis, and Radix Paeoniae Alba

and

- herbs that clear Heat and quell Fire, such as Radix Scutellariae, Rhizoma Coptidis and Cortex Phellodendri.

— The representative formula is *Dang Gui Liu Huang Tang* (**Dang Gui and Six-Yellow Decoction**).

2. Formulae that astringe the intestines and stop diarrhoea

— These formulae consist primarily of herbs that astringe and stop diarrhoea. They are indicated for chronic diarrhoea and faecal incontinence due to Spleen and Stomach Deficiency with stagnation of Cold. Possible signs and symptoms include lassitude, abdominal pain which is alleviated by pressure, reduced appetite, a pale tongue with white coating and a deep, slow pulse.
— In formulating prescriptions, herbs that astringe the intestines are combined with:

- herbs that tonify Qi, such as Radix Ginseng, Radix Astragali seu Hedysari and Rhizoma Atractylodis Macro-cephalae

and

- herbs that warm the Interior and dispel Cold, such as Radix Aconiti Praeparata, Rhizoma Zingiberis, Fructus Evodiae and Cortex Cinnamomi.

— An example is *Si Shen Wan* (**Four-Miracle Pill**) in which Fructus Psoraleae and Semen Myristicae are combined with Fructus Schisandrae and Fructus Evodiae to warm and tonify the Spleen and Kidneys, astringe the intestines and stop diarrhoea.
— Because chronic diarrhoea can lead to Qi and Blood Deficiency, one should also add herbs that nourish Blood and harmonize the Nutritive Qi, such as Radix Angelicae Sinensis, Radix Paeoniae Alba and Colla Corii Asini. In addition, Spleen and Kidney Deficiency with stagnation of Cold can lead to obstruction of Qi in the intestinal tract, which must be treated with herbs that regulate Qi, such as Radix Aucklandiae, Pericarpium Citri Reticulatae and Fructus Amomi. The representative formula is *Zhen Ren Yang Zang Tang* (**True Man's Decoction**

to Nourish the Organs), which consists of Pericarpium Papaveris, Semen Myristicae and Fructus Chebulae to astringe the intestines and stop diarrhoea; Radix Ginseng, Rhizoma Atractylodis Macrocephalae and Radix Glycyrrhizae to tonify Qi and invigorate the Spleen; Radix Angelicae Sinensis and Radix Paeoniae Alba to nourish Blood and harmonize the Nutritive Qi; Cortex Cinnamomi to warm the Interior and dispel Cold; and Radix Aucklandiae to activate Qi circulation and resolve stagnation.
— This formula is effective in treating chronic diarrhoea and faecal incontinence.

3. Formulae that astringe the Essence and stop enuresis

— These formulae consist primarily of herbs that astringe and consolidate the Essence to stop enuresis. They are indicated for spermatorrhoea and urinary incontinence due to Kidney Deficiency with impairment of the Kidney functions of storing Essence and controlling urine. Accompanying signs and symptoms include soreness of the lumbar region, lassitude, poor memory, dizziness, tinnitus, a pale tongue with white coating and a thready, weak pulse.
— Formulae consist primarily of astringent herbs that tonify the Kidneys and consolidate the Essence, such as Semen Astragali Complanati, Semen Euryales, Fructus Corni, Fructus Rubi, Ootheca Mantidis, Fructus Alpiniae Oxyphyllae and Rhizoma Dioscoreae.
— Examples of such formulae include *Jin Suo Gu Jing Wan* (**Metal Lock Pill to Stabilize the Essence**) and *Shui Lu Er Xian Dan* (**Water and Earth Immortals Special Pill**).
— Because prolonged Kidney Deficiency leads to Qi and Blood Deficiency, herbs that tonify Qi and nourish Yin and Blood are often included in the treatment. An example is *Sang Piao Xiao San* (**Mantis Egg-Case Powder**), in which Radix Ginseng tonifies Qi, Radix Angelicae Sinensis nourishes Blood and Plastrum Testudinis invigorates Yin.

4. Formulae that stop uterine bleeding and leucorrhoea

— These formulae consist primarily of astrin-gent herbs that stop bleeding or leucorrhoea.

They are indicated for persistent uterine bleeding and for persistent vaginal discharge due to Deficiency.

— Leucorrhoea stems from deficiency of the Liver, Spleen and Kidneys, impairment of the function of the Dai channel in controlling vaginal discharge, and downward movement of pathogenic Dampness. Persistent leucorrhoea indicates a decline of Upright Qi. Accompanying signs and symptoms commonly include palpitations, dyspnoea, pallor, lumbar soreness, lassitude, a pale tongue and a thready pulse.

— Formulae that stop leucorrhoea are based on astringent herbs that stop leucorrhoea such as Semen Euryales, Semen Ginkgo, Stamen Nelumbinis, calcined Os Sepiellae seu Sepiae and calcined Concha Ostreae.

— For Spleen Deficiency, add herbs that tonify Qi, such as Radix Ginseng, Rhizoma Atractylodis Macrocephalae and Rhizoma Dioscoreae. For Dampness, add herbs that dry Dampness and invigorate the Spleen such as Rhizoma Atractylodis, or herbs that drain Dampness such as Poria, Semen Plantaginis and Rhizoma Alismatis. The representative formula is *Wan Dai Tang* (**End Discharge Decoction**).

— For Heat, add herbs that clear Heat such as Cortex Phellodendri and Rhizoma Coptidis. The representative formula is *Yi Huang Tang* (**Change Yellow [Discharge] Decoction**).

— Uterine bleeding is linked to the Chong and Ren channels. It may be acute and severe, or chronic and mild with a thin pinkish discharge, accompanied by pallor, palpitations, dyspnoea, a pale tongue and a thready or weak pulse, or a large, deficient pulse.

— It is treated primarily with astringent herbs that stop bleeding, such as Os Sepiellae seu Sepiae, Cortex Ailanthi, charred Cacumen Biotae, Herba Agrimoniae, Colla Corii Asini, charred Folium Artemisiae Argyi and Halloysitum Rubrum.

— For Spleen Qi Deficiency and weakness of the Chong and Ren channels, add herbs that tonify Qi such as Radix Astragali seu Hedysari, Radix Ginseng and Rhizoma Atractylodis Macrocephalae to control Blood. The representative formula is *Gu Chong Tang* (**Stabilize Gushing Decoction**).

— In cases of long-term uterine bleeding, the Chong and Ren channels become deficient, and Qi and Blood are greatly damaged. For this condition, herbs that nourish Yin and Blood should be added to stop bleeding. An example is *Jiao Ai Tang* (**Ass-Hide Gelatin and Mugwort Decoction**).

— If uterine bleeding is accompanied by Heat signs, herbs that clear Heat should be added, such as Radix Scutellariae and Cortex Phellodendri in *Gu Jing Wan* (**Stabilize the Menses Pill**).

C. POINTS TO REMEMBER IN FORMULATING ASTRINGENT PRESCRIPTIONS

1. It is essential to determine the cause and location of the disease before formulating a prescription. In most cases, deficiency of Upright Qi is the underlying cause.

— Astringing treats only the Biao, and herbs must be added to formulae according to the degree of consumption of Qi, Blood, Yin, Yang, Essence and Body Fluids.

2. Astringent formulae are indicated for deficiency of Upright Qi giving rise to an excessive loss of Blood, Essence and Body Fluids. Many of the same signs and symptoms may be caused by external pathogenic factors, e.g. profuse sweating in febrile disease, cough due to retention of Phlegm-Fluid, spermatorrhoea due to Empty Fire, diarrhoea due to overeating and uterine bleeding due to Heat in the Blood. These formulae are not appropriate in such cases.

— *The Complete Collection of Jin Yue's Treatises* says, 'The method of astringing is adopted for deficiency conditions. If this method is used in an excess condition, you close the door to keep the devils in.'

— If external pathogenic factors are present, astringents are not used until they have been cleared.

D. A COMPARISON OF COMMONLY USED ASTRINGENT FORMULAE (TABLE 39.1)

1. – *Yu Ping Feng San*
   Jade Wind-Screen Powder
   – *Mu Li San*
   Oyster Shell Powder
   – *Dang Gui Liu Huang Tang*
   Dang Gui and Six-Yellow Decoction

— All three formulae consolidate the Exterior

Table 39.1 Comparison of Astringent formulae

Formula	Actions	Indications
Jade Wind-Screen Powder	Tonifies Qi Consolidates the Exterior Expels Wind	Deficiency of Defensive Qi
Oyster Shell Powder	Stops sweating Tonifies Qi Suppresses hyperactive Yang	Deficiency of Defensive Qi complicated with hyperactive Heart Yang
Dang Gui and Six-Yellow Decoction	Nourishes Yin Quells Fire Stops sweating	Nights sweats due to Yin Deficiency

and stop sweating and are indicated for spontaneous sweating or night sweats.

— **Jade Wind-Screen Powder** and **Oyster Shell Powder** are indicated for spontaneous sweating.

— **Jade Wind-Screen Powder** primarily tonifies Qi, consolidates the Exterior and stops sweating and secondarily expels Wind. It is thus indicated for exterior patterns of the Deficiency type due to deficiency of Defensive Qi, characterized by spontaneous sweating, aversion to wind, pale complexion, lassitude, a pale tongue, a slow pulse and susceptibility to the common cold.

— **Oyster Shell Powder** primarily stops sweating and secondarily tonifies Qi, consolidates the Exterior and suppresses hyperactive Yang. It is also indicated for exterior patterns of the Deficiency type due to deficiency of Defensive Qi, but complicated with hyperactive Heart Yang, characterized by spontaneous sweating that is more severe at night, palpitations, dyspnoea and a thready, weak pulse.

— The first formula focuses on treating the Ben, while the second primarily treats the Biao.

— **Dang Gui and Six-Yellow Decoction** nourishes Yin, quells Fire and stops sweating. It is thus indicated for night sweats due to Yin Deficiency with Empty Fire, characterized by restlessness, five-palm Heat, flushed face, afternoon fever, deep-yellow urine, a red tongue and a rapid pulse.

Part 5:
The treatment of common diseases based on differentiation of syndromes

This section describes the treatment of some common diseases which respond well to traditional herbal medicine. The diseases are categorized for ease of reference, some under their Chinese names and some under their Western names, according to common usage.

Diseases in internal medicine **40**

A. Seasonal and respiratory diseases

1. THE COMMON COLD

GENERAL DESCRIPTION

— The common cold is caused by invasion of external pathogenic factors; it corresponds to various acute infectious diseases of the respiratory tract such as influenza. It occurs throughout the year, but especially in Winter and Spring.
— Clinical manifestations include nasal obstruction and/or discharge, headache, aversion to cold, fever and cough.
— The pathogenesis is invasion of external Wind-Cold or Wind-Heat impairing the dispersing function of the Lungs; the pattern may be complicated by Summer Heat or Dampness. The treatment principle is to Release the Exterior and eliminate the pathogenic factors.

DIFFERENTIATION AND TREATMENT

a. Wind-Cold

— This pattern is due to invasion of the body surface by external pathogenic Wind-Cold impairing the dispersing function of the Lungs. Clinical manifestations include severe aversion to cold, mild fever, absence of sweating, headache, general aching, nasal obstruction, hoarseness, clear nasal discharge, itching of the throat, cough with thin white sputum and a superficial, tense pulse.
— The treatment principle is to Release the Exterior with pungent and warm herbs.
— The recommended formula is a variation of *Jing Fang Bai Du San* (**Schizonepeta and Ledebouriella Powder to Overcome Pathogenic Influences**):

Herba Schizonepetae	10 g
Radix Ledebouriellae	10g
Folium Perillae	6g
Radix Angelicae Dahuricae	10g
Semen Sojae Praeparata	10g
Radix Peucedani	10g
Radix Platycodi	6g
Rhizoma Zingiberis Recens	2 slices

— Modifications:

- If exterior Cold is severe, add Herba Ephedrae (3 g) and Ramulus Cinnamomi (5 g).
- If the pattern is complicated with Dampness, giving rise to a white sticky tongue coating and a heavy distending sensation in the head as if it were tightly wrapped, add Rhizoma seu Radix Notopterygii (10 g), Radix Angelicae Pubescentis (10 g) and Rhizoma Atractylodis (5 g).

CASE STUDY 40.1
THE COMMON COLD

Female, age 32

The patient complained of a heavy sensation in her head as if it were tightly wrapped in cloth, stuffiness of the chest, loss of taste and poor appetite. She had a sticky white tongue coating and a weak-floating and slow pulse.

Pathogenesis: Invasion by External Cold with Retention of Damp in the Interior. Cold and Damp combined in the Spleen and Stomach, hindering Yang Qi.

Western diagnosis: Common cold.

Treatment principle: Disperse Cold, Release the Exterior, Resolve Damp and harmonize the Middle Burner.

The formula used was a variation of *Xiang Ru Yin* (**Elscholtzia Decoction**) and **Agastache Upright Qi Powder**:

Herba Elscholtzia seu Moslae	4.5 g
Cortex Magnoliae Officinalis	4.5 g

Herba Agastachis (*fresh*)	9 g
Folium Perillae	9 g
Rhizoma Atractylodis Macrocephalae (*stir-baked*)	9 g
Poria	9 g
Pericarpium Arecae	9 g
Radix Angelicae Dahuricae	3 g
Rhizoma Pinelliae	9 g
Pericarpium Citri Reticulatae	3 g

After the first dose, the patient experienced mild sweating and the heavy sensation in her head was immediately relieved. Herba Elsholtzia was then removed from the prescription and Semen Coicis (10 g) and Fructus Amomi (3 g) were added, Amomi being added at the end of the decoction. All signs and symptoms disappeared after two doses of this formula.

b. Wind-Heat

— This pattern is due to invasion of the Lungs by external pathogenic Wind-Heat which impairs the Lungs' dispersing function. Clinical manifestations include severe fever, mild aversion to cold, sweating, headache, flushed face, mild thirst, turbid nasal discharge, sore throat, cough with yellow sputum, a thin pale-yellow tongue coating and a superficial, rapid pulse.
— The treatment principle is to Release the Exterior with pungent and cool herbs.
— The recommended formula is a variation of *Yin Qiao San* (**Honeysuckle and Forsythia Powder**):

Flos Lonicerae	10–15 g
Fructus Forsythiae	10 g
Herba Menthae	5 g
(*added at end of decoction*)	
Folium Mori	10 g
Flos Chrysanthemi	10 g
Semen Sojae Praeparata	10 g
Radix Peucedani	10 g
Fructus Arctii	10 g
Radix Platycodi	6 g
Radix Glycyrrhizae	3 g

— Modifications:

  – For influenza with severe Fire Poison, add Radix or Folium Isatidis (15 g).
  – If Heat is complicated with Cold, with symptoms of aversion to cold and absence of sweating, add Herba Schizonepetae (10 g).
– For cough with thick sputum, dyspnoea

and chest pain, combine with *Ma Xing Shi Gan Tang* (**Ephedra–Prunus–Gypsum–Glycyrrhiza Decoction**).
  – For sore throat, add Lasiosphaera seu Calvatia (10 g) and Radix Achyranthis Bidentatae (15 g).
  – If Heat consumes Body Fluids, giving rise to thirst, dry lips and nose and a red tongue with scanty coating, add Radix Adenophorae (10 g), Radix Trichosanthis (10 g) and Rhizoma Phragmitis (15 g). – If the pattern is complicated with pathogenic Dampness, add Rhizoma seu Radix Notopterygii (10 g) and Herba Agastachis (10 g).

c. Summer Heat and Dampness

— This pattern is due to invasion of the body surface by Summer Heat and Dampness, which impair the Lungs' dispersing function. Clinical manifestations include a feverish sensation, mild sweating which does not relieve the fever, irritability, restlessness, thirst, stuffiness of the chest, nausea or abdominal pain, diarrhoea, a sticky yellow tongue coating and a soft, rapid pulse.
— The treatment principle is to Release the Exterior, clear Summer Heat and resolve Dampness.
— The recommended formula is a variation of *Xin Jia Xiang Ru Yin* (**Newly-Augmented Elsholtzia Decoction**):

Herba Elsholtziae seu Moslae	3 g
Semen Glycine Germinatus (*Dou Juan*)	15 g
Herba Agastachis	10 g
Herba Eupatorii	10 g
Herba Artemisiae Chinghao	15 g
Semen Dolichoris Album	15 g
Flos Lonicerae	10 g
Fructus Forsythiae	10 g
and	
Liu Yi San (**Six-to-One Powder** which is made up of Talcum and Radix Glyeyrrizae by 6 to 1) or *Ji su San* (**Six-to-One Powder** is added to Herba Menthae)	10 g

— Modifications:

  – If Summer Heat is more pronounced, remove Herba Elsholtziae seu Moslae from the prescription and add Rhizoma Coptidis and Fructus Gardeniae.
  – If pathogenic Dampness is more pronounced, add Rhizoma Atractylodis and Cortex Magnoliae Officinalis.

2. EPIDEMIC ENCEPHALITIS B

GENERAL DESCRIPTION
— This disease often occurs in Summer or the beginning of Autumn and is caused by exposure to encephalitis B virus. Clinical manifestations include abrupt onset of symptoms, high fever, headache, sweating, restlessness, thirst, and possibly coma and convulsion.
— Diseases caused by Summer Heat and pestilence are differentiated and treated according to the Four Levels. The transmission and progression of this disease is extremely rapid and it enters the Qi level immediately. Persistent Summer Heat tends to affect the Pericardium, thus giving rise to patterns of Heat at the Nutritive and Blood levels.

DIFFERENTIATION AND TREATMENT
— The initial stage of the disease (Summer Heat at the Qi level) is treated by clearing Heat from the Qi level and quelling Fire. If Summer Heat is complicated with Dampness, and Tai Yin is affected, it is treated by clearing Summer Heat and resolving Dampness. If pathogenic factors have entered the Nutritive and Blood levels, causing coma and convulsion, it is treated by clearing Heat from the Nutritive level, cooling Blood, calming Wind and opening the orifices. The sequelae of the disease are treated by resolving Phlegm and removing obstruction from the collaterals.

a. Initial stage

— This pattern presents in the first 3 days after the onset of the disease. It manifests as body temperature of 38–39°C with a feverish sensation, headache, lethargy, nausea, vomiting, mild rigidity of the neck and a flushed face.
— The treatment principle is to Release the Exterior and clear Heat and Summer Heat.
— The recommended formula is a variation of **Honeysuckle and Forsythia Powder** and **Newly-Augmented Elsholtzia Powder**:

Flos Lonicerae	15 g
Fructus Forsythiae	10 g
Folium Isatidis	15 g
Radix Isatidis	15 g
Herba Artemisiae Chinghao	15 g

Semen Sojae Praeparata	10 g
Gypsum Fibrosum *(decocted first)*	30 g

— Modifications:
  - For pronounced exterior symptoms such as headache, aversion to cold and absence of sweating, add Herba Menthae (5 g) *(decocted later)* and Herba Elsholtzia seu Moslae (3 g).
  - If Summer Heat and Dampness combine, giving rise to stuffiness of the chest, epigastric distress and a sticky tongue coating, add Herba Agastachis (10 g) and Herba Eupatorii (10 g).
  - For high fever and profuse sweating, increase the dosage of Gypsum Fibrosum to 50–60 g and add Rhizoma Anemarrhenae (10 g).
  - For constipation and a yellow tongue coating, add Radix et Rhizoma Rhei (6–10 g).

b. Advanced stage

— This pattern develops 4–10 days after the onset of the disease. Clinical manifestations include high fever (over 40°C), flushed face, coarse breathing, restlessness, thirst, profuse sweating, lethargy or coma, convulsion and spastic paralysis.
— There are three sub-stages:

i. Damage to Qi by Summer Heat
— This corresponds to Yang Ming Syndrome, i.e. invasion of Yang Ming by Heat, with consumption of Body Fluids. Clinical manifestations include high fever, restlessness, thirst, profuse sweating, flushed face, coarse breathing, a yellow tongue coating and a surging, rapid pulse. The treatment principle is to clear Summer Heat, nourish Yin and promote Body Fluids.
— The recommended formula is a variation of *Bai Hu Tang* (**White Tiger Decoction**):

Gypsum Fibrosum	50–100 g
Rhizoma Anemarrhenae	12 g
Radix Glycyrrhizae *(raw)*	3 g
Flos Lonicerae	15 g
Fructus Forsythiae	10 g
Radix Scutellariae	10 g
Radix Isatidis	20 g
Rhizoma Paris Polyphagae *(Zao Xiu)*	15 g
Herba Lophatheri	10 g
Herba Dendrobii	15 g

— Modifications:
  - If the fever has subsided but sweating

continues, with shortness of breath and a large but weak pulse, this suggests Collapse of Qi and Body Fluids. In this case, add *Sheng Mai San* (**Generating the Pulse Powder**) to benefit Qi and promote Body Fluids.

ii. Invasion of the Nutritive level of the Heart by Summer Heat

— This pattern is due to inward transmission of Summer Heat to the Nutritive and Blood levels of the Pericardium. Clinical manifestations include high fever, lethargy, coma, convulsion, a deep-red tongue with a burnt coating and a rapid, thready, large pulse. The treatment principle is to clear Heat from the Nutritive level, open the orifices and calm Wind. The recommended formula is a variation of *Qing Ying Tang* (**Clear the Nutritive Level Decoction**) and *Qing Wen Bai Du Yin* (**Clear Epidemics and Overcome Toxin Decoction**):

Cornu Rhinoceri Asiatici	0.5 g
(*ground to a powder and taken separately with water*)	
or Cornu Bubali	30 g
(*decocted with other ingredients*)	
Radix Rehmanniae	30 g
Flos Lonicerae	30 g
Fructus Forsythiae	15 g
Herba Lophatheri	10 g
Folium Isatidis	15 g
Rhizoma Coptidis	5–10 g
Radix Ophiopogonis	15 g
Rhizoma Acori Graminei	5–10 g
(*added at end of decoction*)	
Radix Curcumae	10 g
Ramulus Uncariae cum Uncis	15 g
(*added at end of decoction*)	

— Modifications:

– For delirium and coma, add 1–2 pills of *An Gong Niu Huang Wan* (**Calm the Palace Pill with Cattle Gallstone**) or *Zhi Bao Dan* (**Greatest Treasure Special Pill**), to be taken in three doses.
– For stirring of Wind with convulsion, add 0.3–1.5 g of powdered Cornu Antelopis, to be taken separately.
– For severe convulsions, add 1–2 g of powdered Scorpio and Scolopendra in equal amounts, to be taken with the prepared decoction.
– For severe internal Heat with a burnt-yellow tongue coating, add Gypsum Fibrosum (50 g), Rhizoma Anemarr-

henae (12 g) and Radix et Rhizoma Rhei (6 g).
– For circulatory failure, add Radix Ginseng (10 g) to benefit Qi and rescue Collapse.

CASE STUDY 40.2
ENCEPHALITIS B

Male, age 5

The patient was admitted to hospital after having had fever (39.7° C) and convulsion for 5 days. He presented with coma, convulsion, gurgling due to sputum in the throat, shortness of breath, cold limbs, constipation, a thick yellow tongue coating and a rapid, rolling pulse.

Pathogenesis: Invasion of Jue Yin by pathogenic factors; Phlegm-Heat in the Interior disturbing the Pericardium.

Western diagnosis: Encephalitis B

Treatment principle: Clear Heat from the Heart, open the orifices, resolve Phlegm, relieve constipation and subdue Liver Wind.
The herbs used were:

a. One pill of **Calm the Palace Pill with Cattle Gallstone**, taken with fresh Succus Bambusae, to clear Heat, resolve Phlegm and open the orifices.

b. Gypsum Fibrosum (*raw*)	50 g
(*decocted first*)	
Flos Lonicerae	30 g
Fructus Forsythiae	10 g
Fructus Gardeniae	10 g
Bamboo juice	10 g
Radix et Rhizoma Rhei (*raw*)	6 g
(*added at end*)	
Natrii Sulfas	10 g
(*taken separately with water*)	
Semen Pharbitides	10 g
Ramulus Uncariae cum Uncis	12 g
(*added at end*)	
Scorpio	3 g
Carapax Eretmochaelydis (*Dai Mao*)	10 g
(*decocted first*)	
Concha Haliotidis	20 g
(*decocted first*)	
Rhizoma Phragmitis	15 g
Radix Glycyrrhizae (*raw*)	3 g

After administration of three doses, the fever gradually subsided and convulsions stopped; the patient had two bowel motions with black sticky stool; gurgling in the throat improved and the patient's mental state became clear.

Two doses of herbs that clear Heat and resolve Phlegm were then administered, after which the boy was discharged from hospital.

iii. Recovery stage
— In the recovery stage, the body temperature gradually subsides and the various signs and symptoms improve. The main clinical manifestations at this stage are a low-grade fever which is more pronounced at night, flushed face, thirst, a red tongue and a rapid, thready pulse. The pattern at this point consists of deficiency of Qi and Yin, complicated with residual Summer Heat.
— The treatment principle is to nourish Yin and clear Heat. The recommended formula is **Qing Hao Bie Jia Tang (Artemisia Annua and Soft-shelled Turtle Shell Decoction)**:

Herba Artemisiae Chinghao	15 g
Carapax Trionycis	15 g
(decocted first)	
Radix Rehmanniae	15 g
Radix Ophiopogonis	15 g
Radix Adenophorae	15 g
Rhizoma Anemarrhenae	10 g
Radix Cynanchi Atrati	10 g
Herba Dendrobii	15 g

— Modifications:

  – For delirium, add Arisaema cum Bile (10 g), Rhizoma Acori Graminei (6 g) (added at end of decoction) and Radix Curcumae (10 g) to clear Heat, resolve Phlegm and open the orifices.
  – For spasm of the limbs and tremor of the hands and feet, add Plastrum Testudinis (15 g) and Concha Ostreae (20 g) (both decocted first) to nourish Yin and calm Wind.

d. Sequelae

— If neurological symptoms are still present 6 months after the onset, they are caused by blockage of the collaterals and misting of the Heart by Phlegm and Stagnant Blood due to Fire Poison damaging the Yin and condensing Body Fluids into Phlegm.
— The main signs and symptoms at this stage include delirium, dementia, aphasia, dysphagia and paralysis of the limbs. The treatment principle is to promote Upright Qi, resolve Phlegm and remove obstruction from the collaterals.
— The recommended formula is:

Carapax Trionycis	15 g
(decocted first)	
Squama Manitis	12 g
(decocted first)	
Eupolyphaga seu Steleophaga	10 g

Lumbricus	10 g
Arisaema cum Bile	10 g
Rhizoma Acori Graminei *(decocted first)*	3 g
Radix Polygalae	10 g

— Modifications:

  – For tremor of the hands and feet and a dry red tongue, add Plastrum Testudinis (15 g) (decocted first), Radix Rehmanniae (20 g) and Herba Dendrobii (15 g) to nourish Yin, calm Wind and remove obstruction from the collaterals.
  – For paralysis of the limbs, add Radix Astragali seu Hedysari (20 g), Radix Angelicae Sinensis (10 g), Semen Persicae (10 g) and Flos Carthami (3 g).

3. TRACHEITIS AND PNEUMONIA

GENERAL DESCRIPTION
— The main symptom of both tracheitis and pneumonia is cough, possibly accompanied by fever. In their acute form, both diseases are caused by the invasion of external pathogenic Wind-Cold or Wind-Heat, while chronic tracheitis results from invasion of the Lungs by Phlegm Damp or Liver Fire, the retention of Phlegm-Fluid in the Lungs or Yin Deficiency with Empty Heat.

DIFFERENTIATION AND TREATMENT

a. Cough due to invasion of external pathogenic factors (acute tracheitis and pneumonia).

i. Wind-Cold
— This pattern is due to invasion of the Lungs by pathogenic Wind-Cold, which impairs the Lungs' dispersing function. Clinical manifestations include cough with thin white sputum, nasal obstruction and discharge and a thin, white tongue coating. The treatment principle is to eliminate Wind-Cold, promote the dispersing function of the Lungs and stop cough. The recommended formula is a variation of *Zhi Ke San* (**Stop Coughing Powder**) and *San Ao Tang* (**Three-Unbinding Decoction**):

Herba Ephedrae	3–6 g
Herba Schizonepetae	10 g
Folium Perillae	3–6 g
Fructus Perillae	10 g
Radix Peucedani	10 g
Radix Platycodi	5 g
Semen Armeniacae Amarum	10 g

| Radix Stemonae | 10 g |
| Radix Asteris | 10 g |

CASE STUDY 40.3
TRACHEITIS

Male, age 32

The patient complained of a cough, becoming worse in Autumn and Winter over the past 10 years. The most recent aggravation was caused by exposure to rain and cold. Clinical manifestations included frequent cough with scanty sputum, shortness of breath which was worse when lying down, general aching, reduced appetite, thirst, a red tongue and a slightly wiry pulse.

Pathogenesis: Constitutional Lung Heat with retention of Phlegm in the Lung channel, complicated with invasion by pathogenic Cold, resulting in impairment of the Lungs' function of dispersing and descending.

Western diagnosis: Tracheitis

Treatment principle: Promote the Lungs' dispersing function, eliminate Cold, resolve Phlegm and relieve cough.

The formula used was a variation of *San Ao Tang* (**Three-Unbinding Decoction**) and *Zhi Shi San* (**Stop Coughing Powder**):

Herba Ephedrae (*treated*)	4.5g
Semen Armeniacae Amarum	9g
Radix Glycyrrhizae (*raw*)	4.5g
Radix Peucedani	9g
Folium Mori	9g
Cortex Mori Radicis	9g
Radix Asteris (*treated*)	15g
Radix Stemonae (*treated*)	9g
Radix Scutellariae	4.5g
Pericarpium Citri Reticulatae	4.5g
Concha Metetricis seu Cyclinae (*Ge Ke*)	15g

After administration of three doses, the cough improved. At this point, the tongue was red with a thin, sticky coating, and the pulse was slightly wiry, indicating that the Lungs' descending function was not yet restored. Bulbus Fritillariae Thunbergii (9 g) was therefore added to the formula.

After three doses of the new formula, the cough was further improved, the general aching had disappeared and the patient's appetite had increased. The tongue tip was not red, and the tongue coating was thin and white. Herba Ephedrae and Radix Scutellariae were then removed from the prescription and treated Rhizoma Cynanchi Stauntonii (9 g) and Fructus Trichosanthis (9 g) were added. After three doses of this formula, all signs and symptoms disappeared.

ii. Wind-Heat

— This pattern is due to invasion of the Lungs by Wind-Heat which impairs the Lungs' descending function. Signs and symptoms include cough with yellow sputum which is difficult to expectorate, sore throat, fever, dyspnoea and chest pain.

— The treatment principle for a mild case is to eliminate Wind, clear Heat, promote the descending function of the Lungs; for a severe case, it is to promote the dispersing function of the Lungs and clear Heat. The recommended formula for a mild case is a variation of *Sang Ju Yin* (**Folia Mori–Flos Chrysanthemi Decoction**):

Folium Mori	10 g
Fructus Arctii	10–15 g
Herba Menthae	2–3 g
(*added at end of decoction*)	
Flos Chrysanthemi	10 g
Flos Lonicerae	10 g
Fructus Forsythiae	10 g
Semen Armeniacae Amarum	10 g
Radix Peucedani	10 g
Radix Platycodi	5 g

— The recommended formula for a severe case is a variation of Ephedra-Prunus-Gypsum-Glycyrrhiza Decoction:

Herba Ephedrae	3–6 g
Gypsum Fibrosum	15–30 g
(*decocted first*)	
Rhizoma Anemarrhenae	10–12 g
Semen Armeniacae Amarum	10 g
Flos Lonicerae	10–15 g
Fructus Forsythiae	10 g
Herba Houttuyniae	15 g
Radix Scutellariae	10 g

CASE STUDY 40.4
PNEUMONIA

Male, age 21

The patient complained of fever for 3 days, with cough, chest pain and shortness of breath. He was not sweating. The tip and border of his tongue were red, with a thin, yellow coating; the pulse was rolling and rapid. Chest X-rays showed a large shadow of increased density in the right lower lung.

Pathogenesis: Invasion by pathogenic Wind, complicated with retention of Lung Heat impairing the Lungs' function of dispersing.

Western diagnosis: Lobar pneumonia

Treatment principle: Promote the Lung's function

of dispersing with pungent and cool herbs, clear Lung Heat and relieve cough.

The formula used was a variation of **Ephedra–Prunus–Gypsum–Glycyrrhiza Decoction** and **Reed Decoction:**

Herba Ephedrae	4.5 g
Gypsum Fibrosum (*raw*)	30 g
(*decocted first*)	
Semen Armeniacae Amarum	9 g
Radix Glycyrrhizae (*raw*)	4.5 g
Semen Benincasae (*Dong Gua Zi*)	18 g
Semen Coicis (*raw*)	15 g
Rhizoma Phragmitis	
(*fresh, with the joint removed*)	30 g
Semen Persicae	4.5 g
Flos Lonicerae	30 g
Fructus Forsythiae	15 g

After administration of two doses the fever subsided and shortness of breath was relieved. After another 15 doses, X-rays showed complete absorption of the shadow in the right lower lung.

b. Cough due to internal injury (chronic tracheitis)

i. Invasion of the Lungs by Phlegm-Damp
— The clinical manifestations of this pattern include cough with profuse white sticky sputum, stuffiness of the chest and a sticky tongue coating.
— The treatment principle is to invigorate the Spleen, dry Dampness, and resolve Phlegm. The recommended formula is a variation of *Er Chen Tang* (**Two-Cured Decoction**):

Rhizoma Pinelliae	10 g
Rhizoma Arisaematis	10 g
Semen Sinapis Albae	2–3 g
Rhizoma Atractylodis	5–10 g
Rhizoma Atractylodis	
Macrocephalae	10 g
Cortex Magnoliae Officinalis	2–5 g
Semen Ziziphi Spinosae	10 g
Fructus Aurantii	5 g
Pericarpium Citri Reticulatae	5 g

ii. Retention of Phlegm and Fluid in the Lungs
— The clinical manifestations of this pattern include cough with profuse thin sputum, a white tongue coating and a rolling pulse. The treatment principle is to warm the Lungs and resolve retained fluid. The recommended formula is a variation of *Xiao Qing Long Tang* (**Small Green Dragon Decoction**) and *Ling Gui Zhu Gan Tang* (**Poria–Ramulus**

Cinnamomi   Atractylodes–Glycyrrhiza Decoction):

Herba Ephedrae	3–6 g
Ramulus Cinnamomi	2–5 g
Rhizoma Atractylodis	
Macrocephalae	10 g
Poria	10 g
Rhizoma Zingiberis	2–5 g
Herba Asari	1–2 g
Fructus Schisandrae	2 g
Radix Glycyrrhizae	3 g

iii. Invasion of the Lungs by Liver Fire
— This pattern is due to invasion of the Lungs by Liver Fire, with retention of Heat in the Lungs and impairment of the Lungs' descending function. Clinical manifestations include cough with thick yellow sputum and hypochondriac pain, flushed face and haemoptysis.
— The treatment principle is to sedate the Liver, clear Lung Heat and stop cough.
— The recommended formula is a variation of *Xie Bai San* (**Expelling Whiteness Powder**) and *Dai Ge San* (**Indigo Naturalis–Concha Meretricis Powder**):

Cortex Mori Radicis	10 g
Radix Scutellariae	10 g
Cortex Lycii Radicis	10 g
Rhizoma Anemarrhenae	10 g
Bulbus Fritillariae Thunbergii	10 g
Fructus Gardeniae	10 g
Concha Meretricis seu Cyclinae	15 g
Fructus Trichosanthis	10–15 g
Cortex Moutan Radicis	10 g
Radix Curcumae	10 g
Herba Agrimoniae	10–12 g

iv. Yin Deficiency
— The clinical manifestations of this pattern include dry cough with scanty sputum, dry throat, dysphonia, tidal fever, haemoptysis, a dry red tongue and a rapid, thready pulse. The treatment principle is to nourish Yin, moisten the Lungs, and stop cough.
— The recommended formula is a variation of *Sha Shen Mai Dong Tang* (**Glehnia–Ophiopogon Decoction**):

Radix Adenophorae	10–15 g
Radix Ophiopogonis	10–15 g
Radix Asparagi	10–15 g
Bulbus Lilii	10 g
Colla Corii Asini	10 g
(*melted and taken separately*)	
Bulbus Fritillariae Thunbergii	10 g
Fructus Trichosanthis	10 g

4. ASTHMA

GENERAL DESCRIPTION

— The main symptoms of asthma are shortness of breath and wheezing. It often presents as bronchial asthma and asthmatic bronchitis. The pathogenesis is a combination of Phlegm and Qi blocking the air passages and impairing the dispersing and descending functions of the Lungs.

— During an acute attack, the pattern is of the Excess type and may involve either Cold or Heat. The treatment principle is to promote the dispersing function of the Lungs, conduct Rebellious Qi downward, resolve Phlegm and soothe wheeze.

— However, the root of the pattern is in Deficiency, and in the remission stage the treatment principle is to tonify the Lungs, invigorate the Spleen and benefit the Kidneys.

DIFFERENTIATION AND TREATMENT

a. During an attack

i. Cold type

— This pattern is due to retention of Cold and Fluid in the Lungs and a combination of Phlegm and Qi impairing the Lung's dispersing and descending functions. It occurs most often in Autumn and Winter.

— The main signs and symptoms include wheeze, cough with profuse frothy white sputum, gurgling in the throat, stuffiness of the chest, a slippery or sticky white tongue coating and a rolling pulse. Exterior symptoms such as aversion to cold and headache may be present.

— The treatment principle is to warm the Lungs, resolve Phlegm-Fluid, stimulate the Lungs' dispersing function and soothe wheeze.

— The recommended formula is a variation of **Small Green Dragon Decoction** and *She Gan Ma Huang Tang* (**Belamcanda and Ephedra Decoction**):

Herba Ephedrae	3–10 g
Semen Armeniacae Amarum	10 g
Fructus Perillae	10 g
Herba Asari	2–3 g
Rhizoma Zingiberis	2–5 g
Fructus Schisandrae	2 g
Rhizoma Pinelliae	10 g
Radix Asteris	10 g
Flos Farfarae	10 g
Rhizoma Belamcandae	5–10 g
Fructus Aurantii	5 g
Radix Platycodi	5 g

CASE STUDY 40.5
ASTHMA

Female, age 6

The patient had had asthma for 3 weeks. Clinical manifestations included cough, wheeze, dyspnoea and gurgling of sputum in the throat, all of which were worse at night. Dyspnoea was aggravated when lying down. Other signs included profuse sweating, sticky white sputum, pallor, loss of body weight, a pale tongue with a thin, white coating and a weak, floating pulse.

The patient was initially treated with aminophylline and ephedrine, which were not effective.

Pathogenesis: Invasion by pathogenic Wind-Cold and retention of Phlegm-Fluid in the Lungs complicated with dysfunction of the Kidneys' reception of Qi.

Western diagnosis: Bronchial asthma

Treatment principle: Primarily, warm the Lungs, disperse Cold, resolve Phlegm and soothe wheeze; secondarily, assist the Kidneys' reception of Qi.

The formula used was a variation of **Small Green Dragon Decoction** and **Kidney Qi Pill**:

Herba Ephedrae (*treated*)	4.5 g
Semen Armeniacae Amarum	9 g
Herba Asari	3 g
Fructus Schisandrae	3 g
Rhizoma Zingiberis	3 g
Flos Farfarae	9 g
Rhizoma Pinelliae (*prepared*)	9 g
Radix Glycyrrhizae (*treated*)	3 g
plus **Kidney Qi Pill** (*decocted wrapped*)	9 g

The asthma improved after the first dose. On the second day, Semen Lepidii seu Descurainiae (9 g) was added to the prescription, and there was a further improvement the next day. All signs and symptoms disappeared after another three doses.

---

ii. Heat type

— This pattern results from the combination of retained Phlegm-Heat in the Interior, and pathogenic factors invading the Exterior; both factors act to impair the Lungs' descending function. Clinical manifestations include shortness of breath, gurgling in the throat, a choking cough with thin, sticky yellow sputum which is difficult to expectorate, stuffiness of the chest and diaphragm, restlessness, thirst, a red tongue with sticky yellow coating and a rapid, rolling pulse. Fever and headache may be present as well.

— The treatment principle is to clear Heat, resolve Phlegm, conduct Rebellious Qi downward and soothe wheeze.

— The recommended formula is a variation of *Ding Chuan Tang* (**Arrest Wheezing Decoction**), *Ting Li Da Zao Xie Fei Tang* (**Descurainia and Jujube Decoction to Drain the Lungs**) and **Belamcanda and Ephedra Decoction**:

Herba Ephedrae (*treated*)	3–6 g
Radix Scutellariae	10 g
Rhizoma Anemarrhenae	12 g
Cortex Mori Radicis	10 g
Arisaema cum Bile or Rhizoma Pinelliae (*treated with Succus Bambusae*)	10 g
Rhizoma Belamcandae	5–10 g
Semen Armeniacae Amarum	10 g
Bulbus Fritillariae Cirrhosae	10 g
Fructus Trichosanthis	10 g
Radix Glycyrrhizae (*raw*)	3 g

— Modifications:

- For gurgling in the throat and dyspnoea, add Semen Lepidii seu Descurainiae (6 –16 g) and Lumbricus (10 g).
- For thick purulent yellow sputum, add Herba Houttuyniae (15 g), Rhizoma Phragmitis (15 g) and Radix Platycodi (10 g).
- For fever, add Gypsum Fibrosum (30 g) (decocted first) and Flos Lonicerae (15 g).
- For thirst and a red tongue with scant coating, add Radix Adenophorae (15 g) and Radix Trichosanthis (15 g).
- For invasion of the body surface by Wind-Cold, with symptoms of fever and aversion to cold, use raw Herba Ephedrae (3–6 g) combined with Herba Schizonepetae (10 g) and Ramulus Cinnamomi (5 g).

b. During the remission stage

i. *Deficiency of Lung and Spleen Qi*

— This pattern results from a deficiency of Lung Qi (and thus Defensive Qi) and Spleen Qi (with production of Phlegm in the Interior). Signs and symptoms include susceptibility to the common cold, wheeze induced by changes in weather, aversion to cold, spontaneous sweating, reduced appetite, lassitude, loose stools and profuse sputum.

— The treatment principle is to benefit Qi, consolidate Defensive Qi, invigorate the Spleen and resolve Phlegm.

— The recommended formula is a variation of *Yu Ping Feng San* (**Jade Wind-Screen Powder**) and *Liu Jun Zi Tang* (**Six Gentleman Decoction**):

Radix Astragali seu Hedysari	10 g
Radix Codonopsis Pilosulae	10 g
Rhizoma Atractylodis Macrocephalae	10 g
Poria	10 g
Fructus Schisandrae	2–3 g
Radix Asteris	10 g
Flos Farfarae	10 g
Rhizoma Pinelliae	10 g
Pericarpium Citri Reticulatae	5 g
Radix Ledebouriellae	5 g
Fructus Chebulae	10 g

ii. *Lung and Kidney Deficiency*

— This patterns results from deficiency of Lung Qi and impairment of the Kidney function of reception of Qi. Clinical manifestations include chronic asthma, shortness of breath and palpitations on exertion, lumbar soreness and tinnitus.

— The treatment principle is to tonify the Lungs and Kidneys, assist reception of Qi and soothe asthma.

— The recommended formula is a variation of *Shen Qi Wan* (**Kidney Qi Pill**), *Ren Shen Ge Jie San* (**Ginseng and Gecko Powder**) and *Ren Shen Hu Tao Tang* (**Ginseng and Walnut Decoction**):

Radix Rehmanniae Praeparata	10–15 g
Fructus Corni	10 g
Semen Juglandis	10 g
Umbilical cords	1–2
Placenta Hominis	10 g
Lignum Aquilariae Resinatum	2–3 g
Radix Ginseng, or Radix Codonopsis Pilosulae	10 g
Fructus Schisandrae	3–5 g
Radix Asteris	10 g
Flos Farfarae	10 g

— Modifications:

- For Yang Deficiency with cold limbs, pallor and thin sputum, add Radix Aconiti Praeparata (2–5 g), Cortex Cinnamomi (2–3 g) and Fructus Psoraleae (10 g).

- For Yin Deficiency with scanty sticky sputum, dry mouth and throat, malar flush, a red tongue with scanty coating and a rapid, thready pulse, remove Lignum Aquilariae Resinatum from the prescription and add Radix Adenophorae (10–15 g), Radix Ophiopogonis (10–15 g), Bulbus Fritillariae Cirrhosae (10 g) and Cordyceps (2–3 g) (ground to powder and taken separately).
  - For dyspnoea, spontaneous sweating and palpitations, add powdered Gecko (2–3 g) and powdered Radix Ginseng (2–3 g), to be taken separately.

— The following is a prescription for external application; it is to be used during the Summer, in order to prevent asthmatic attacks during the Winter:

Semen Sinapis	20 g
Rhizoma Corydalis	10 g
Radix Euphorbiae Kansui	9 g
Herba Asari	9 g

— The herbs are ground to a powder and mixed with Moschus (0.6 g) and sufficient ginger juice to make a paste, which is then applied to acupuncture points such as *Feishu* (UB 13), *Gaohuang* (UB 43), and *Bailao* (extra: 2 cm above and lateral to *Dazhui*, Du 14). The paste is removed from the points after 2–3 hours. Treatment is given once every 10 days.

---

5. DYSPHONIA

GENERAL DESCRIPTION

— Dysphonia consists of hoarseness or loss of the voice. The Excess type results from invasion of the throat by pathogenic Wind-cold or retention of Phlegm-Heat. The Deficiency type results from Lung Fire due to Lung and Kidney Yin Deficiency, or from a deficiency of Lung Qi and Yin due to excessive speaking or singing.

DIFFERENTIATION AND TREATMENT

a. Dysphonia of the Excess type

i. Wind-Cold

— This pattern results from invasion of the Lungs by pathogenic Wind-Cold, which impairs the Lungs' function of opening and closing the vocal cords. Clinical manifestations include sudden onset of aphonia or hoarseness, cough, stuffiness of the chest, nasal obstruction, headache and possible fever and aversion to cold.
— The treatment principle is to disperse Wind-Cold and promote the smooth circulation of Lung Qi.
— The recommended formula is:

Herba Ephedrae	2–3 g
Herba Schizonepetae	10 g
Radix Peucedani	10 g
Semen Armeniacae Amarum	10 g
Bulbus Fritillariae Thunbergii	10 g
Radix Platycodi	6 g
Semen Sterculiae Scaphigerae (*Pang Da Hai*)	3–5 pieces

ii. Phlegm-Heat

— This pattern results from invasion of the Lungs by Wind-Heat, which condenses Body Fluids into Phlegm. Phlegm and Heat then combine to block the air passage. Clinical manifestations include hoarseness, cough with thick yellow sputum, a dry or sore throat and a sticky yellow tongue coating.
— The treatment principle is to clear Heat, resolve Phlegm, and ease the voice.
— The recommended formula is:

Cortex Mori Radicis	10 g
Radix Peucedani	10 g
Bulbus Fritillariae Thunbergii	10 g
Cortex Trichosanthis	10 g
Fructus Gardeniae	10 g
Radix Scutellariae	10 g
Fructus Arctii	10–15 g
Radix Platycodi	6 g
Periostracum Cicadae	2–3 g
Radix Glycyrrhizae (raw)	3 g

b. Dysphonia of the Deficiency type

i. Yin Deficiency with Dryness and Heat

— This pattern results from Dryness and Heat damaging Yin, or from Lung and Kidney Yin Deficiency due to prolonged illness. In either case, Yin Deficiency produces internal Heat, which prevents the production of normal vocal sound. Clinical manifestations include chronic hoarseness, sore throat, dry throat and mouth, dry cough with little sputum, tinnitus, tidal fever, night sweats, a red tongue with scanty coating and a rapid, thready pulse. The treatment principle is to nourish Yin, reduce Fire and moisten Dryness.
— The recommended formula is a variation of

Bai He Gu Jing Tang (**Lily Bulb Decoction to Preserve the Metal**):

Radix Adenophorae	10–15 g
Radix Ophiopogonis	10–15 g
Radix Rehmanniae	10–15 g
Radix Scrophulariae	10–15 g
Radix Platycodi	6 g
Folium Mori	10 g
Semen Armeniacae Amarum	10 g
Fructus Chebulae	10 g
Semen Oroxyli (*Mu Hu Die*)	2 g

CASE STUDY 40.6
HOARSENESS

Female, age 36

The patient complained of recurrent attacks of hoarseness over the past 10 years, the most recent attack having occurred 3 months previously following a common cold with cough. Other possible precipitating factors were sudden changes of weather, emotional stress and speaking in a loud voice (the patient was a teacher). Clinical manifestations of the recent attack included hoarseness, dry throat, sore throat following excessive use of the voice, a slightly red throat, dizziness and vertigo, lumbar soreness, weak knees, a red tongue with a thin, white and slightly sticky coating, and a deep, thready pulse.

Pathogenesis: Lung and Kidney Yin Deficiency, Phlegm combining with stagnant Qi in the throat, and failure of Body Fluids to nourish the upper body.

Western diagnosis: Chronic laryngitis

Treatment principle: Nourish Lung and Kidney Yin and subdue Fire.

The formula used was a variation of *Shen Mai Di Huang Tang* (**Six-Flavour Rehmannia Decoction with Adenophora, Glehnia and Ophiopogon**):

Radix Adenophorae	10 g
Radix Glehniae	10 g
Radix Asparagi	10 g
Radix Ophiopogonis	10 g
Radix Rehmanniae	12 g
Rhizoma Polygonati Odorati	10 g
Radix Scrophulariae	15 g
Rhizoma Anemarrhenae	10 g
Rhizoma Dioscoreae	10 g
Fructus Corni	10 g
Semen Oroxyli	3 g
Radix Glycyrrhizae (*raw*)	3 g
Fructus Citri Sarcodactylis	3 g

On subsequent visits to the clinic, Semen Juglandis (10 g) and Fructus Chebulae (10 g) were added to the prescription and the patient was instructed to take honey with water separately.

After 42 doses of this formula, the patient was still only capable of whispering.

At this point, the treatment method was altered to include relieving depression and stagnation, and **Free and Relaxed Powder** (30 g) and **Great Tonify the Yin Pill** (5 g) were added to the prescription; the former was decocted wrapped with the other ingredients while the latter was taken separately with water twice daily.

After another month of treatment, her condition was somewhat improved, but she still could not speak loudly and overuse of her voice resulted in shortness of breath. Treated Herba Ephedrae (1.5 g) was then added to the formula to promote the smooth circulation of Lung Qi, and after three doses her voice suddenly returned to normal.

---

ii. *Damage to Lung Qi due to overuse of the voice*
— Overuse of the voice damages Lung Qi and the vocal cords, thus producing hoarseness, low voice and fatigue. The treatment principle is to tonify Lung Qi and ease the throat and voice.
— The recommended formula is *Huang Shi Xiang Sheng Wan* (**Huang's Pill for Promoting the Voice**):

Radix Astragali seu Hedysari	10–12 g
Fructus Chebulae	10 g
Bulbus Fritillariae Thunbergii	10 g
Semen Sterculiae Scaphigerae	5 pieces
Radix Platycodi	6 g
Radix Glycyrrhizae	10 g
Periostracum Cicadae	2–3 g

B. Diseases of the digestive system

1. EPIGASTRIC PAIN

GENERAL DESCRIPTION
— Epigastric pain corresponds to the Western medical categories of acute gastritis, chronic gastritis and gastric and duodenal ulcer. Excess types of epigastric pain include retention of food, retention of Cold, retention of Dampness, retention of Heat and stagnation of Qi. Deficiency types of epigastric pain include Qi Deficiency, deficiency of Spleen Yang and deficiency of Stomach Yin.

DIFFERENTIATION AND TREATMENT

a. Acute epigastric pain

i. Retention of Food

— Retention of Food produces pain, distension and fullness in the epigastrium, foul belching, acid regurgitation, loss of appetite, a thick tongue coating and a rolling pulse.
— The treatment principle is to promote digestion and harmonize the Stomach.
— The recommended formula is a variation of *Bao He Wan* (**Preserving and Harmonizing Pill**):

Fructus Crataegi	10–15 g
Massa Fermentata Medicinalis	12 g
Fructus Oryzae Germinatus	12 g
Fructus Hordei Germinatus	12 g
Fructus Aurantii Immaturus	10 g
Rhizoma Pinelliae	10 g
Fructus Forsythiae	10 g
Rhizoma Coptidis	2–3 g

ii. Retention of Cold and Qi Stagnation

— This pattern results from invasion of the Stomach by pathogenic Cold, leading to retention of Cold and stagnation of Qi. Clinical manifestations include epigastric pain which is alleviated by warmth, reflux of clear fluid, a white tongue coating and a wiry pulse.
— The treatment principle is to warm the Middle Burner and regulate Qi.
— The recommended formula is a variation of *Liang Fu Wan* (**Galangal and Cyperus Pill**):

Rhizoma Alpiniae Officinalis	2–5 g
Ramulus Cinnamomi	2–5 g
Rhizoma Zingiberis or Rhizoma Zingiberis Recens	2–5 g
Fructus Evodiae	1–3 g
Rhizoma Cyperi	10 g
Radix Aucklandiae	3–5 g
Fructus Amomi *(added at end of decoction)*	2–3 g
Rhizoma Pinelliae	10 g

iii. Fire and Damp-Heat in the Stomach

— Invasion of the Middle Burner by Damp-Heat impairs the descending function of the Stomach and produces symptoms of vomiting soon after eating, foul breath, a bitter taste in the mouth, distending pain in the epigastrium, a yellow and sticky tongue coating and a rolling and rapid pulse. The treatment principle is to clear Heat, resolve Dampness, reduce Fire and harmonize the Stomach.

— The recommended formula is a variation of *Xie Xin Tang* (**Drain the Epigastrium Decoction**) and *Huo Xiang Zheng Qi San* (**Agastache Upright Qi Powder**):

Rhizoma Coptidis	2–3 g
Fructus Aurantii Immaturus	5–10 g
Herba Agastachis	10 g
Cortex Magnoliae Officinalis	2–5 g
Rhizoma Pinelliae (*alum treated*)	10 g
Rhizoma Atractylodis	5–10 g
Pericarpium Citri Reticulatae	5 g
Fructus Gardeniae	10 g
Fructus Meliae Toosendan	10 g
Rhizoma Corydalis	10 g

— Modifications:

  – For abdominal distension and constipation, add Radix et Rhizoma Rhei (3–6 g).

b. Chronic epigastric pain

i. Disharmony between the Liver and Stomach

— Stagnation of Liver Qi impairs the Stomach's function of descending. Clinical manifestations include distending epigastric pain which extends to the hypochondrium, belching, acid regurgitation, aggravation of symptoms with emotional stress, a thin tongue coating and a wiry pulse.
— The treatment principle is to soothe the Liver and harmonize the Stomach.
— The recommended formula is a variation of *Chai Hu Shu Gan San* (**Bupleurum Soothing the Liver Decoction**):

Radix Bupleuri	5 g
Fructus Aurantii Immaturus *or* Fructus Aurantii	10 g
Radix Paeoniae Alba	10 g
Rhizoma Ligustici Chuanxiong	5–10 g
Rhizoma Cyperi	10 g
Pericarpium Citri Reticulatae Viride	5 g
Pericarpium Citri Reticulatae	5 g
Fructus Meliae Toosendan	10 g
Rhizoma Coydalis	10 g

— Modifications:

  – For Stagnant Liver Qi turning to Heat, with symptoms of a bitter taste in the mouth and a red tongue with yellow coating, add Cortex Moutan Radicis (10 g) and Fructus Gardeniae (10 g).
  – For acid regurgitation, add Os Sepiellae seu Sepiae (10–15 g) and Concha Areae (10–15 g).

- If belching is pronounced, add Rhizoma Pinelliae (10 g), Fructus Amomi (2–3 g) (added at end of decoction) and Haematitum (15–20 g) (decocted first).

CASE STUDY 40.7
EPIGASTRIC PAIN

Female, age 40

The patient had recently suffered from depression, which caused distension and pain in the epigastrium, referred to the hypochondrium on both sides. Other clinical manifestations included sighing and belching, which slightly alleviated the distension, but not the pain. She also had acid regurgitation, a red tongue with a thin coating, and a wiry pulse.

Pathogenesis: Stagnant Liver Qi turned to Fire, which then invaded the Stomach.

Western diagnosis: Chronic gastritis

Treatment principle: Primarily, soothe the Liver and harmonize the Stomach; secondarily, clear Heat with bitter herbs.

The formula used was a variation of **Bupleurum Soothing the Liver Decoction** and **Left Metal Pill**:

Radix Bupleuri	3 g
Rhizoma Cyperi	9 g
Radix Curcumae	9 g
Rhizoma Corydalis	9 g
Pericarpium Citri Reticulatae Viride	4.5 g
Fructus Meliae Toosendan	9 g
Fructus Gardeniae (burnt)	4.5 g
Radix Scutellariae	4.5 g
plus **Left Metal Pill**	3 g
(taken separately with water)	

After administration of two doses, epigastric distension improved and the pain became less severe. All signs and symptoms disappeared after another three doses.

---

ii. *Deficiency of the Spleen and Stomach with stagnation of Cold*
— Yang Deficiency produces Internal Cold; deficiency of Spleen Yang means impairment of the Spleen's functions of transportation and transformation, which causes disharmony of Stomach Qi. Clinical manifestations include dull epigastric pain which is alleviated by eating, warmth and pressure; lassitude, reduced appetite and loose stools.

— The treatment principle is to benefit Qi and warm the Middle Burner.
— The recommended formula is a variation of *Huang Qi Jian Zhong Tang* (**Astragalus Decoction to Construct the Middle**) and *Li Zhong Wan* (**Regulating the Middle Decoction**):

Radix Codonopsis Pilosulae	10 g
Radix Astragali seu Hedysari	10–15 g
Rhizoma Atractylodis Macrocephalae	10 g
Ramulus Cinnamomi or Cortex Cinnamomi	2–5 g
Rhizoma Zingiberis	2–5 g
Radix Paeoniae Alba	10 g
Radix Glycyrrhizae (treated)	3 g

— Modifications:

– For deficiency of the Middle Burner complicated by retention of fluid, with symptoms of reflux of clear fluid and splashing sounds in the Stomach, add Poria (12 g), Fructus Evodiae (2 g) and Pericarpium Zanthoxyli (2 g).

iii. *Deficiency of the Middle Burner and stagnation of Qi*
— Deficiency of the Spleen and Stomach means weakness in transportation and transformation, thus producing stagnation of Qi. Clinical manifestations include dull or distending epigastric pain, especially after eating and alleviated by belching, and reduced appetite and lassitude.
— The treatment principle is to tonify the Middle Burner and regulate Qi.
— The recommended formula is a variation of *Xiang Sha Liu Jun Zi Tang* (**Six Gentlemen Decoction with Aucklandia and Amomum**) and *Zhi Zhu Wan* (**Aurantia Immaturus–Atractylodis Macrocephalae Pill**):

Radix Codonopsis Pilosulae	10 g
Radix Astragali seu Hedysari	10 g
Rhizoma Atractylodis Macrocephalae	10 g
Fructus Aurantii Immaturus	10 g
Radix Aucklandiae	5 g
Fructus Amomi (added at end of decoction)	2–3 g
Rhizoma Pinelliae	10 g
Pericarpium Citri Reticulatae	5 g
Rhizoma Cyperi	10 g
Poria	10 g
Radix Glycyrrhizae (treated)	3 g
Fructus Oryzae Germinatus	10 g

CASE STUDY 40.8
EPIGASTRIC PAIN

Male, age 39

The patient complained of epigastric pain tending to occur in the Autumn and Winter over the past 6 years. The most recent attack had begun 1 month previously. The pain usually occurred about an hour after meals or at midnight, and could be alleviated by heat or pressure, or by eating small amounts of food. Eating more than a small amount would cause distension. His appetite was poor. His tongue coating was thin and sticky, and his pulse thready and wiry.

2 years ago he had passed black stools, and the diagnosis of duodenal ulcer was established by barium meal fluoroscopy.

Pathogenesis: Spleen and Stomach Deficiency with retention of Cold, complicated by stagnation of Qi.

Western diagnosis: Duodenal ulcer

Treatment principle: Invigorate the Spleen, harmonize the Stomach, activate Qi circulation and harmonize the Middle Burner.

The formula used was a variation of **Six Gentlemen Decoction with Aucklandia and Amomum**:

Radix Codonopsis Pilosulae *(stir-baked)*	9 g
Rhizoma Atractylodis Macrocephalae *(stir-baked)*	9 g
Poria	9 g
Radix Glycyrrhizae *(treated)*	3 g
Radix Aucklandiae	9 g
Rhizoma Pinelliae	9 g
Pericarpium Citri Reticulatae	4.5 g
Fructus Amomi	3 g
Pericarpium Zanthoxyli	3 g
Flos Magnoliae Officinalis *(Chuan Po Hua)*	4.5 g

After administration of three doses, epigastric pain was less and the patient's appetite improved, but he complained of stuffiness of the chest and insomnia. His tongue coating was thin and sticky and his pulse was thready and wiry. Pericarpium Zanthoxyli and Fructus Amomi were then removed from the prescription; Radix Salviae Miltiorrhizae (9 g), Radix Paeoniae Rubra (9 g), aged Fructus Chaenomelis (3 g) and Fructus Ziziphi Jujubae (5 pieces) were added.

After five doses of this new formula the symptoms were relieved, and the patient was given another five doses to consolidate the therapeutic results.

iv. Retention of Dampness in the Spleen and Stomach
— Improper diet impairs the Spleen's functions of transportation and transformation, producing Turbid Damp in the interior which blocks Qi circulation. Clinical manifestations include distending epigastric and abdominal pain, reduced appetite and a sticky tongue coating.
— The treatment principle is to resolve Dampness and harmonize the Middle Burner.
— The recommended formula is a variation of *Xiang Sha Ping Wei San* (**Regulate the Stomach Decoction with Aucklandia and Amomum**):

Rhizoma Atractylodis	6–10 g
Rhizoma Atractylodis Macrocephalae	10 g
Cortex Magnoliae Officinalis	2–5 g
Poria	10 g
Radix Aucklandiae	3–5 g
Fructus Amomi *(added at end of decoction)*	2–3 g
Rhizoma Pinelliae	10 g
Pericarpium Citri Reticulatae	5 g
Fructus Aurantii Immaturus	5–10 g

v. Yin Deficiency with Empty Fire
— Constitutional Yin Deficiency produces Empty Fire, which eventually consumes Stomach Yin. Clinical manifestations include dull or burning epigastric pain, an empty and uncomfortable sensation in the stomach, dryness and a bitter taste in the mouth, retching, a red tongue without coating or with a thin yellow coating, and a rapid, thready pulse.
— The treatment principle is to nourish Yin, reduce Fire and benefit the Stomach.
— The recommended formula is a variation of *Yi Guan Jian* (**Linking Decoction**):

Radix Glehniae	10–15g
Herba Dendrobii	10–15g
Radix Ophiopogonis	10–15g
Radix Paeoniae Alba	10g
Radix Glycyrrhizae	3g
Fructus Meliae Toosendan	10g
Rhizoma Corydalis	10g
Fructus Aurantii Immaturus	5–10g
Fructus Gardeniae	10g

— Modifications:

– For lack of gastric acid, add Fructus Mume (3–5 g) and fresh Fructus Crataegi (10–15 g).

- If Liver Qi Stagnation is pronounced, add Radix Bupleuri (5 g), Rhizoma Cyperi (10 g) and Fructus Citri Sarcodactylis (5 g).
- For constipation with dry stool, add Fructus Cannabis (10 g), Radix Angelicae Sinensis (10 g) and Semen Biotae (10 g).

vi. Blood Stagnation with damage to the vessels
— Chronic epigastric pain damages the blood vessels and produces Blood Stagnation. Clinical manifestations include boring epigastric pain, possibly melaena or haematemesis, a purple tongue and a wiry, hesitant pulse.
— The treatment principle is to resolve Blood Stasis and harmonize the collaterals.
— The recommended formula is a variation of *Huo Luo Xiao Ling Dan* (**Fantastically Effective Pill to Invigorate the Collaterals**) and *Shi Xiao San* (**Sudden Smile Powder**):

Radix Salviae Miltiorrhizae	10–15 g
Radix Angelicae Sinensis	10 g
Radix Paeoniae Rubra	10 g
Radix Paeoniae Alba	10 g
Resina Olibani	2–3 g
Resina Myrrhae	2–3 g
Os Sepiellae seu Sepiae	10–15 g
Rhizoma Corydalis	10 g
Corium Erinacei	10 g
Faeces Trogopterorum	10 g

— Modifications:

- For melaena or haematemesis, remove Resina Olibani and Resina Myrrhae from the prescription and add Cacumen Biotae (10–15 g) and Radix et Rhizoma Rhei (5–10 g); also administer a powder of 1.5–2 g each of Radix Notoginseng and Rhizoma Bletillae, to be taken separately.

---

2. DIARRHOEA AND DYSENTERY

GENERAL DESCRIPTION
— Diarrhoea and dysentery principally affect the Spleen, Stomach, Small and Large Intestines. They are caused by the invasion of external Cold-Damp, Summer Heat and Dampness, improper diet and violent emotions, all of which impair the Spleen's functions of transportation and transformation and the Large Intestine's function of transmission.

DIFFERENTIATION AND TREATMENT

a. Retention of Food

— Improper diet or ingestion of contaminated food damages the Spleen and Stomach, thus causing retention of Food in the Interior. Clinical manifestations include epigastric and abdominal distension and fullness, abdominal pain, borborygmus, foul belching, loss of appetite, smelly stool, a thick tongue coating and a rolling pulse.
— The treatment principle is to promote digestion, harmonize the Middle Burner and stop diarrhoea and dysentery.
The recommended formula is a variation of **Preserving and Harmonizing Pill** and *Mu Xiang Bing Long Wan* (**Aucklandia and Betel Nut Pill**):
— For simple diarrhoea:

Fructus Crataegi *(burnt)*	10–15 g
Massa Fermentata Medicinalis	12–15 g
Fructus Oryzae Germinatus	10–15 g
Fructus Hordei Germinatus	10–15 g
Rhizoma Pinelliae	10 g
Pericarpium Citri Reticulatae	5 g
Rhizoma Coptidis	2 g
Poria	10 g

— For dysentery, remove Rhizoma Pinelliae, Pericarpium Citri Reticulatae and Poria, and add:

Radix Aucklandiae	5 g
Semen Arecae	5–10 g
Radix et Rhizoma Rhei	5–10 g

b. Cold-Damp

— Invasion of the Spleen by Cold-Damp impairs the Spleen's functions of transportation and transformation and the Large Intestine's function of transmission. Clinical manifestations include abdominal distension and pain, diarrhoea with watery stool or dysentery with white mucus, tenesmus, borborygmus and a sticky white tongue coating.
— The treatment principle is to warm the Middle Burner and resolve Dampness.
— The recommended formula is a variation of **Agastache Upright Qi Powder** and *Ping Wei San* (**Calm the Stomach Powder**):

Rhizoma Atractylodis	6–10 g
Cortex Magnoliae Officinalis	2–3 g
Herba Agastachis	10 g
Radix Aucklandiae	5 g

Pericarpium Citri Reticulatae	5 g
Massa Fermentata	10 g
Poria	10 g

— Modifications:

- For severe diarrhoea accompanied by exterior symptoms, add Herba Schizonepetae (10g), Radix Ledebouriellae (10g) and Folium Perillae (3g).
- For diarrhoea with watery stool, add Semen Plantaginis (10g) (decocted wrapped).
- For severe dysentery, add Semen Arecae (5–10g).
- For prolonged diarrhoea and dysentery, add Rhizoma Atractylodis Macrocephalae (10g), Rhizoma Zingiberis (2–3g) and Pericarpium Granati (10g).

c. Damp-Heat

— Damage to the Middle Burner by Summer Heat and Dampness, or invasion of the Spleen by Damp-Heat, impairs the Large Intestine's function of transmission. Clinical manifestations include diarrhoea with abdominal pain and tenesmus, a burning sensation in the anus, foul stool with blood or mucus, scanty, deep-yellow urine, a sticky yellow tongue coating and a rapid, soft pulse.
— The treatment principle is to clear Heat from the Intestines and resolve Dampness.
— The recommended formula is a variation of *Ge Gen Qin Lian Tang* (**Kudzu, Coptis and Scutellaria Decoction**), *Xiang Lian Wan* (**Aucklandia and Coptis Pill**), and *Shao Yao Tang* (**Peony Decoction**):

Radix Scutellariae	10 g
Rhizoma Coptidis	3–10 g
Radix Paeoniae Alba	10 g
Radix Aucklandiae	5 g
Radix Puerariae	10 g
Herba Portulacae	15 g

— Modifications:

- For diarrhoea, add Poria (10 g) and Semen Plantaginis (10 g) (decocted wrapped).
- For dysentery, add Radix Angelicae Sinensis (10 g) and Cortex Fraxini (10 g).
- For bloody dysentery due to Fire Poison, add Radix Pulsatillae (10–15 g).

CASE STUDY 40.9
DYSENTERY
Female, age 54

This patient had had chronic bacillary dysentery for 3 years. For the past 3 days she had experienced abdominal pain with blood and mucus in the stool, tenesmus, seven to eight bowel motions daily, loss of body weight, reduced appetite, irritability, five-palm Heat, a bitter taste in her mouth and deep-yellow urine. She had a deep-red tongue with no coating, and a thready, rapid pulse.

Pathogenesis: Combination of Damp and Heat in the Large Intestine; damage to Yin and Blood due to prolonged dysentery.

Western diagnosis: Chronic bacillary dysentery

Treatment principle: Primarily, clear Damp-Heat; secondarily, nourish Yin and Blood.
The formula used was a variation of *Bai Tou Weng Tang* (**Pulsatilla Decoction**):

Radix Pulsatillae	9 g
Cortex Fraxini	9 g
Cortex Phellodendri	6 g
Rhizoma Coptidis	4.5 g
Colla Corii Asini	9 g
Radix Angelicae Sinensis	9 g
Radix Aucklandiae	4.5 g
Rhizoma Zingiberis *(charred)*	3 g
Fructus Crataegi *(charred)*	12 g
Radix et Rhizoma Rhei *(prepared)*	9 g

After two doses, the abdominal pain and tenesmus were slightly improved, as was the bitter taste. All other symptoms remained unchanged. Radix et Rhizoma Rhei was removed from the prescription.

After three more doses, both the abdominal pain and tenesmus had disappeared. There was some mucus, but no blood in the stool. Her irritability and five-palm Heat were reduced and her urine was not such a deep yellow. The bitter taste persisted. At this point, Rhizoma Zingiberis was removed from the prescription and another five doses were prescribed.

By her next visit, her stool had become formed and contained no mucus, with bowel motions occurring once or twice daily. Both the irritability and the bitter taste had substantially improved, as had her appetite. Her tongue was red with a scanty coating, and her pulse was thready and rapid. The prescription was modified to clear residual pathogens as follows:

Radix Pulsatillae	9 g
Cortex Fraxini	6 g
Cortex Phellodendri	6 g
Rhizoma Coptidis	3 g
Colla Corii Asini	9 g

Radix Angelicae Sinensis	9 g
Radix Rehmanniae	9 g
Fructus Crataegi *(stir-baked)*	9 g
Fructus Oryzae Germinatus *(stir-baked)*	9 g
Fructus Hordei Germinatus *(stir-baked)*	9 g
Pericarpium Citri Reticulatae	4.5 g

A follow-up visit 2 years later revealed no relapse.

d. Spleen Deficiency

— Chronic diarrhoea or dysentery means deficiency of Spleen Qi with impairment of the functions of transportation and transformation. Clinical manifestations include reduced appetite, loose stool with undigested food, lassitude and anal prolapse.
— The treatment principle is to benefit Qi and invigorate the Spleen.
— The recommended formula is a variation of *Shen Ling Bai Zhu San* (**Panax–Poria–Atractylodes Powder**) and *Bu Zhong Yi Qi Tang* (**Tonifying the Middle and Benefiting Qi Decoction**):

Radix Codonopsis Pilosulae	10 g
Rhizoma Atractylodis Macrocephalae	10 g
Rhizoma Dioscoreae	10–15 g
Semen Dolichoris	10–15 g
Semen Coicis	12 g
Poria	10 g
Radix Aucklandiae	5 g
Fructus Amomi	2–3 g
(added at end of decoction)	

— Modifications:

 – For Spleen Yang Deficiency, add Rhizoma Zingiberis (2–5 g), Radix Aconiti Praeparata (2–5 g) and Fructus Alpiniae Oxyphyllae (10 g).
 – For Sinking of Central Qi, add Rhizoma Cimicifugae (2 g), Radix Bupleuri (2 g) and Radix Astragali seu Hedysari (10 g).
 – For chronic dysentery, add Fructus Chebulae (10 g) and Pericarpium Granati (10 g).

e. Spleen and Kidney Yang Deficiency

— Chronic dysentery leads to Spleen and Kidney Yang Deficiency, which means an inability to digest food. Clinical manifestations include daybreak diarrhoea, dysentery with white mucus or undigested food, faecal

incontinence, cold limbs, a pale tongue and a deep, thready pulse.
— The treatment principle is to warm the Kidneys and Spleen.
— The recommended formula is a variation of *Si Shen Wan* (**Four-Miracle Pill**), *Fu Zi Li Zhong Wan* (**Prepared Aconite Pill to Regulate the Middle**), and *Zhen Ren Yang Zang Tang* (**True Man's Decoction for Nourishing the Organs**):

Fructus Psoraleae	10 g
Fructus Alpiniae Oxyphyllae	10 g
Fructus Evodiae	2–3 g
Fructus Schisandrae	3–5 g
Fructus Chebulae	10 g
Fructus Mume	3–5 g
Semen Myristicae	10 g
Cortex Ailanthi	10 g
Rhizoma Atractylodis Macrocephalae	10 g
Rhizoma Zingiberis	2–5 g

— Modifications:

 – For dysentery, add Radix Angelicae Sinensis (10 g) and Radix Paeoniae Alba (10 g).
 – For Food Stagnation, remove Fructus Chebulae, Semen Myristicae and Fructus Schisandrae from the prescription and add Fructus Aurantii Immaturus (6 g), Radix et Rhizoma Rhei (5–10 g) and Fructus Crataegi (10–15 g).

CASE STUDY 40.10
DIARRHOEA

Male, age 44

The patient complained of loose stools for the past 6 years, with between five and ten motions each day. He felt more comfortable after taking warm drinks. He had a sallow complexion, a thin, white tongue coating and a weak-floating, thready and rapid pulse.

Pathogenesis: Deficiency of Kidney Yang and of the Spleen and Stomach.

Treatment principle: Primarily warm and invigorate the Spleen and Kidneys and secondarily tonify Qi and astringe the intestines.

The formula used was a variation of **Four-Miracle Pill** and **Prepared Aconite Pill to Regulate the Middle**):

Radix Codonopsis Pilosulae *(stir-baked)*	9g
Rhizoma Atractylodis Macrocephalae *(stir-baked)*	12g

Rhizoma Zingiberis	3g
Halloysitum Rubrum	12g
Radix Linderae	6g
Pericarpium Papaveris *(Ying Su Ke)*	9g
Fructus Evodiae	3g
plus	
Four-Miracle Pill	9g
Powdered sulphur 0.9g	
(both to be taken separately with water)	

After 2 weeks of treatment, the frequency of bowel motions decreased, but the looseness of the stool remained unchanged. The patient also noted stuffiness of the chest, belching, abdominal distension and a cold sensation in the abdomen. At this point, the dosage of Rhizoma Zingiberis and powdered sulphur were increased to 4.5 g and 1.5 g respectively.

After another seven doses, the frequency of the motions had further decreased, but the stool remained loose, with weakness of the body and limbs, dizziness and shortness of breath, indicating deficiency of both the Spleen and Kidneys. Treatment was continued as follows:

4.5 g each of **Prepared Aconite Pill to Warm the Middle** and **Four-Miracle Pill** to be taken twice daily with 0.6 g of powdered sulphur.

After another month, the stool began to be formed and the patient became more energetic. After a total of 3 months of treatment, all signs and symptoms had disappeared.

vi. Yin Deficiency
— In this pattern, long-term dysentery due to Damp-Heat is complicated with Yin Deficiency resulting from the dysentery itself.
— Clinical manifestations include chronic dysentery with blood and mucus in the stool, abdominal pain, mild tenesmus, a red tongue with scanty moisture and a rapid, thready pulse.
— The treatment principle is to nourish Yin, clear Heat from the Intestines and stop dysentery.
— The recommended formula is a variation of *Zhu Ji Wan* (**Zhu Ji Pill**):

Rhizoma Coptidis	3–5 g
Colla Corii Asini	10 g
(melted and taken separately)	
Radix Sanguisorbae	10–15 g
Radix Angelicae Sinensis	10 g
Radix Paeoniae Alba	10 g
Fructus Mume	5 g
Cortex Ailanthi	10 g
Semen Nelumbinis	10–15 g

vii. Unregulated emotions
— Invasion of the Spleen by Liver Qi impairs the Spleen's functions of transportation and transformation. Clinical manifestations include diarrhoea which is related to the patient's emotional state, stuffiness of the chest, hypochondriac distension, borborygmus, abdominal pain immediately alleviated by bowel motion, and a wiry pulse.
— The treatment principle is to soothe the Liver and promote the function of the Spleen.
— The recommended formula is a variation of *Tong Xie Yao Fang* (**Important Formula for Painful Diarrhoea**):

Radix Paeoniae Alba	10 g
Radix Ledebouriellae	5–10 g
Rhizoma Atractylodis Macrocephalae	12 g
Radix Bupleuri	5 g
Radix Aucklandiae	5 g
Pericarpium Citri Reticulatae	5 g
Fructus Mume	3 g
Radix Codonopsis Pilosulae	10 g
Rhizoma Dioscoreae	15 g
Radix Glycyrrhizae	3 g

CASE STUDY 40.11
DIARRHOEA

Male, age 30

The patient complained of loose stools for nearly 5 years, with three to five motions daily. He frequently had abdominal pain before each motion. Other clinical manifestations included distension in the right hypochondrium and epigastrium which was worse after eating, poor appetite, pallor, lassitude, aversion to cold, a pale tongue with a thin sticky coating, and a wiry pulse. X-rays showed chronic colitis.

Pathogenesis: Hyperactivity of the Liver and deficiency of the Spleen; Yang Deficiency of the Middle Burner.

Western diagnosis: Chronic colitis

Treatment principle: Invigorate the Spleen, calm the Liver and warm the Yang of the Middle Burner. The formula used was a variation of **Important Formula for Painful Diarrhoea** and *Huang Qi Jian Zhong Tang* (**Astragalus Decoction to Construct the Middle**):

Radix Astragali seu Hedysari (treated)	9 g
Rhizoma Atractylodis Macrocephalae *(stir-baked)*	9 g
Radix Paeoniae Alba	9 g
Radix Ledebouriellae *(stir-baked)*	15 g
Radix Glycyrrhizae *(treated)*	15 g

Poria	9 g
Ramulus Cinnamomi	2.4 g
Fructus Crataegi *(charred)*	12 g
Rhizoma Zingiberis *(baked)*	9 g
Fructus Ziziphi Jujubae	5 pieces
Saccharum Granorum	120 g
(taken separately with water)	

After four doses, the stool become less loose and frequency of motions decreased to three times daily. Abdominal pain before each motion decreased and the patient felt more energetic, but suffered from flatulence. At this point, Radix Glycyrrhizae and Poria were removed from the prescription and Pericarpium Citri Reticulatae (6 g) and roasted Radix Aucklandiae (9 g) were added.

After seven doses of this formula, the stool was formed and frequency of motions was normal (once or twice daily). There was still occasional abdominal pain, but this disappeared after a total of 48 doses of the prescription.

3. VIRAL HEPATITIS

GENERAL DESCRIPTION
— Icteric hepatitis falls into the TCM category of jaundice, while anicteric hepatitis is classified as hypochondriac pain. Viral hepatitis is caused by invasion of the interior of the body by pathogenic Damp-Heat, or by stagnation of Liver Qi, with resultant disharmony of the Liver and Spleen. In prolonged cases, Spleen Qi Deficiency, stagnation of Qi and Blood, and Liver and Kidney Yin Deficiency eventually result.
— Acute viral hepatitis is usually of the Excess type and presents as Damp-Heat, Fire Poison, Liver Qi Stagnation and/or invasion of the Spleen and Stomach by Dampness. Chronic viral hepatitis is usually of the Deficiency type and presents as Spleen Deficiency with stagnation of Liver Qi, Qi and Blood Stagnation and/or Liver and Kidney Yin Deficiency.

DIFFERENTIATION AND TREATMENT

a. Retention of Damp-Heat

— Retention of Damp-Heat causes disorders of the Liver and Gall Bladder. Clinical manifestations include yellow sclera, yellow skin, deep-yellow urine, distension and fullness in the epigastrium and abdomen, a bitter taste in the mouth, poor appetite and a sticky yellow tongue coating. This pattern is often present in acute icteric hepatitis, or anicteric hepatitis with severe Damp-Heat.
— The treatment principle is to clear Heat, eliminate Dampness, soothe the Liver and invigorate the Spleen.
— The recommended formula is a variation of *Yin Chen Hao Tang* (**Artemisia Yinchenhao Decoction**) and **Calm the Stomach Powder**:

Herba Artemisiae Scopariae	15–30 g
Fructus Gardeniae	10 g
Radix Bupleuri	6–10 g
Radix Scutellariae	10 g
Rhizoma Atractylodis	5–10 g
Cortex Magnoliae Officinalis	2–5 g
Poria	10 g
Rhizoma Polygoni Cuspidati	15 g
Radix et Rhizoma Rhei	5–10 g

— Modifications:

  – If Fire Poison is pronounced, add Radix Isatidis (15 g), Folium Isatidis (15 g) and Herba Taraxaci (15 g).
  – For severe Dampness with loose stools, remove Radix et Rhizoma Rhei and Fructus Gardeniae from the prescription and add Fructus Amomi (2–3 g) (added at end of decoction), Rhizoma Zingiberis (2–5 g) and Semen Plantaginis (10 g) (decocted wrapped).

CASE STUDY 40.12
HEPATITIS

Male, age 35

This patient had had yellow skin and sclera for 2 weeks, with deep-yellow urine, lassitude, poor appetite, a sticky yellow tongue coating and a wiry, rolling pulse. Liver function test showed icteric index 20 units and GPT 400 units.

Pathogenesis: Accumulation of Damp and Heat in the Liver, Gall Bladder, Spleen and Stomach, spreading the bile to the muscles and skin.

Western diagnosis: Acute icteric infectious hepatitis.

Treatment principle: Clear Damp-Heat from the Liver and Gall Bladder.

The formula used was a variation of **Artemisia Yinchenhao Decoction**:

Herba Artemisiae Scopariae	30 g
Radix Isatidis	30 g
Cortex Phellodendri	10 g
Fructus Gardeniae	10 g
Radix et Rhizoma Rhei	10 g

Semen Plantaginis	10 g
(decocted wrapped)	
Poria	10 g
Rhizoma Alismatis	10 g
Herba Taraxaci	15 g
Cortex Magnoliae Officinalis	3g

After five doses, the jaundice disappeared; after another 10 days of treatment, liver function returned to normal. Treatment was continued for another 2 weeks based on the principles of soothing the Liver and invigorating the Spleen, and the patient was discharged from the hospital free of all signs and symptoms.

b. Liver Qi Stagnation and Spleen Deficiency

— Liver Qi Stagnation and Spleen Deficiency result in disharmony between the Liver and Spleen. Clinical manifestations include distending or dull pain in the costal and hypochondriac regions, percussion pain in the Liver area, mild enlargement of the Liver, reduced appetite, lassitude, depression or irritability and restlessness, and a wiry pulse. This pattern is often present in acute anicteric hepatitis or chronic hepatitis.
— The treatment principle is to soothe the Liver, relieve stagnation, benefit Qi and invigorate the Spleen.
— The recommended formula is a variation of *Xiao Yao San* (**Free and Relaxed Powder**):

Radix Bupleuri	5 g
Radix Paeoniae Alba	10 g
Fructus Aurantii	5 g
Rhizoma Cyperi	10 g
Radix Curcumae	10 g
Fructus Meliae Toosendan	10 g
Rhizoma Corydalis	10 g
Radix Codonopsis Pilosulae	10 g
Rhizoma Atractylodis	
Macrocephalae	10 g
Poria	10 g
Radix Glycyrrhizae	3 g

— Modifications:

  – For Damp-Heat, add Herba Artemisiae Scopariae (10–15 g), Fructus Gardeniae (10 g), Rhizoma Polygoni Cuspidati (15 g), Rhizoma Atractylodis (5–10g) and Cortex Magnolia Officinalis (2–5 g).
  – For Blood Stagnation, add Radix Salviae Miltiorrhizae (15 g), Rhizoma Ligustici Chuanxiong (10 g) and **Sudden Smile Powder** (10 g).
  – For severe Blood Stagnation, add Rhizoma Sparganii (5–10 g), Rhizoma

Zedoariae (5–10 g) and 15 g of Carapax Trionycis in the form of *Bie Jia Jian Wan* (**Decocted Turtle Shell Pill**).

c. Liver and Kidney Yin Deficiency

— Chronic illness leads to deficiency of Blood and Yin, and of Liver and Kidneys. Clinical manifestations include dull hypochondriac pain, dizziness and vertigo, tinnitus, five-palm Heat, bleeding gums, a red, cracked tongue with a thin, clean coating, and a thready, wiry pulse.
— The treatment principle is to nourish the Kidneys and Liver and harmonize the collaterals.
— The recommended formula is a variation of **Linking Decoction**:

Radix Rehmanniae	10–15 g
Radix Rehmanniae Praeparata	10–15 g
Radix Angelicae Sinensis	10 g
Fructus Lycii	10 g
Radix Adenophorae	10–15 g
Radix Ophiopogonis	10–15 g
Fructus Meliae Toosendan	10 g
Radix Curcumae	10 g
Fructus Aurantii	5 g
Fructus Citri Sarcodactylis	5 g

— Modifications:

  – For bleeding due to Heat in the Blood, add Cortex Moutan Radicis (10 g), Fructus Gardeniae (burnt) (10 g), Radix Rubiae (10 g) and Indigo Naturalis (5 g) (mixed with water and taken separately).
  – For Spleen Deficiency, add Radix Codonopsis Pilosulae (10 g), Radix Astragali seu Hedysari (10–15 g) and Rhizoma Atractylodis Macrocephalae (10 g).

4. CHOLECYSTITIS AND CHOLELITHIASIS

GENERAL DESCRIPTION
— The key symptom of cholecystitis and cholelithiasis is right hypochondriac pain, which typically radiates to the shoulder and back and may be accompanied by fever.
— The pathogenesis of the disease is retention of Damp-Heat in the Interior, leading to disorders of the Liver and Gall Bladder.
— The treatment principle is to soothe the Liver, ease the Gall Bladder, clear Heat and eliminate Dampness.

DIFFERENTIATION AND TREATMENT

a. Damp-Heat in the Liver and Gall Bladder

— Retention of Damp-Heat in the Interior impairs the Liver's function of promoting the free flow of Qi and causes disorders of the biliary tract. Clinical manifestations include distending or colicky pain in the right hypochondrium, which radiates to the shoulder and back, a bitter taste in the mouth, aversion to greasy food, nausea, vomiting, a sticky yellow tongue coating and a wiry pulse.

— The treatment principle is to soothe the Liver, ease the Gall Bladder, clear Heat and eliminate Dampness.

— The recommended formula is:

Radix Bupleuri	10 g
Fructus Aurantii *or* Fructus	
Aurantii Immaturus	5–10 g
Fructus Meliae Toosendan	10 g
Rhizoma Corydalis	10 g
Herba Artemisiae Scopariae	15–30 g
Fructus Gardeniae	10 g
Herba Taraxaci	15–30 g
Rhizoma Polygoni Cuspidati	10 g
Radix Curcumae	10 g

— Modifications:

– For stones, add Herba Lysimachiae (15 g), Spora Lygodii (15 g) (decocted wrapped), Radix et Rhizoma Rhei (5–10 g) and Endothelium Corneum Gigeriae Galli (10 g).

– For stagnation of Qi and Blood, add Rhizoma Ligustici Chuanxiong (10 g), Radix Paeoniae Rubra (10 g), Semen Persicae (10 g) and Faeces Trogopterorum (10 g).

– For Fire which consumes Yin, add Radix Adenophorae (10 g), Radix Ophiopogonis (10g) and Radix Paeoniae Alba (10 g).

CASE STUDY 40.13
CHOLECYSTITIS AND CHOLEITHIASIS

Male, age 64

This patient had suffered from recurrent attacks of right upper abdominal pain for 10 years. He was hospitalized 2 days after an acute attack of pain with fever. Clinical manifestations included violent pain in the right hypochondrium, vomiting, a bitter taste in the mouth, yellow urine, constipation, a yellow tongue coating and a wiry, rapid pulse. B mode ultrasonic wave examination showed the gall bladder 3.2 × 5.6 cm in size, its wall 0.3 cm thick and coarse, and a few pointed strong light beams. Blood test showed a white cell count of $11 \times 10^7/mm^3$, in which the neutrophils accounted for 80%. Body temperature was 38°C.

Pathogenesis: Accumulation of Damp-Heat in the Liver and Gall Bladder.

Western diagnosis: Acute aggravation of chronic cholecystitis with sandy gallstones.

Treatment principle: Clear Heat, eliminate Fire, benefit the Gall Bladder and expel stones.

The formula consisted of:

Herba Lysimachiae	30 g
Radix Scutellariae	15 g
Fructus Gardeniae	15 g
Radix Gentianae	6 g
Rhizoma Polygoni Cuspidati	15 g
Radix et Rhizoma Rhei	12 g
Radix Curcumae	12 g
Fructus Aurantii	12 g
Radix Aucklandiae	10 g
Radix Paeoniae Rubra	12 g

After ten doses, the fever subsided and the pain improved. After another five doses, the patient saw a few stones in his stool, the largest being 0.3 X 0.5 cm in size.

The patient took a total of 30 doses of this prescription, after which further ultrasound examination showed no stones and normal contraction of the gall bladder.

A follow-up visit 6 months later showed no relapse.

---

b. Shao Yang Syndrome

— This pattern is found in acute cholecystitis or acute exacerbations of chronic cholecystitis and cholelithiasis. It manifests as aversion to cold, fever or alternating chills and fever, right hypochondriac pain, a bitter taste in the mouth and nausea.

— The treatment principle is to harmonize Shao Yang, soothe the Liver and ease the Gall Bladder.

— The recommended formula is a variation of *Xiao Chai Hu Tang* (**Small Bupleurum Decoction**):

Radix Bupleuri	10–15 g
Radix Scutellariae	10 g
Fructus Gardeniae	10 g
Rhizoma Pinelliae	10 g
Radix Curcumae	10 g
Rhizoma Polygoni Cuspidati	15 g
Herba Taraxaci	15 g

— Modifications:

  – For stones or constipation, add Radix et Rhizoma Rhei (10 g), Natrii Sulfas (10 g) and Fructus Aurantii Immaturus (10 g).

---

5. CONSTIPATION

GENERAL DESCRIPTION

— Habitual constipation may be caused by dryness of the Large Intestine due to Liver Fire, deficiency of Blood and Body Fluids, deficiency of Qi and/or deficiency of Yang.

DIFFERENTIATION AND TREATMENT

a. Dryness of the Large Intestine due to Liver Fire

— Hyperactivity of Liver Fire consumes Body Fluids and dries the Large Intestine. Clinical manifestations include constipation, irritability, restlessness, headache, red eyes and a red tongue with yellow coating.
— The treatment principle is to clear Liver Heat and moisten the Large Intestine.
— The recommended formula is a variation of *Dang Gui Long Hui Wan* (**Angelica, Gentian and Aloe Pill**) and *Geng Yi Wan* (**Pill Requiring a Change of Clothes**):

Radix Gentianae	2–3 g
Fructus Gardeniae	10 g
Radix Angelicae Sinensis	10 g
Radix Rehmanniae	10–20 g
Aloe	1 g
(ground to a powder and taken as a capsule)	
Semen Cassiae	10–15 g

b. Dryness of the Large Intestine due to deficiency of Body Fluids and Blood.

— Deficiency of Body Fluids and Blood – whether constitutional, as in old age, or as the result of a serious illness – causes dryness of the Large Intestine and leads to constipation. Clinical manifestations include constipation, dry mouth, a pale tongue or a red tongue with scanty moisture, and a thready hesitant pulse.
— The treatment principle is to nourish Blood and Yin, moisten the Large Intestine and relieve constipation.
— The recommended formula is a variation of

Run Chang Wan (**Moisten the Intestines Pill**):

Radix Angelicae Sinensis	10 g
Radix Rehmanniae	10–20 g
Radix Scrophulariae	10–15 g
Semen Biotae	10 g
Radix Polygoni Multiflori	10–15 g
Fructus Cannabis	10 g
Semen Pruni	10 g

c. Qi Deficiency

— Deficiency of Spleen Qi means weakness in transportation. Clinical manifestations include constipation, reduced appetite and lassitude.
— The treatment principle is to benefit Qi, invigorate the Spleen, moisten the intestines and relieve constipation.
— The recommended formula is:

Rhizoma Atractylodis Macrocephalae	15–20 g
Radix Codonopsis Pilosulae	10 g
Radix Rehmanniae	15 g
Radix Angelicae Sinensis	10 g
Semen Biotae	10 g
Fructus Aurantii Immaturus	6 g

d. Yang Deficiency

— Kidney Yang Deficiency results in a lack of Body Fluids and Blood in the intestinal tract. This pattern occurs most often in the elderly. Clinical manifestations include constipation, cold limbs, a pale tongue and a deep and thready pulse.
— The treatment principle is to warm the Kidneys and relieve constipation.
— The recommended formula is:

Herba Cistanchis	10 g
Semen Juglandis	10–15 g
Radix Polygoni Multiflori	10–15 g
Radix Angelicae Sinensis	10 g
Herba Cynomorii	10 g
Fructus Cannabis	10 g

C. Cardiovascular disease

1. CORONARY HEART DISEASE

GENERAL DESCRIPTION

— Coronary heart disease is classified in TCM as Chest Bi syndrome, palpitation or real cardiac pain. The Excess type of the disease is caused by stagnation of Qi and Blood and retention of Phlegm; these factors block Chest Yang and lead to disorders of the cardiac vessels. The Deficiency type is caused by deficiency of the Heart, Spleen, Liver and Kidneys. Complicated cases of combined Excess and Deficiency are often seen clinically.

DIFFERENTIATION AND TREATMENT

a. Stagnation of Qi and Blood

— Stagnant Blood blocks the circulation of Qi and causes disorders of the cardiac vessels. The key symptom is intermittent stabbing chest pain which is fixed in location and may be accompanied by a sensation of suffocation; in severe cases, the pain may radiate to the back. Other clinical manifestations include sweating, cold limbs, cyanosis of the lips, a purple or dull tongue with purple spots and thin, white coating, and a wiry, hesitant or intermittent pulse.
— The treatment principle is to activate Blood circulation and resolve Stasis, regulate Qi and remove obstruction from the vessels.
— The recommended formula is a variation of *Xue Fu Zhu Yu Tang* (**Blood Mansion Eliminating Stasis Decoction**):

Radix Salviae Miltiorrhizae	15 g
Rhizoma Ligustici Chuanxiong	10 g
Radix Angelicae Sinensis	10 g
Semen Persicae	10 g
Flos Carthami	5–10 g
Radix Curcumae	10 g
Rhizoma Corydalis	10 g
Resina Olibani	2–5 g
Resina Myrrhae	2–5 g
Faeces Trogopterorum	10 g

— Modifications:

  – For severe Blood Stasis, add Rhizoma Sparganii (5–10 g) and Rhizoma Zedoariae (5–10 g).
  – If signs of Cold are pronounced, add Ramulus Cinnamomi (2–5 g) and Radix Aconiti Praeparata (2–5 g).
  – For Qi Deficiency, add Radix Ginseng (5–10g) or Radix Codonopsis Pilosulae (15 g), and Radix Astragali seu Hedysari (15 g).

b. Stagnation of Phlegm and Blood

— Retention of Turbid Phlegm in the Interior blocks Chest Yang and the blood vessels.

Clinical manifestations include a sensation of suffocation or tightness in the chest, paroxysmal pain in the heart, obesity, a purple tongue with a sticky white coating, and a wiry, rolling pulse.
— The treatment principle is to eliminate Phlegm, invigorate Yang, resolve Blood Stasis and remove obstruction from the vessels.
— The recommended formula is a variation of *Gua Lou Xie Bai Ban Xia Tang* (**Trichosanthes–Allium–Pinellia Decoction**):

Fructus Trichosanthis	15 g
Bulbus Allii Macrostemi	10 g
Rhizoma Pinelliae	10 g
Fructus Aurantii Immaturus	5–10 g
Ramulus Cinnamomi	2–5 g
Radix Salviae Miltiorrhizae	15 g
Rhizoma Ligustici Chuanxiong	10 g
Radix Curcumae	10 g

— Modifications:

  – If Phlegm turns to Heat, manifesting as thirst, irritability, restlessness and a red tongue with yellow coating, remove Ramulus Cinnamomi from the prescription and add Rhizoma Coptidis (2–3 g) and Arisaema cum Bile (10 g).

CASE STUDY 40.14
CORONARY HEART DISEASE

Male, age 54

This patient complained of chest pain radiating to the back, shoulder and neck. He had shortness of breath, especially when lying down, and expectorated a small amount of white sputum. His tongue was pale with purple spots and a sticky white coating; his pulse was wiry and thready.

Pathogenesis: Deficiency of Chest Yang and retardation of Qi, complicated with retention of Turbid Phlegm (Chest Bi syndrome).

Western diagnosis: Coronary heart disease

Treatment principle: Invigorate Yang with pungent and warm herbs; regulate Qi and open the chest.

The formula used was a variation of **Trichosanthes-Allium-Pinellia Decoction** and **Styrax Pill**:

Fructus Trichosanthis	9g
Bulbus Allii Macrostemi (stir-baked in wine)	12g
Rhizoma Pinelliae *(ginger-treated)*	9g
Radix Curcumae	9g

Lignum Santalum   1.5g
   (added at end)
plus
Styrax Pill   1 pill
   (taken separately with water)

After administration of two doses, the chest pain disappeared, but the patient still felt a sensation of pressure in the chest. After taking another five doses, all symptoms had disappeared.

---

c. Yin Deficiency

— Heart and Kidney Yin Deficiency leads to Liver Yang Rising. Clinical manifestations include a feeling of suffocation, cardiac pain, dizziness, tinnitus, thirst, a red tongue and a thready, wiry pulse.
— The treatment principle is to nourish Yin, calm the Liver, soothe the Heart and remove obstruction from the vessels.
— The recommended formula is a variation of *Qi Ju Di Huang Wan* (**Lycium Fruit, Chrysanthemum and Rehmannia Pill**):

Radix Polygoni Multiflori
   (treated)   15g
Fructus Lycii   15g
Radix Rehmanniae Praeparata   15g
Fructus Corni   10g
Radix Salviae Miltiorrhizae   15g
Radix Paeoniae Alba   10g

— Modifications:

– For hypertension with symptoms of dizziness, vertigo and red eyes, add Ramulus Uncariae cum Uncis (10–15 g) (added at end of decoction), Rhizoma Gastrodiae (10 g), Cortex Moutan Radicis (10 g), Spica Prunellae (15 g) and Concha Haliotidis (15 g) (decocted first).
– For Heart Yin Deficiency with symptoms of restlessness and insomnia, add Radix Ophiopogonis (15 g), Fructus Schisandrae (3 g), Semen Ziziphi Spinosae (10 g) and Os Draconis (15 g) (decocted first).

d. Deficiency of both Qi and Yin

— Heart Qi Deficiency causes disorders of the cardiac vessels while deficiency of Yin and Blood leads to restlessness. Clinical manifestations include palpitation, shortness of breath, a feeling of suffocation, lassitude, cardiac pain, a red tongue with tooth-prints, and a thready and rapid or weak pulse, or an intermittent pulse.

— The treatment principle is to benefit Qi, nourish Yin, remove obstruction from the vessels and soothe the Heart.
— The recommended formula is a variation of *Sheng Mai Yin* (**Generating the Pulse Decoction**) and *Zhi Gan Cao Tang* (**Glycyrrhiza Decoction**):

Radix Ginseng *(decocted separately)*   5–10g
or Radix Codonopsis Pilosulae   15g
Radix Pseudostellariae   15g
Radix Astragali seu Hedysari   12g
Radix Ophiopogonis   15g
Rhizoma Polygonati Odorati   15g
Fructus Schisandrae   5g
Radix Glycyrrhizae *(treated)*   5g
Radix Polygoni Multiflori   15g
Radix Salviae Miltiorrhizae   15g
Semen Ziziphi Spinosae   10g
Semen Biotae   10g
Os Draconis   15g
   (decocted first)

— Modifications:

– For pronounced deficiency of Heart Qi with symptoms of spontaneous sweating and an intermittent pulse, increase the dosage of Radix Glycyrrhizae Praeparata to 10 g and add Ramulus Cinnamomi (5 g).

e. Yang Deficiency

— This pattern is due to Heart and Kidney Yang Deficiency, and deficiency of Heart Qi. Clinical manifestations include palpitation, shortness of breath, a feeling of suffocation, cardiac pain, lumbar soreness, lassitude, aversion to cold, cold limbs, pallor, a pale or purplish tongue and a deep, thready or intermittent pulse.
— The treatment principle is to benefit Qi, warm Yang and remove obstruction from the vessels.
— The recommended formula is *Shen Fu Tang* (**Panax-Aconitum Decoction**) with additions:

Radix Ginseng *(decocted separately)*   5–10 g
Radix Aconiti Praeparata   5 g
Ramulus Cinnamomi   5 g
Rhizoma Zingiberis   5 g
Radix Rehmanniae Praeparata   15 g
Herba Epimedii   10 g
Radix Morindae Officinalis   10 g
Radix Glycyrrhizae *(treated)*   5 g
Radix Salviae Miltiorrhizae   15 g
Fructus Schisandrae   5 g

2. PALPITATION

GENERAL DESCRIPTION

— The term palpitation refers to arrhythmia, which can derive from a variety of causes. Constitutional deficiency of Qi, Blood, Yin or Yang can produce palpitation as the Heart is deprived of nourishment. Mental and emotional excesses such as worry, over-thinking, fear and fright can also produce palpitation. A third possible cause is invasion of the Heart by external pathogenic factors, which consumes Heart Qi and Yin and blocks the cardiac vessels.

DIFFERENTIATION AND TREATMENT

a. Heart and Spleen Deficiency

— Deficiency of Heart Blood and Qi, and of Spleen Qi, deprives the Heart of nourishment. Clinical manifestations include palpitation, restlessness, shortness of breath, spontaneous sweating, lassitude, poor memory, insomnia, pallor, a slightly red tongue and a thready, weak pulse.
— The treatment principle is to tonify the Heart and Spleen, soothe the Heart and calm the Mind.
— The recommended formula is a variation of *Gui Pi Tang* (**Tonifying the Spleen Decoction**):

Radix Codonopsis Pilosulae	10g
Radix Astragali seu Hedysari	10g
Radix Glycyrrhizae *(treated)*	3g
Fructus Schisandrae	3–5g
Radix Angelicae Sinensis	10g
Radix Rehmanniae Praeparata	10g
Arillus Longan	10–15g
Semen Biotae	10g
Semen Ziziphi Spinosae	10g
Os Draconis	15g
(decocted first)	

— Modifications:

– For Heart Yin Deficiency, add Radix Ophiopogonis (15 g) and Rhizoma Polygonati Odorati (15 g).
– For an intermittent pulse, suggesting retarded blood circulation in the cardiac vessels, add Ramulus Cinnamomi (5 g) and increase the dosage of Radix Glycyrrhizae to 10 g.

b. Yin Deficiency with Empty Fire

— Heart and Kidney Yin Deficiency produces Empty Fire, which then disturbs the Heart and Mind. Clinical manifestations include palpitation which is aggravated by mental and emotional stress, restlessness, insomnia, dizziness, tinnitus, a flushed face, a red tongue with yellow coating, and a thready, rapid pulse.
— The treatment principle is to nourish Yin, reduce Fire, soothe the Heart and calm the Mind.
— The recommended formula is a variation of *Tian Wang Bu Xin Dan* (**Heavenly Emperor Tonifying the Heart Pill**):

Radix Rehmanniae	15 g
Radix Ophiopogonis	15 g
Rhizoma Polygonati Odorati	15 g
Rhizoma Coptidis	2–3 g
Fructus Gardeniae	10 g
Fructus Schisandrae	5 g
Semen Ziziphi Spinosae	10 g
Semen Biotae	10 g
Magnetitum	15–30 g
(decocted first)	
Os Draconis	15 g
(decocted first)	
Poria cum Ligno Hospite	
(Cinnabaris coated)	10 g

— Modifications:

– For Kidney Yin Deficiency, add Radix Rehmanniae Praeparata (15 g), Rhizoma Anemarrhenae (10 g) and Plastrum Testudinis (15 g) (decocted first).
– For Liver Yang Rising, add Concha Ostreae (15–20 g) (decocted first), Cortex Moutan Radicis (10 g) and Flos Chrysanthemi (10 g).

c. Phlegm-Fire

— Phlegm-Fire disturbs the Heart and Mind. Clinical manifestations include palpitation which is likely to be induced by anxiety or fright, stuffiness of the chest, restlessness, insomnia, dream-disturbed sleep, thick sticky sputum, a sticky yellow tongue coating and a rapid, rolling pulse.
— The treatment principle is to clear Fire, resolve Phlegm, soothe the Heart and calm the Mind.
— The recommended formula is a variation of *Wen Dan Tang* (**Warming the Gall Bladder Decoction**):

Rhizoma Coptidis	2–3 g
Fructus Gardeniae	10 g
Caulis Bambusae in Taeniam	10 g

Arisaema cum Bile	10 g
Rhizoma Pinelliae *(treated with Succus Bambusae)*	10 g
Poria	10 g
Fructus Aurantii Immaturus	5 g
Radix Polygalae	10 g
Semen Ziziphi Spinosae	10 g
Cortex Albiziae	15 g

CASE STUDY 40.15
PALPITATION

Male, age 53

This patient complained of frequent episodes of palpitations, which could become very severe at times; he had also suffered from dizziness, blurred vision, timidity and insomnia over the past 3 months. Other clinical manifestations included profuse sputum, poor appetite, hypertension (160/100), a white sticky tongue coating and a wiry pulse.

Pathogenesis: Disturbance by Phlegm-Heat in the Interior.

Western diagnosis: Hypertension

Treatment principle: Clear Heat, resolve Phlegm and calm the Mind with heavy substances.

The formula used was a variation of **Warming the Gall Bladder Decoction** and **Magnetite and Cinnabar Pill**:

Rhizoma Pinelliae	
(ginger-treated)	9 g
Pericarpium Citri Reticulatae	4.5 g
Fructus Aurantii Immaturus	
(stir-baked)	4.5 g
Caulis Bambusae in Taeniam	9 g
Poria	9g
Os Draconis	15 g
Concha Ostreae	30 g
(decocted first)	
Rhizoma Arisaematis *(prepared)*	4.5 g
Radix Glycyrrhizae *(treated)*	3 g
plus	
Magnetite and Cinnabar Pill	4.5 g

After ten doses of this prescription, all symptoms had disappeared.

---

d. Stagnation of Heart Blood

— Stagnant Qi and Blood blocks the cardiac vessels. Clinical manifestations include palpitation, a feeling of suffocation, intermittent boring chest pain, a purple tongue or a tongue with purple spots, and a hesitant or intermittent pulse.
— The treatment principle is to resolve Blood

Stasis, remove obstruction from the vessels and soothe the Heart.
— The recommended formula is a variation of **Blood Mansion Eliminating Stasis Decoction**:

Radix Angelicae Sinensis	10 g
Radix Paeoniae Rubra	10 g
Radix Salviae Miltiorrhizae	15 g
Rhizoma Ligustici Chuanxiong	10 g
Semen Persicae	10 g
Flos Carthami	5–10 g
Radix Curcumae	10 g
Poria cum Ligno Hospite	10 g
Succinum	2 g
(ground to a powder and taken separately)	
Os Draconis	15 g
Semen Biotae	10 g

e. Heart Yang Deficiency

— Deficiency of Heart Qi and Yang allows the Heart and Mind to be disturbed. Clinical manifestations include palpitation which is worse on exertion, shortness of breath, stuffiness of the chest, aversion to cold, cold limbs, dizziness, a pale tongue and a deep, thready or intermittent pulse.
— The treatment principle is to warm Yang, benefit Qi, soothe the Heart and calm the Mind.
— The recommended formula is a combination of **Panax–Aconitum Decoction** and *Gui Zhi Gan Cao Long Gu Mu Li Tang* (**Cinnamon Twig, Licorice, Dragon Bone and Oyster Shell Decoction**), with additions:

Radix Aconiti Praeparata	3–5 g
Ramulus Cinnamomi	5 g
Radix Ginseng	5–10 g
or Radix Codonopsis Pilosulae	15 g
Astragali seu Hedysari	15 g
Radix Glycyrrhizae *(treated)*	5 g
Fructus Schisandrae	5 g
Os Draconis	15 g
(decocted first)	
Concha Ostreae	20 g
(decocted first)	

— Modifications:

  – For retention of Phlegm and Fluid, add Poria (10 g), Rhizoma Pinelliae (10 g), Rhizoma Atractylodis Macrocephalae (10 g) and Rhizoma Alismatis (10 g).
  – For oedema, remove Fructus Schisandrae, Os Draconis and Concha Ostreae from the prescription and add Rhizoma Atractylodis Macrocephalae

(10 g), Poria (10 g) and Semen Plantaginis (10 g) (decocted wrapped).
- For deficiency of both Yin and Yang, add Radix Ophiopogonis (15 g), Radix Paeoniae Alba (10 g) and Rhizoma Polygonati Odorati (15 g).

D. Diseases of the urogenital system

1. ACUTE AND CHRONIC NEPHRITIS

GENERAL DESCRIPTION

— The oedematous stage of acute nephritis falls into the TCM category of oedema while the other stages of the disease are categorized as consumption. The external causes of nephritis include invasion of pathogenic Wind, inward transmission of Water and Dampness, and Damp toxins. Internal causes include dysfunction of the Lungs, Spleen and Kidneys in regulating the water passages, transporting and transforming Water and Dampness, and dominating Water metabolism respectively. In any case, the root cause of the disease lies in the Kidneys.

DIFFERENTIATION AND TREATMENT

a. Wind-Water

— Invasion of the Lungs by pathogenic Wind impairs the Lungs' function of regulating the water passages. Wind and Water combine to produce oedema of sudden onset which is more pronounced in the head and face; pitting disappears quickly when pressure is removed. Other clinical manifestations include scanty urine, and possibly cough, dyspnoea and aversion to wind or cold.
— The treatment principle is to eliminate Wind, promote the dispersing function of the Lungs and promote diuresis.
— The recommended formula is:

Herba Ephedrae	3–10 g
Radix Ledebouriellae	10 g
Folium Perillae	3 g
Ramulus Cinnamomi	5 g
Semen Armeniacae Amarum	10 g
Radix Platycodi	5 g
Polyporus Umbellatus	10 g

Poria	10 g
Semen Plantaginis	10 g
(decocted wrapped)	

— Modifications:

- If cough and dyspnoea are pronounced, add Cortex Mori Radicis (10 g) and Semen Lepidii seu Descurainiae (6 g).
- For inward transmission of Wind-Heat and Dampness with symptoms of sore throat and oozing skin ulcers, remove Ramulus Cinnamomi from the prescription and add Fructus Forsythiae (10 g), Semen Phaseoli (15 g), Cortex Phellodendri (10 g) and Herba Violae (15 g).

b. Spleen Deficiency and invasion of Dampness

— Invasion of the Spleen by Cold-Damp impairs the functions of transportation and transformation. Clinical manifestations include oedema of the face, limbs and body, distension and fullness in the epigastrium and abdomen, reduced appetite, loose stool, sallow complexion, lassitude, a sticky white tongue coating and a soft or deep, thready, weak pulse.
— The treatment principle is to invigorate the Spleen, resolve Dampness and promote diuresis.
— The recommended formula is a variation of *Wei Ling San* (**Calm the Stomach and Poria Decoction**) and *Wu Pi San* (**Five-Peel Powder**):

Rhizoma Atractylodis	5–10 g
Rhizoma Atractylodis Macrocephalae	10 g
Cortex Magnoliae Officinalis	2–3 g
Ramulus Cinnamomi	2–5 g
Poria	10 g
Polyporus Umbellatus	10 g
Rhizoma Alismatis	10 g
Radix Stephaniae Tetrandrae	10 g
Pericarpium Arecae	10 g
Pericarpium Citri Reticulatae	5 g

— Modifications:

- For Qi Deficiency with spontaneous sweating and aversion to Wind, add (raw) Radix Astragali seu Hedysari (10 g) and Radix Ledebouriellae (10 g).
- For cough, dyspnoea and oedema of the

upper body, add Semen Lepidii seu Descurainiae (6 g), Semen Armeniacae Amarum (10 g) and Herba Ephedrae (3–5 g).

- For abdominal distension and fullness, a sensation of heat, restlessness, thirst and constipation, remove Ramulus Cinnamomi from the prescription and add Semen Zanthoxyli (3 g), Semen Lepidii seu Descurainiae (6 g) and Radix et Rhizoma Rhei (5 g).

— *NB*: If the patient's blood pressure is high, Herba Ephedrae should not be used in the treatment of the two patterns discussed above.

c. Spleen and Kidney Yang Deficiency

— Spleen and Kidney Yang Deficiency means an inability to resolve Water and Dampness. This is a chronic pattern, and clinical manifestations include pitting oedema which is more pronounced in the lower body, lumbar soreness, cold limbs, lassitude, pallor, a pale tongue and a deep, thready pulse.
— The treatment principle is to warm the Kidneys, invigorate the Spleen and promote diuresis.
— The recommended formula is a variation of *Fu Zi Li Zhong Wan* (**Prepared Aconite Pill to Regulate the Middle**) and *Wu Ling San* (**Five-Ingredient Powder with Poria**):

Radix Aconiti Praeparata	2–5 g
Ramulus Cinnamomi	2–5 g
Rhizoma Zingiberis	2–5 g
Rhizoma Atractylodis	
Macrocephalae	10 g
Poria	10 g
Polyporus Umbellatus	10 g
Rhizoma Alismatis	10 g
Radix Achyranthis Bidentatae	10 g
Herba Leonuri	10–15 g

— Modifications:

- For Qi Deficiency, add (raw) Radix Astragali seu Hedysari (12 g).
- If oedema is not present, remove the diuretic herbs and add Radix Rehmanniae Praeparata (10 g), Semen Cuscutae (15 g), Rhizoma Dioscoreae (15 g) and Radix Morindae Officinalis (10 g) to tonify the Spleen and Kidneys.

CASE STUDY 40.16
NEPHRITIS
Male, age 35

This patient presented with oedema of the face and lower limbs, pallor, palpitation and shortness of breath on exertion, lumbar soreness and a bearing-down sensation in the anus. He had a white tongue coating and a weak-floating and thready pulse.

Pathogenesis: Spleen and Kidney Deficiency resulting in retention of Water and Damp which spread to the muscles.

Western diagnosis: Acute aggravation of chronic nephritis

Treatment principle: Invigorate the Spleen and Kidneys' function of controlling Water and Damp.

The formula used was a variation of **Five 'Ling' Powder** and **Five-Peel Powder**:

Ramulus Cinnamomi	3 g
Pericarpium Citri Reticulatae	9 g
Polyporus Umbellatus	15 g
Poria *(with skin)*	30 g
Rhizoma Alismatis	9 g
Radix Stephaniae Tetrandrae	9 g
Pericarpium Arecae	9 g
Peel of Rhizoma Zingiberis	
Recens	4.5 g
Cortex Magnoliae Officinalis	3 g
Red bean	15 g

After administration of ten doses, the oedema had lessened markedly. Cortex Magnoliae Officinalis was then removed from the prescription and Qi and Yang tonics such as Radix Astragali seu Hedysari, Radix Aconiti Praeparata and Rhizoma Atractylodis Macrocephalae were added.

Treated was continued for over 2 months, by which time the oedema had subsided; lumber soreness, palpitations and dyspnoea had improved as well and the patient was in better spirits.

---

d. Kidney Deficiency and retention of Damp-Heat

— Deficiency of Kidney Yin encourages the retention of Damp-Heat. Clinical manifestations include absence of oedema or indistinct oedema, lumbar soreness, weak limbs, dizziness and vertigo, tinnitus, five-palm Heat, scanty deep-yellow urine, a red tongue with a slightly sticky, thin, yellow coating, and a deep and thready or rapid pulse.
— The treatment principle is to nourish the Kidneys and clear Damp-Heat.

— The recommended formula is a variation of *Zhi Bai Di Huang Wan* (**Anemarrhena, Phellodendron and Rehmannia Pill**):

Radix Rehmanniae	15 g
Radix Rehmanniae Praeparata	15 g
Fructus Corni	10 g
Rhizoma Dioscoreae	15 g
Semen Cuscutae	15 g
Rhizoma Anemarrhenae	10 g
Cortex Phellodendri	10 g
Cortex Moutan Radicis	10 g
Rhizoma Alismatis	10 g
Radix Achyranthis Bidentatae	10 g
Poria	10 g

2. URINARY TRACT INFECTION AND URINARY LITHIASIS

GENERAL DESCRIPTION

— Urinary tract infection and urinary lithiasis are categorized in TCM as 'urinary disturbance'; this category includes disturbance due to strain, urolithiasis, dysfunction of the urinary bladder, chyluria or haematuria. If the primary symptom is lumbago, and difficult or painful urination is not pronounced, the pattern is categorized as lower back pain; the cause is Kidney Deficiency complicated with Damp-Heat and the treatment principle is to tonify the Kidneys and clear Damp-Heat.

DIFFERENTIATION AND TREATMENT

a. Damp-Heat

— Downward movement of Damp-Heat impairs the bladder's function of controlling urine. Clinical manifestations include frequent, urgent, dribbling and/or painful urination with a burning sensation, a bearing-down sensation in the lower abdomen, a sticky tongue coating and a soft, rapid pulse. There may also be low back pain, aversion to cold, fever, thirst and a bitter taste in the mouth.

— The treatment principle is to clear Heat, eliminate Dampness and ease urination.

— The recommended formula is a variation of *Ba Zheng San* (**Eight-Herb Powder for Rectification**):

Caulis Akebiae	2–5 g
Cortex Phellodendri	10 g
Fructus Gardeniae	10 g
Radix Rehmanniae	10 g
Herba Dianthi	10 g

Herba Plantaginis	15 g
Semen Plantaginis *(decocted wrapped)*	12 g
Rhizoma Polygoni Cuspidati	15 g
Talcum	10 g
Radix Glycyrrhizae *(raw)*	3 g
Radix et Rhizoma Rhei	5 g

— Modifications:

– For fever and aversion to cold, add Radix Bupleuri (10–15 g) and Radix Scutellariae (10 g).

– For distending pain in the lower abdomen, add Radix Linderae (10 g) and Fructus Meliae Toosendan (10 g).

– If Damp-Heat injures Yin, remove Radix et Rhizoma Rhei from the prescription and add Rhizoma Anemarrhenae (10 g).

– For haematuria, add Radix Rubiae (12 g) and Herba Cephalanoploria (15 g).

– For urolithiasis, add Folium Pyrrosiae (12 g), Herba Lysimachiae (15–30 g) and Spora Lygodii (15 g) (decocted wrapped).

CASE STUDY 40.17
URINARY TRACT INFECTION
Female, age 31

5 days previously, this patient had experienced sudden distending pain in the lower abdomen with urgency, frequency and burning pain on urination. Her urine was deep-yellow in colour and she passed urine more than 20 times daily. The pain radiated from the umbilicus down to the urethra, and the middle of the lower abdomen was tender. Urinalysis showed yellow and mildly turbid urine, a small amount of protein, white blood cells +++, and red blood cells ++. Urine culture revealed *Escherichia coli*.

Pathogenesis: Downward movement of Damp-Heat.

Western diagnosis: Acute cystitis

Treatment principle: Clear Damp and Heat.

The prescription used consisted of:

Radix Rehmanniae	12 g
Cortex Phellodendri	9 g
Herba Dianthi	9 g
Caulis Akebiae	6 g
Semen Plantaginis	9 g
Herba Polygoni Avicularis	9 g
Fructus Gardeniae *(raw)*	9 g
Talcum	9 g
Radix Glycyrrhizae *(tips only)*	4.5 g
Medulla Junci *(Deng Xin Cao)*	2 bundles

Succinum	6 g

(to be taken separately with water three times daily)

After two doses, the pain on urination disappeared and frequency decreased from more than 20 times to 10 times daily. There was still some mild distending pain and tenderness in the lower abdomen. Urinalysis showed clear, yellow urine with a small quantity of white blood cells.

The same prescription was continued, and after another three doses all symptoms had disappeared and urinalysis was normal.

b. Spleen and Kidney Deficiency

— Long-term urinary infection and urinary lithiasis leads to Spleen Deficiency, Sinking of Spleen Qi and weakness of Kidney Qi. Clinical manifestations include recurrent episodes of difficult and dribbling urine with haematuria, lumbar soreness and listlessness. Aggravations are often induced by overwork or stress. If there is concurrent Yin Deficiency, symptoms will also include restlessness, five-palm Heat or low-grade fever, and tidal flushing of the face.
— The treatment principle is primarily to benefit Qi and tonify the Kidneys and secondarily to clear Damp-Heat.
— The recommended formula for Spleen Deficiency is a variation of **Tonifying the Middle and Benefiting Qi Decoction**:

Radix Codonopsis Pilosulae	10 g
Radix Astragali seu Hedysari	10 g
Rhizoma Atractylodis Macrocephalae	10 g
Rhizoma Cimicifugae	3 g
Radix Bupleuri	3 g
Radix Dipsaci	10 g
Semen Astragali Complanati	15 g
Poria	10 g
Radix Achyranthis Bidentatae	10 g

— The recommended formula for Kidney Yin Deficiency is a variation of **Anemarrhena, Phellodendron and Rehmannia Pill**:

Radix Dipsaci	10 g
Cortex Eucommiae	10 g
Radix Rehmanniae	15 g
Rhizoma Anemarrhenae	10 g
Cortex Phellodendri	10 g
Fructus Rosae Laevigatae	10 g
Semen Cuscutae	15 g
Fructus Schisandrae	2 g
Rhizoma Alismatis	10 g
Cortex Moutan Radicis	10 g

3. SPERMATORRHOEA, IMPOTENCE AND INFERTILITY

GENERAL DESCRIPTION

— Spermatorrhoea is caused by a dysfunction of the Kidneys in storing Essence. There are two types. Nocturnal emission is often of the Excess type and is caused by disturbance of the seminal chamber by Heart and Kidney Fire or by Damp-Heat in the Lower Burner; the treatment principle is primarily to clear Fire or Heat. Spontaneous emission is often of the Deficiency type and is caused by weakness of the seminal gate due to Kidney Deficiency; the treatment principle is to tonify the Kidneys and consolidate the Essence.
— Impotence is usually caused by decline of Ming Men Fire; in some patients it is the result of downward movement of Damp-Heat causing relaxation of the penis.
— Female infertility results from deficiency of Essence and Blood with stagnation of Cold in the uterus, or from Damp-Heat in the Lower Burner, stagnation of Liver Qi or retention of Phlegm-Damp. The treatment principles are accordingly to provide warmth and tonify Essence, to clear Heat and eliminate Dampness, to relieve stagnation of Liver Qi and regulate menstruation or to dry Dampness and resolve Phlegm.

DIFFERENTIATION AND TREATMENT

a. Yin Deficiency with Empty Fire

— The seminal chamber is disturbed by Empty Fire due to Kidney Yin Deficiency, or by Heart Fire. Clinical manifestations include nocturnal emissions with dreams, excessive erection or premature ejaculation, tinnitus, lumbar soreness, restlessness and insomnia.
— The treatment principle is to nourish Yin and reduce Fire.
— The recommended formula is a variation of **Anemarrhena, Phellodendron and Rehmannia Pill**:

Radix Rehmanniae	15 g
Radix Rehmanniae Praeparata	15 g
Fructus Corni	10–15 g
Fructus Ligustri Lucidi	10 g
Rhizoma Dioscoreae	15 g
Cortex Moutan Radicis	10 g
Rhizoma Anemarrhenae	10 g
Cortex Phellodendri	10 g
Fructus Rosae Laevigatae	10 g

Fructus Rubi	10 g
Fructus Schisandrae	5 g
Semen Ziziphi Spinosae	10 g
Os Draconis	15 g
(decocted first)	

— Modifications:

- For hyperactivity of Empty Kidney Fire and Heart Fire, add Rhizoma Coptidix (2 g) and Radix Gentianae (2 g).

b. Downward movement of Damp-Heat

— This pattern is caused by Damp-Heat in the Liver channel moving down to the Lower Burner. Clinical manifestations include nocturnal emission with or without dreams, impotence, premature ejaculation, dampness of the scrotum, thick yellow and foul leucorrhoea, lower abdominal pain, soreness and sluggishness of the lower limbs, a sticky yellow tongue coating and a wiry and rolling or soft and rapid pulse.
— The treatment principle is to clear Heat, eliminate Dampness and reduce Liver Fire.
— The recommended formula is a variation of *Long Dan Xie Gan Tang* (**Gentiana Draining the Liver Decoction**):

Radix Gentianae	2–5 g
Cortex Moutan Radicis	10 g
Cortex Phellodendri	10 g
Radix Bupleuri	5 g
Fructus Gardeniae	10 g
Caulis Akebiae	2–5 g
Rhizoma Anemarrhenae	10 g
Radix Atractylodis	5 g
Rhizoma Alismatis	10 g
Semen Plantaginis	10 g
Rhizoma Dioscoreae Septemlobae	10 g

CASE STUDY 40.18
IMPOTENCE

Male, age 40

For over a year this patient had suffered from impotence, lumbar soreness and weak legs. He had yellow urine, a red tongue with a thick, sticky yellow coating, and a rapid, wiry pulse.

Pathogenesis: Deficiency of Kidney Yin and Yang, complicated with downward movement of Damp-Heat.

Treatment principle: Tonify Kidney Yin and Yang and clear Damp-Heat.

The formula used was a variation of **Restoring the Right Pill**:

Radix Rehmanniae	12 g
Radix Rehmanniae Praeparata	12 g
Semen Cuscutae	12 g
Radix Dipsaci	10 g
Radix Morindae Officinalis	10 g
Herba Epimedii	15 g
Herba Cynomorii	15 g
Cortex Moutan Radicis	8 g
Cortex Phellodendri	10 g
Rhizoma Alismatis	10 g

After ten doses, the impotence was improved; after another five doses, it was cured.

---

c. Decline of Ming Men Fire

— Decline of the Fire of Ming Men due to Kidney Deficiency means insufficient Essence and Blood. Clinical manifestations include spontaneous emission, thin clear and cold semen, impotence, a prolonged menstrual cycle with scanty flow, hyposexuality, sore and weak lumbar region and knees, aversion to cold, cold limbs, a pale tongue and a deep, thready pulse.
— The treatment principle is to warm and tonify Ming Men, invigorate Yang and benefit Essence.
— The recommended formula is a variation of *You Gui Wan* (**Restoring the Right [Kidney] Pill**):

Radix Rehmanniae Praeparata	10–20 g
Fructus Corni	15 g
Fructus Lycii	10–15 g
Herba Epimedii	10 g
Herba Cistanchis	10 g
Semen Cuscutae	15 g
Radix Morindae Officinalis	10 g
Fructus Schisandrae	5 g
Cornu Cervi Pantotrichum	1–3 g
(ground to powder and taken separately)	

— Modifications:

- For spermatorrhoea, add Fructus Rosae Laevigatae (12 g), Stamen Nelumbinis (10 g) and Os Draconis (15 g) (decocted first).
- For infertility due to retention of Cold in the uterus, add Radix Angelicae Sinensis (10 g), Rhizoma Ligustici Chuanxiong (6 g), Cortex Eucommiae (12 g), Colla Corii Asini (10 g) (melted and taken separately) and Folium Artemisiae Argyi (10 g).

d. Retention of Phlegm-Damp

— Obesity produces Phlegm-Damp in the Interior, which blocks Qi and hinders the Chong and Ren channels. This is a common cause of female infertility. Clinical manifestations include prolonged menstrual cycle with scanty pale and thin flow or amenorrhoea, leucorrhoea, obesity, dizziness, lassitude, stuffiness of the chest, a pale tongue with a sticky white coating, and a deep, rolling pulse.

— The treatment principle is to dry Dampness, resolve Phlegm, activate Qi and invigorate the Spleen.

— The recommended formula is a variation of *Cang Fu Dao Tan Wan* (**Atractylodis and Cyperi Pill for Eliminating Phlegm**):

Rhizoma Atractylodis	10g
Rhizoma Atractylodis Macrocephalae	10g
Rhizoma Pinelliae	10g
Pericarpium Citri Reticulatae	10g
Rhizoma Arisaematis	10g
Rhizoma Cyperi	10g
Fructus Aurantii Immaturus	10g
Poria1	2g

— Modifications:

- For Cold, add Ramulus Cinnamomi (2–5 g).
- For stagnation of Blood, add Rhizoma Ligustici Chuanxiong (6–10 g), Radix Angelicae Sinensis (10 g) and Radix Achyranthis Bidentatae (10g).
- For Qi stagnation, add Radix Bupleuri (5 g) and Cortex Albiziae (10–15 g).

E. Diseases of the motor and nervous systems

1. BI SYNDROMES (PAINFUL JOINTS)

GENERAL DESCRIPTION

— Bi syndrome refers to pain and limited movement of the body, limbs, joints and muscles. It corresponds to the Western diagnostic categories of rheumatoid arthritis and osteoarthritis and is caused by invasion of the channels, collaterals, joints and muscles by pathogenic Wind, Cold, Dampness and Heat.

DIFFERENTIATION AND TREATMENT

a. Wind, Cold and Dampness

— When body resistance is weak, pathogenic Wind, Cold and Dampness are able to invade the channels and collaterals, thus inhibiting mobility of the joints. Clinical manifestations include intermittent pain in the joints and muscles which is aggravated in damp weather, a thin white tongue coating and a wiry or soft pulse.

— The treatment principle is to eliminate Wind, Cold and Dampness and remove obstruction from the collaterals.

— The recommended formula is a variation of *Yi Yi Ren Tang* (**Coix Decoction**):

Rhizoma seu Radix Notopterygii	5–10 g
Radix Angelicae Pubescentis	5–10 g
Ramulus Cinnamomi	2–5 g
Radix Gentianae Macrophyllae	10 g
Semen Coicis	15 g
Rhizoma Atractylodis	10 g

— Modifications:

- If Wind predominates, causing wandering joint pain, add Radix Ledebouriellae (10 g), Radix Clematidis (10 g) and Agkistrodon Acutus or Zaocys (5–10 g).
- If Cold predominates, causing a sensation of cold and joint pain which is worse on exposure to cold, add (treated) Rhizoma Aconitum Carmichaeli (2–5 g), Herba Asari (2–6 g) and Herba Ephedrae (3–10 g).
- If Dampness predominates, causing a soreness and heaviness of the joints which is fixed in location, add Radix Stephaniae Tetrandrae (10 g) and Rhizoma Atractylodis Macrocephalae (10 g).
- In chronic cases with deficiency of Qi and Blood and of Liver and Kidneys, add Radix Astragali seu Hedysari (10 g), Radix Angelicae Sinensis (10 g), Ramulus Loranthi (15 g) and Rhizoma Cybotii (10 g).

CASE STUDY 40.19
BI SYNDROME

Male, age 49

This patient complained of soreness and pain in the left leg and foot for the past 4 months. He had received acupuncture, cupping, plasters and

Chinese patent medicines for 2 months, with poor therapeutic results. He presented with intolerable pain between the muscles and bones with no redness or swelling in the painful area. He was thirsty, with a preference for hot drinks. His tongue was red with a sticky white coating, and his pulse was weak-floating and slow.

Pathogenesis: Accumulation of Cold in the channels and collaterals impairing the function of the joints.

Western diagnosis: Sciatica

Treatment principle: Warm Yang, remove obstruction from the channels, disperse Cold and relieve pain.

The formula used was a variation of **Yang-Heartening Decoction**:

Radix Rehmanniae Praeparata	15 g
Herba Ephedrae	6 g
Semen Sinapis Albae	5 g
Lumbricus	10 g
Colla Cornus Cervi	10 g
Rhizoma Zingiberis	3 g
Radix Aconiti *(raw)*	3 g
Radix Aconiti Kusnezoffii *(raw)*	3 g
Rhizoma Atractylodis	10 g
Ramulus Cinnamomi	3 g

After 11 doses of this prescription the pain disappeared.

b. Wind, Dampness and Heat

— Wind-Damp can combine with Heat to block the channels. This pattern has an acute onset and clinical manifestations include redness, swelling and pain of joints with limitation of movement, and/or fever, sweating, restlessness, thirst, a red tongue with a sticky yellow coating, and a rapid pulse.
— The treatment principle is to eliminate Wind-Damp, clear Heat and remove obstruction from the collaterals.
— The recommended formula is a combination of *Bai Hu Jia Gui Zhi Tang* (**White Tiger Ramulus Cinnamomi Decoction**) and *Si Miao San* (**Four-Marvel Pill**):

Ramulus Cinnamomi	2–5 g
Rhizoma Atractylodis	10 g
Gypsum Fibrosum *(decocted first)*	15–30 g
Rhizoma Anemarrhenae	12 g
Radix Stephaniae Tetrandrae	10 g
Cortex Phellodendri	10 g
Semen Coicis *(raw)*	15 g

— Modifications:
  – For fever and aversion to cold with minimal sweating, remove Rhizoma Anemarrhenae from the prescription and add Herba Ephedrae (5–10 g).
  – For constitutional Yin Deficiency, or damage to Yin due to Heat, with symptoms of persistent low-grade fever and a red tongue with scanty coating, remove Rhizoma Atractylodis, Ramulus Cinnamomi and Gypsum Fibrosum from the prescription and add Radix Gentianae Macrophyllae (12 g), Radix Rehmanniae (15–30 g) and Radix Paeoniae Alba (10 g).

CASE STUDY 40.20
BI SYNDROME
Female, age 15

This patient had had painful joints and low-grade fever for 2 weeks. 4 days before she was admitted to hospital, she developed a high fever and aggravated pain and swelling of the knees and ankles.

Enquiry revealed that the illness had begun with a sore throat; two weeks later she developed a low-grade fever and pain in both knees that wandered to the ankles. After another 2 weeks, she had high fever that was not relieved by sweating, irritability, thirst with desire to drink and redness, swelling and pain of the knees and ankles so severe she could not walk. ESR was 97 mm/h.

Pathogenesis: Invasion of the channels, collaterals and joints by Wind, Dampness and Heat, causing retardation of the circulation of Qi and Blood and hyperactivity of Heat in the Interior.

Western diagnosis: Acute rheumatoid arthritis

Treatment principle: Eliminate Wind, Heat and Dampness

The formula used was a variation of **White Tiger Ramulus Cinnamomi Decoction**:

Ramulus Cinnamomi	6 g
Gypsum Fibrosum *(raw)* *(decocted first)*	30 g
Rhizoma Anemarrhenae	10 g
Radix Paeoniae Rubra	10 g
Rhizoma Polygoni Cuspidati	15 g
Radix Achyranthis Bidentatae	10 g
Semen Coicis *(raw)*	15 g
Caulis Lonicerae *(Ren Dong Teng)*	30 g
Radix Gentianae Macrophyllae	10 g
Excrementum Bombycis Mori *(Can Sha) (decocted wrapped)*	12 g
Radix Glycyrrhizae *(raw)*	5 g

After two doses, the fever, swelling and pain subsided. The prescription was then modified according to the remaining symptoms, and the patient was discharged from hospital 6 days later free of all symptoms. She continued treatment for a short time to consolidate the therapeutic results until she was fully recovered.

c. Kidney Deficiency with stagnation of Phlegm and Blood

— Long-term rheumatism leads to stagnation of Phlegm and Blood, and deficiency of the Liver and Kidneys. This is a chronic pattern. Clinical manifestations include swelling, rigidity, deformity and restricted movement of the joints, and intermittent pain.
— The treatment principle is to tonify the Liver and Kidneys, resolve Phlegm and Blood Stasis, eliminate Wind and remove obstruction from the collaterals.
— The recommended formula is:

Radix Angelicae Pubescentis	10 g
Ramulus Loranthi	15 g
Cortex Acanthopanacis Radicis	10 g
Radix Rehmanniae	15 g
Semen Sinapis Albae	2–3 g
Radix Paeoniae Rubra	10 g
Agkistrodon Acutus	5–10 g
or Zaocys	15 g
Scolopendra	2–5 g
Eupolyphaga seu Steleophaga	10 g
Herba Tripterygii *(Lei Gong Teng)*	10 g

— Modifications:

  – For Cold, add Ramulus Cinnamomi (5 g), Rhizoma Aconitum Carmichaeli or Radix Aconiti Praeparata (2–5 g), and Radix Morindae Officinalis (10 g).
  – For Heat, add Rhizoma Anemarrhenae (12 g), Radix Gentianae Macrophyllae (12 g) and Lumbricus (10 g).

---

2. WEI SYNDROMES (PARALYSIS)

GENERAL DESCRIPTION

— Wei syndrome refers to weakness, motor impairment and muscular atrophy of the limbs and body. It corresponds to the Western diagnostic categories of severe multiple neuritis, poliomyelitis, progressive muscular atrophy, myasthenia gravis, myodystrophy and periodic paralysis.
— These patterns are variously caused by Lung Heat consuming Body Fluids, Damp-Heat

affecting the tendons and channels, and Liver and Kidney Deficiency.
— The treatment principles are to clear Heat, nourish Yin, benefit the Lungs and Stomach, clear Damp-Heat and tonify the Liver and Kidneys.

DIFFERENTIATION AND TREATMENT

a. Lung Heat consuming Body Fluids

— Pathogenic Damp-Heat and toxins act on the Lungs and Stomach to consume Body Fluids, thus depriving the tendons and channels of moisture. Clinical manifestations include fever at the onset of the disease, weakness of the limbs and body when the fever subsides, dryness of the throat, thirst, a red tongue and a thready, rapid pulse.
— The treatment principle is to clear Heat, nourish Yin and benefit the Lungs and Stomach.
— The recommended formula is a variation of *Sha Shen Mai Dong Tang* (**Glehnia–Ophiopogon Decoction**):

Radix Adenophorae	10–15 g
Radix Ophiopogonis	10–15 g
Herba Dendrobii	10–15 g
Rhizoma Anemarrhenae	10 g
Radix Trichosanthis	10 g
Radix Rehmanniae	10 g
Folium Mori	10 g
Rhizoma Polygonati	10–15 g

— Modifications:

  – If Heat is severe and accompanied by thirst and sweating, add Gypsum Fibrosum (15 g) (decocted first), Flos Lonicerae (10 g) and Caulis Trachelospermi (10 g).
  – For dry throat with a choking cough, add Cortex Trichosanthis (10 g) and Cortex Mori Radicis (10 g).
  – For reduced appetite and lassitude when the fever subsides, remove Rhizoma Anemarrhenae from the prescription and add Rhizoma Dioscoreae (15 g), Semen Coicis (15 g) and Fructus Ziziphi Jujubae (5 pieces).

b. Damp-Heat affecting the tendons and channels

— When Damp-Heat is retained in the Interior, it affects the tendons and channels,

manifesting primarily as progressive weakness and paralysis of the body and limbs, particularly the lower limbs. Other signs include slight swelling and numbness of the limbs, a sticky yellow tongue coating and a soft, rapid pulse.
— The treatment principle is to clear Heat and eliminate Dampness.
— The recommended formula is a variation of **Four-Marvel Powder**:

Cortex Phellodendri	10 g
Rhizoma Atractylodis	10 g
Radix Achyranthis Bidentatae	15 g
Radix Stephaniae Tetrandrae	10 g
Rhizoma Dioscoreae Septemlobae	10 g
Cortex Acanthopanacis Radicis	10 g
Fructus Chaenomelis	10 g

— Modifications:
  – For chronic cases presenting with Liver and Kidney Yin Deficiency, remove Rhizoma Atractylodis from the prescription and add Radix Rehmanniae (15 g), Plastrum Testudinis (15 g) (*decocted first*) and Herba Dendrobii (15 g).
  – For Blood Stasis with numbness or pain in the body and limbs and a purple tongue, add Radix Paeoniae Rubra (10 g), Squama Manitis (10 g) and Eupolyphaga seu Steleophaga (10 g).
  – If Heat signs are absent, but there is a localized sensation of cold, remove Cortex Phellodendri from the prescription and add Ramulus Cinnamomi (2–5 g) and Herba Epimedii (10 g).

c. Liver and Kidney Deficiency

— Clinical manifestations include weakness or paralysis of the body and limbs, sore and weak lumbar region and knees, dizziness and vertigo, tinnitus, nocturnal enuresis and urinary incontinence.
— The treatment principle is to tonify the Liver and Kidneys and strengthen the tendons and bones.
— The recommended formula is a variation of *Hu Qian Wan* (**Hidden Tiger Pill**):

Radix Rehmanniae	15 g
Radix Rehmanniae Praeparata	15 g
Herba Dendrobii	15 g
Rhizoma Polygonati	15 g
Fructus Lycii	15 g
Plastrum Testudinis	15 g
Cortex Acanthopanacis Radicis	15 g

Ramulus Loranthi	15 g
Cortex Eucommiae	10 g

— Modifications:
  – For pronounced Yin Deficiency marked by a red tongue with scanty coating, remove Cortex Eucommiae from the prescription and add Rhizoma Anemarrhenae (10 g) and Cortex Phellodendri (10 g).
  – For pronounced Yang Deficiency with coldness of the paralysed limbs, add Cornu Cervi (5–10 g), Herba Epimedii (10–15 g) and Radix Morindae Officinalis (10 g).
  – For Spleen and Stomach Deficiency with muscular atrophy, reduced appetite and loose stool, add Radix Astragali seu Hedysari (15 g), Radix Codonopsis Pilosulae (10 g), Rhizoma Atractylodis Macrocephalae (10 g) and Rhizoma Dioscoreae (15 g).

CASE STUDY 40.21
WEI SYNDROME

Male, age 52

This patient had suffered paroxysmal paralysis of his lower limbs for over 2 years and a diagnosis of hypokalaemia was established (0.9 m g/100 ml). The paralysis was worse on rainy days. In May he had an aggravation and could not get up; he was treated with an intravenous drip of potassium chloride and improved slightly. On his way to the hospital he fell to the ground six times due to weakness of the legs. His legs were cold, he had an aversion to cold generally and he had frequent nocturia.

Pathogenesis: Spleen Deficiency leading to frequent urination and weakness of the lower limbs.

Western diagnosis: Hypokalaemia
Treatment principle: Primarily to invigorate the Middle Burner and benefit Qi; secondarily to promote Yin with sour and sweet herbs.

Initially, the method of warming and tonifying Kidney Yang was adopted, but with poor results. On his second visit, the patient presented with thirst, a sticky sensation in his mouth, reduced appetite, frequent urination, weakness of the lower limbs, a thin tongue coating and a soft pulse.

At this point, the treatment principle was revised and the following formula was prescribed:

Codonopsis Pilosulae	12 g

Rhizoma Atractylodis	
Macrocephalae	10 g
Rhizoma Cimicifugae *(treated)*	3 g
Rhizoma Dioscoreae	12 g
Fructus Alpiniae Oxyphyllae	10 g
Fructus Schisandrae	5 g
Fructus Mume	6 g
Concha Ostreae *(calcined)*	30 g
(decocted first)	
Radix Glycyrrhizae *(treated)*	3 g
Fructus Ziziphi Jujubae	5 pieces

After taking four doses, the patient walked to the hospital without falling down, indicating an improvement in his lower limbs. Frequency of urination was reduced by half and his appetite improved.

On subsequent visits to the hospital, Fructus Mume was replaced by Fructus Chaenomelis in the prescription. Treatment was continued for a month until the patient could walk to the market to do his shopping and suffered no new attack on rainy days.

3. HEADACHE

GENERAL DESCRIPTION
— Headache may occur as a symptom of various acute and chronic diseases. Headache due to external invasion is often the result of pathogenic Wind which combines with Cold, Heat or Dampness. Headache due to internal imbalance is often the result of Blood Deficiency, hyperactive Liver Yang or Liver Fire, Phlegm-Damp or stagnation of Blood.

DIFFERENTIATION AND TREATMENT

a. Invasion of the head by pathogenic Wind

— This pattern is variously caused by invasion of the channels and collaterals by Wind-Cold, invasion of the clear cavity by Wind-Heat or disturbance of the clear Yang by Wind-Damp. The invasion gives rise to temporal or occipital headache, which may be accompanied by aversion to cold, fever, nasal obstruction, general aching, a thin tongue coating and a superficial pulse. It often corresponds to the Western diagnostic categories of acute chronic rhinitis, accessory nasal sinusitis and certain types of trigeminal neuralgia.
— The treatment principle is to eliminate Wind and relieve pain.
— The recommended formula is **Ligusticum–**

Green Tea Regulating Powder:

Rhizoma Ligustici Chuanxiong	5–10 g
Herba Schizonepetae	10 g
Radix Ledebouriellae	10 g
Radix Angelicae Dahuricae	10 g
Fructus Viticis	10 g

— Modifications:

- If Wind-Cold predominates, add Rhizoma seu Radix Notopterygii (5–10 g) and Herba Asari (1.5–3 g).
- If Wind-Heat predominates, remove Herba Schizonepetae and Radix Ledebouriellae from the prescription and add Folium Mori (10 g), Flos Chrysanthemi (10 g), Fructus Tribuli (10–15 g) and Gypsum Fibrosum (15 g) (decocted first).
- For turbid nasal discharge, add Flos Magnoliae (2–5 g) and Fructus Xanthii (10 g).
- If pathogenic Wind is complicated with Dampness, giving rise to a feeling as if the head is tightly wrapped, heaviness of the limbs and a sticky tongue coating, add Rhizoma seu Radix Notopterygii (5 –10 g) and Rhizoma Atractylodis (5–10 g).

CASE STUDY 40.22
HEADACHE

Male, age 27

This patient complained of left temporal headache for over 10 years, with attacks becoming more frequent in Winter. Other clinical manifestations included aversion to cold, cold limbs, a thin, white tongue coating and a fine, thready pulse.

Pathogenesis: Invasion of pathogenic Wind-Cold, complicated by Yang Deficiency.

Western diagnosis: Neurovascular headache

Treatment principle: Eliminate Wind and Cold, warm Yang and relieve pain.

The formula used was a variation of **Ligusticum–Green Tea Regulating Powder** and **Lead to Symmetry Powder**:

Rhizoma Ligustici Chuanxiong	4.5 g
Radix Angelicae Dahuricae	6 g
Bombyx Batryticatus *(prepared)*	9 g
Herba Schizonepetae	9 g
Radix Ledebouriellae	9 g
Rhizoma seu Radix Notopterygii	4.5 g
Scorpio	3 g
Herba Asari	1.5 g

| Radix Glycyrrhizae *(treated)* | 3 g |
| Radix Aconiti Praeparata | 9 g |

After two doses of this formula the headache improved; after another two doses it disappeared.

b. Liver Yang Rising

— Hyperactive Liver Yang and Liver Fire disturb the clear cavity, giving rise to headache, red eyes, dizziness and vertigo and (in severe cases) referred pain. Other signs and symptoms include thirst, a bitter taste in the mouth, a red tongue and a wiry pulse. All symptoms are aggravated by emotional stress.
— This pattern corresponds to the Western diagnostic categories of hypertension and neurosis.
— The treatment principle is to suppress hyperactive Liver Yang.
— The recommended formula is a variation of **Gastrodia–Uncaria Decoction**:

Rhizoma Gastrodiae	10 g
Ramulus Uncariae cum Uncis	10–15 g
Folium Mori	10 g
Flos Chrysanthemi	10 g
Fructus Tribuli	10–15 g
Semen Cassiae	10–15 g
Concha Ostreae	15–20 g
(decocted first)	

— Modifications:

  – For hyperactive Liver Fire, add Spica Prunellae (15 g) and Fructus Gardeniae (10 g).
  – For Liver and Kidney Yin Deficiency, add Fructus Lycii (10–15 g), treated Radix Polygoni Multiflori (10–15 g) and Radix Rehmanniae (15 g).

c. Blood Deficiency

— Deficiency of Blood deprives the head of nourishment. Clinical manifestations include headache, dizziness, a hollow sensation in the head, blurred vision, palpitation, a pale tongue and a thready pulse. This pattern is seen in anaemia, neurosis and debilitation due to long-term illness or excessive loss of blood in childbirth.
— The treatment principle is to nourish the Blood, eliminate Wind and relieve pain.
— The recommended formula is **Four-Substance Decoction** with additions:

| Rhizoma Ligustici Chuanxiong | 10 g |

Radix Paeoniae Alba	10 g
Radix Rehmanniae Praeparata	15 g
Radix Angelicae Sinensis	10 g
Radix Polygoni Multiflori *(treated)*	10–15 g
Fructus Lycii	10–15 g
Flos Chrysanthemi	10 g
Fructus Vitici	10 g

— Modifications:

  – For palpitations, add Magnetitum (15–20 g) (decocted first), Semen Biotae (10 g) and Semen Ziziphi Spinosae (10 g).
  – For Qi Deficiency with shortness of breath and sweating, add Radix Codonopsis Pilosulae (10 g) and Radix Astragali seu Hedysari (10 g).

d. Blood Stagnation

— Stagnant Blood blocks the vessels. Clinical manifestations include recurrent stabbing pain which is fixed in location. There may be a history of trauma.
— The treatment principle is to activate Blood circulation, resolve Stasis and relieve pain.
— The recommended formula is:

Radix Angelicae Sinensis	10 g
Rhizoma Ligustici Chuanxiong	10 g
Semen Persicae	10 g
Flos Carthami	5–10 g
Radix Paeoniae Rubra	10 g
Radix Angelicae Dahuricae	10 g

— Modifications:

  – If the headache is chronic and severe, add Scorpio (2–5 g), Scolopendra (2–5 g), Bombyx Batryticatus (10 g), Lumbricus (10 g), Resina Olibani (2–3 g) and Resina Myrrhae (2–3 g).

e. Upward disturbance of Turbid Phlegm

— Turbid Phlegm prevents the clear Yang from ascending. Clinical manifestations include headache, dizziness, a heavy sensation in the head, stuffiness of the chest, nausea (and in severe cases vomiting of phlegm), a sticky tongue coating and a rolling pulse.
— The treatment principle is to resolve Phlegm-Damp, eliminate Wind and relieve pain.
— The recommended formula is a variation of **Pinellia–Atractylodes–Gastrodia Decoction**:

| Rhizoma Pinelliae | 10 g |

Rhizoma Gastrodiae	10 g
Radix Angelicae Dahuricae	10 g
Rhizoma Typhonii	10 g
Rhizoma Atractylodis	5–10 g
Rhizoma Atractylodis Macrocephalae	10 g
Fructus Tribuli	10–15 g
Poria	10–12 g
Rhizoma Alismatis	10–15 g

— Modifications:

- For vomiting, add Haematitum (15 g) (decocted first)
- If Phlegm turns to Heat, remove Rhizoma Atractylodis, Rhizoma Atractylodis Macrocephalae and Rhizoma Typhonii from the prescription and add Arisaema cum Bile (10 g), Caulis Bambusae in Taeniam (10 g), Fructus Aurantii Immaturus (10 g), Bombyx Batryticatus (10 g) and Lumbricus (10 g).
- For frontal headache, add Radix Angelicae Dahuricae (10 g).
- For temporal headache, add Rhizoma Ligustici Chuanxiong (10 g) and Radix Bupleuri (5–10 g).
- For parietal headache due to invasion of pathogenic Cold-Damp, add Rhizoma Ligustici (5–10 g).
- For parietal headache which is Cold in nature and due to internal imbalance, add Fructus Evodiae (2–3 g) and Herba Asari (1.5–2 g).
- For occipital headache, add Radix Puerariae (10–15 g).

---

4. DIZZINESS AND VERTIGO

GENERAL DESCRIPTION

— Dizziness and vertigo are often seen in hypertension, aural vertigo and neurosis. Their causes include Stagnant Liver Qi turning to Fire and Liver Yang Rising, Phlegm-Damp misting the Mind, deficiency of Qi and Blood depriving the head of nourishment, and Kidney Deficiency with insufficiency of the Sea of Marrow.

DIFFERENTIATION AND TREATMENT

a. Liver Yang Rising

— Liver Yang Rising disturbs the head and eyes. Clinical manifestations include dizziness and vertigo, headache, irritability, a thin yellow tongue coating and a wiry pulse. All symptoms are aggravated by emotional stress.
— The treatment principle is to suppress Liver Yang and calm Liver Wind.
— The recommended formula is a variation of **Gastrodia–Uncaria Decoction**:

Ramulus Uncariae cum Uncis	10–15 g
Rhizoma Gastrodiae	10 g
Flos Chrysanthemi	10 g
Fructus Tribuli	15 g
Concha Ostreae (decocted first)	15–20 g
Concha Haliotidis (decocted first)	15–20 g

— Modifications:

- For hyperactivity of Liver Fire with a flushed face and a bitter taste in the mouth, add Spica Prunellae (15 g), Fructus Gardeniae (10 g) and Cortex Moutan Radicis (10 g).
- For vomiting, add Haematitum (15 g) (decocted first)
- For Liver and Kidney Yin Deficiency, add Fructus Lycii (15 g), Radix Rehmanniae (15 g) and Radix Polygoni Multiflori (15 g).
- For hypertension, increase the dosage of Ramulus Uncariae cum Uncis and add Herba Siegesbeckiae (15 g) and Folium Apocyni Veneti (15 g).

— The treatment principle is to nourish Blood and eliminate Wind.
— The recommended formula is a variation of **Four-Substance Decoction**:

Radix Angelicae Sinensis	10 g
Radix Rehmanniae	10 g
Radix Paeoniae Alba	10 g
Rhizoma Ligustici Chuanxiong	5 g
Radix Polygoni Multiflori	15–30 g
Herba Schizonepetae	10 g
Radix Ledebouriellae	10 g
Bombyx Batryticatus	10 g

CASE STUDY 40.23
DIZZINESS AND VERTIGO

Male, age 52

This patient presented with dizziness and vertigo, distending pain at the top of the head and back of the neck, tidal flushing, tinnitus, nausea, reflux of clear fluid, closing of the eyes, inability to fall asleep, dream-disturbed sleep, a red tongue with no coating, and a wiry, thready and rapid pulse. His blood pressure was 176/126. Examination of the eye fundus showed mild arteriosclerosis.

Pathogenesis: Liver Yang Rising and upward disturbance of Liver Wind.

Western diagnosis: Hypertension

Treatment principle: Subdue Liver Yang, calm Liver Wind and clear Heat.

The formula used was a variation of **Gastrodia–Uncaria Decoction**:

Rhizoma Gastrodiae	9 g
Fructus Tribuli	9 g
Poria	9 g
Ramulus Uncariae cum Uncis	12 g
Concha Haliotidis	18 g
Ramulus Loranthi	9 g
Concha Margaritifera Usta	30 g
Magnetitum	30 g
Caulis Bambusae in Taeniam	9 g
Fructus Gardeniae *(burnt)*	9 g
Radix Paeoniae Alba *(raw)*	9 g

After two doses, the dizziness, vertigo and vomiting improved. After another three doses, all symptoms further improved, but there was Yin Deficiency in the lower body and hyperactivity of Yang in the upper body, indicating that Fire could not return to its origin because Kidney Yin had not recovered.

Subsequent treatment was thus focused on the underlying cause of the condition and a variation of **Restoring the Left Pill** was prescribed:

Radix Rehmanniae	12 g
Radix Rehmanniae Praeparata	12 g
Fructus Corni	6 g
Fructus Lycii	9 g
Radix Achyranthis Bidentatae	6 g
Fructus Ligustri Lucidi	9 g
Ramulus Loranthi	9 g
Ramulus Uncariae cum Uncis	9 g
Radix Paeoniae Alba *(raw)*	9 g
Herba Ecliptae	9 g
Plastrum Testudinis	18 g
(decocted first)	

After five doses of this formula, all symptoms had disappeared and blood pressure was 140/96. The patient was then asked to take 9 g of **Lycium Fruit, Chrysanthemum and Rehmannia Pill** twice daily. 20 days of treatment comprised a course, with a few days' break between courses. A follow-up visit 30 months later showed no relapse.

b. Retention of Turbid Phlegm

— Turbid Phlegm moves upward and mists the clear cavity of the head. Clinical manifestations include dizziness and vertigo, stuffiness of the chest, nausea, abundant sputum, obesity, a sticky tongue coating and a rolling pulse.
— The treatment principle is to resolve Phlegm-Damp and calm Wind.
— The recommended formula is a variation of **Pinellia–Atractylodis Gastrodia Decoction**:

Rhizoma Gastrodiae	10 g
Rhizoma Atractylodis Macrocephalae	10–12 g
Rhizoma Pinelliae	10 g
Poria	10–12 g
Rhizoma Alismatis	10–15 g

— Modifications:

  – If vomiting is severe, add Haematitum and ginger-treated Caulis Bambusae in Taeniam.
  – For Liver Yang Rising, add herbs that calm Liver Yang.
  – For aural vertigo and labyrinthine hydrops, increase the dosage of Rhizoma Alismatis and Poria and add Semen Plantaginis (12 g) (decocted wrapped).

c. Qi and Blood Deficiency

— Deficiency of Qi and Blood deprives the head and eyes of nourishment. Clinical manifestations include dizziness, vertigo, blurred vision, lassitude, pallor, a pale tongue and a thready pulse.
— The treatment principle is primarily to tonify Qi and Blood and secondarily to subdue Wind.
— The recommended formula is a variation of **Restore the Spleen Decoction**:

Radix Codonopsis Pilosulae	10 g
Radix Astragali seu Hedysari	10 g
Rhizoma Ligustici Chuanxiong	5–10 g
Radix Angelicae Sinensis	10 g
Fructus Lycii	10–15 g
Radix Rehmanniae Praeparata	10–15 g
Radix Paeoniae Alba	10 g
Magnetitum	15–20 g
(decocted first)	
Poria cum Ligno Hospite	10 g

— Modifications:

  – For Spleen Qi Deficiency with loose stool, remove Radix Angelicae Sinensis and Radix Rehmanniae Praeparata from the prescription and add Rhizoma Dioscoreae (15g), Radix Aucklandiae (5g) and Radix Bupleuri (3g).
  – For deficiency of Yin and Blood, remove Radix Codonopsis Pilosulae and Radix

Astragali seu Hedysari from the prescription and add Radix Polygoni Multiflori (15g) and Fructus Ligustici Lucidi (15g).

d. Liver and Kidney Deficiency

— Liver and Kidney Deficiency implies insufficiency of the Sea of Marrow. Clinical manifestations include chronic dizziness and vertigo, tinnitus, blurred vision, lumbar soreness and spermatorrhoea or thin clear leucorrhoea.
— The treatment principle is to tonify the Liver and Kidneys.
— The recommended formula is a variation of *Qi Ju Di Huang Wan* (**Lycium Fruit, Chrysanthemum and Rehmannia Pill**):

Radix Rehmanniae Praeparata	15 g
Fructus Lycii	15 g
Flos Chrysanthemi	10 g
Fructus Corni	10 g
Radix Polygoni Multiflori *(treated)*	15 g
Magnetitum *(decocted first)*	15–30 g
Plastrum Testudinis *(decocted first)*	15 g

— Modifications:

- For hypertension, add Cortex Eucommiae (10–12 g), Ramulus Loranthi (15 g) and Radix Achyranthis Bidentatae (10–15 g).
- If dizziness and vertigo are due to hypertension as part of menopausal syndrome, add Herba Epimedii (10 g), Rhizoma Curculiginis (10 g), Rhizoma Anemarrhenae (10 g) and Cortex Phellodendri (10 g).
- For Liver and Kidney Yin Deficiency complicated with Liver Yang Rising, add Rhizoma Gastrodiae (10 g), Ramulus Uncariae cum Uncis (10–15 g) and Concha Ostreae (15–30 g) (decocted first).
- For spermatorrhoea or leucorrhoea, add Semen Euryales (10–15 g), Os Draconis (15 g) and Rhizoma Dioscoreae (15 g).

5. WIND-STROKE

GENERAL DESCRIPTION
— Wind-Stroke presents with sudden collapse and loss of consciousness, or mental cloudiness and hemiplegia or deviation of the mouth and eye. The former condition is referred to as attack on the Zang-Fu, while the latter is considered to be attack on the channels and collaterals.

— Deviation of the mouth and eye in an attack on the channels and collaterals is caused by facial paralysis. The other conditions are the consequences of cerebrovascular accident, which include cerebral haemorrhage, cerebral thrombosis, cerebrovascular spasm, cerebral embolism and subarachnoid haemorrhage.
— Facial paralysis is caused by invasion of the collaterals by pathogenic Wind mixed with Phlegm. Cerebrovascular accident is caused by Liver and Kidney Yin Deficiency, Liver Yang Rising with stirring of Liver Wind, Liver Wind complicated with Phlegm-Fire, or perversion of Qi and Blood.
— Attack on the Zang-Fu is further differentiated into tense syndrome and flaccid syndrome. The treatment method adopted for tense syndrome is to promote resuscitation; it is also necessary to determine whether Liver Wind, Fire or Phlegm predominates. The treatment method adopted for flaccid syndrome is to rescue Collapse, and it is necessary to determine whether the pattern is one of Yin Collapse or Yang Collapse.
— The treatment method adopted for attack on the channels and collaterals is to subdue Liver Wind, resolve Phlegm and remove obstructions from the collaterals.

DIFFERENTIATION AND TREATMENT

a. Attack on the channels and collaterals (invasion of the collaterals by Wind-Phlegm)

i. Facial paralysis
— When the collaterals are empty and resistance to disease is weak, pathogenic Wind invades and combines with Phlegm-Damp. Clinical manifestations include an abrupt onset of deviation of the mouth and eye, drooling, unclear speech, numbness of the face, possible aversion to cold, a sticky white tongue coating and a wiry, rolling pulse.
— The treatment principle is to eliminate Wind, resolve Phlegm and remove obstruction from the collaterals.
— The recommended formula is a variation of **Lead to Symmetry Powder**:

Rhizoma Typhonii	10 g
Rhizoma Arisaematis	10 g
Bombyx Batryticatus	10 g
Lumbricus	10 g
Scorpio	2-5 g

| Radix Gentianae Macrophyllae | 10 g |
| Radix Ledebouriellae | 10 g |

ii. *Cerebral thrombosis, cerebral embolism and cerebrovascular spasm*

— Yin Deficiency and hyperactive Yang are complicated with acute blockage of the collaterals by Liver Wind, Phlegm and stagnant Blood. Clinical manifestations at the early stage include transient mental confusion, deviation of the mouth and eye, and hemiplegia; later signs include numbness and heaviness of the face and four limbs, contracture and spasm of the hands and feet, dizziness with a heavy sensation in the head, profuse expectoration of sputum, rigidity of the tongue and slurred speech, a thin white tongue coating or a white or yellow sticky tongue coating, and a wiry and rolling or thready pulse.

— The treatment principle is to calm Liver Wind, resolve Phlegm and remove obstruction from the collaterals.

— The recommended formula is a combination of **Gastrodia–Uncaria Decoction** and *Dao Tan Tang* (**Eliminating Phlegm Decoction**):

Rhizoma Gastrodiae	12 g
Ramulus Uncariae cum Uncis	15 g
Concha Haliotidis	15-20 g
Rhizoma Pinelliae	10 g
Arisaema cum Bile	10 g
Fructus Aurantii Immaturus	10 g
Poria	12 g
Bombyx Batryticatus	10 g
Rhizoma Typhonii	5-10 g
Lumbricus	10 g
Herba Siegesbeckiae	10-15 g

— Modifications:

– If Wind-Phlegm is complicated with Blood Stasis, indicated by a purple tongue suggesting cerebrovascular obstructive disorder, add Semen Persicae (10 g), Radix Paeoniae Rubra (10 g), Flos Carthami (10 g) and Hirudo (5 g).

b. Attack on the Zang-Fu

i. *Liver Wind, Liver Yang, Phlegm and Fire (tense syndrome)*

— When constitutional Liver and Kidney Yin Deficiency are aggravated by long-term worry, anxiety or anger, this leads to hyperactivity of Heart and Liver Yang; this in turn produces Fire and stirs up Wind which condenses Body Fluids into Phlegm.

— The combination of Phlegm-Fire with Liver Yang and Wind moves upward, causing rebellious movement of Qi and Blood and resulting in the tense form of Wind Stroke.

— Clinical manifestations include coma, clenched hands, contracture or spasm of the limbs, body and jaw, snoring, coarse breathing, flushed face, a feverish sensation, constipation, a red tongue with sticky yellow coating, and a rapid, wiry and rolling pulse.

— The treatment principle is to subdue Wind, clear Fire, resolve Phlegm and open the orifices.

— The recommended formula is a variation of **Antelope Horn and Uncaria Decoction**:

Cornu Antelopis *(taken separately)*	0.5-1 g
Concha Haliotidis *(decocted first)*	30 g
Ramulus Uncariae cum Uncis *(added at end of decoction)*	12 g
Arisaema cum Bile	10 g
Bulbus Fritillariae Cirrhosae	10 g
Caulis Bambusae in Taeniam	10 g
Rhizoma Acori Graminei *(added at end of decoction)*	3-5 g
Radix Curcumae	10 g
Rhizoma Coptidis	3-6 g

plus one pill of *Zhi Bao Dan* (**Greatest Treasure Special Pill**) or *Niu Huang Qing Xin Wan* (**Cattle Gallstone Pill to Clear the Heart**), to be taken in one or two doses separately.

— Modifications:

– For Yin deficiency with a red tongue and scanty coating, add Radix Rehmanniae (12-20 g), Radix Paeoniae Alba (10-12 g), Radix Ophiopogonis (15 g) and Radix Trichosanthis (10-15 g).

– For Stomach Fire with a yellow tongue coating and constipation, add Radix et Rhizoma Rhei (10 g) (added at end of decoction) and Natrii Sulfas (10 g) (taken separately).

– For Liver Fire with symptoms of restlessness, a flushed face and a feeling of heat, add Radix Gentianae (2-5 g), Fructus Gardeniae (10 g), and Haematitum (15-20 g) (decocted first).

– For cerebral haemorrhage, add Radix Achyranthis Bidentatae (15 g), Cortex Moutan Radicis (10 g), Fructus Gardeniae (1 g) and powdered Radix Notoginseng (1 g) (taken separately).

– If the pattern is Cold in nature, the patient will not be restless and irritable, but will have a pale complexion, purple lips and a sticky white tongue coating. In this case, remove Rhizoma Coptidis and Concha Haliotidis from the prescription and add *Su He Xiang Wan* (**Styrax Pill**), to be taken separately.

ii. Exhaustion of Yin and Collapse of Yang (flaccid syndrome)

— In this pattern, the Upright Qi has failed in its struggle against the pathogenic factors, thus transforming an Excess pattern into one of Deficiency. As a result, both Qi and Yin are injured and both Yin and Yang are collapsing. Clinical manifestations include coma, snoring, closed eyes, open mouth, relaxed hands, incontinence of both urine and faeces, profuse sticky or cold sweating, pallor, cold limbs and a deep and hidden or thready, rapid and fading pulse.

— The treatment principle is to rescue Yin and recapture Yang.

— The recommended formula is a variation of *Sheng Fu Tang* (**Ginseng and Aconite Decoction**) and **Restoring the Pulse Powder**:

Radix Ginseng Rubra *(Hong Shen)* *(decocted separately)*	10 g
Radix Aconiti Praeparata *(decocted at length)*	10 g
Radix Ophiopogonis	15 g
Fructus Schisandrae	5 g
Os Draconis *(decocted first)*	15 g
Concha Ostreae *(decocted first)*	30 g

— Modifications:

  – For shortness of breath, add Fructus Corni (20 g) and Magnetitum (20 g) (decocted first) to rescue Collapse, assist reception of Qi and soothe wheeze.

  – For Collapse of Yin with profuse sticky sweating, flushed face and a thready, rapid and fading pulse, remove Radix Aconiti Praeparata from the prescription and add Radix Glehniae (15 g) or Radix Panacis Quinquefolii (10 g) *(decocted separately)*.

c. Recuperative stage

i. Blockage by Wind, Phlegm and stagnant Blood

— This pattern represents the late stage of Wind-Stroke, manifesting as clear consciousness, hemiplegia, numbness, contracture and pain, and heaviness of the limbs and body.

— The treatment principle is to eliminate Wind, resolve Phlegm and Blood Stasis and remove obstruction from the collaterals.

— The recommended formula is:

Rhizoma Gastrodiae	10 g
Herba Siegesbeckiae	15 g
Lumbricus	10 g
Scorpio	2-5 g
Bombyx Batryticatus	10 g
Semen Persicae	10 g
Flos Carthami	10 g
Eupolyphaga seu Steleophaga	10 g

ii. Deficiency and stagnation of Qi and Blood

— Clinical manifestations include hemiplegia in the aftermath of Wind Stroke; soreness, weakness and motor impairment of the limbs and body, with loss of sensation in severe cases; and dyspnoea and lassitude.

— The treatment principle is to benefit Qi, activate the Blood, resolve Blood Stasis and remove obstruction from the collaterals.

— The recommended formula is a variation of **Tonify the Yang to Restore Five-Tenths Decoction**:

Radix Astragali seu Hedysari	15-30 g
Radix Angelicae Sinensis	10 g
Rhizoma Ligustici Chuanxiong	10 g
Radix Paeoniae Rubra	10 g
Semen Persicae	10 g
Flos Carthami	6-10 g
Lumbricus	10 g
Eupolyphaga seu Steleophaga	10 g

CASE STUDY 40.24
WIND-STROKE

Male, age 40

This patient awoke one morning with numbness in the right side of his face, deviation of the mouth and eye, weakness in the right side of his body and mild difficulty in speaking. He had a pale tongue with a slightly sticky white coating, and a deep, wiry pulse.

Pathogenesis: Deficiency of Qi leading to retarded circulation of Blood and stagnation of Blood in the vessels.

Treatment principle: Tonify Qi and Blood, resolve Blood Stasis and remove obstruction from the vessels.

The formula used was a variation of **Tonify the Yang to Restore Five-tenths Decoction**:

Radix Astragali seu Hedysari	30 g

Radix Paeoniae Rubra	12 g
Radix Angelicae Sinensis	9 g
Lumbricus	9 g
Semen Persicae	9 g
Flos Carthami	9 g
Rhizoma Typhonii	9 g
Bombyx Batryticatus	15 pieces
Scorpio	15 pieces

After ten doses, the patient's face felt more relaxed and his speech became more fluent, but he still could not open and close his mouth and eye freely. His walking was somewhat hindered and his pulse was deep and slow. The dosage of Radix Astragali was then doubled and Herba Asari (1.5 g) was added to the prescription.

After another ten doses, the patient could open and close his mouth and eye freely, but still complained of thirst and dizziness. His pulse was deep and slightly rapid and his tongue coating was thin and white. Herba Asari and Rhizoma Typhonii were then removed from the prescription and Rhizoma Gastrodiae (6 g) and Herba Dendrobii (9 g) were added.

After ten doses of the new prescription, both dizziness and thirst had improved and movement of the leg became almost normal. After a further ten doses, all symptoms had disappeared.

---

iii. Liver and Kidney Deficiency
— Long-term Liver and Kidney Deficiency gives rise to hemiplegia, muscular atrophy, dizziness, tinnitus, rigidity of the tongue, slurred speech, a deep-red or dark purple tongue and a deep, thready and wiry, or hesitant pulse.
— The treatment principle is to tonify the Liver and Kidneys.
— The recommended formula is a variation of *Di Huang Yin Zi* (**Rehmannia Decoction**):

Radix Rehmanniae *or* Radix	
Rehmanniae Praeparata	15-30 g
Fructus Corni	12 g
Herba Dendrobii	15 g
Ramulus Loranthi	15 g
Herba Cistanchis	10 g
Radix Morindae Officinalis	10 g
Rhizoma Acori Graminei	3-5 g
(*added at end of decoction*)	
Radix Polygalae	10 g
Radix Achyranthis Bidentatae	15 g
Eupolyphaga seu Steleophaga	10 g

— Modifications:
  – For Yin Deficiency, remove Radix Morindae Officinalis from the prescription and add Radix Ophiopogonis (15 g)

and Fructus Lycii (15 g).
  – For Yang Deficiency, add Cortex Eucommiae (12 g) and Rhizoma Cibotii (12 g).
  – For Blood Stagnation, add Semen Persicae (10 g), Flos Carthami (10 g) and Lumbricus (10 g).

---

6. EPILEPSY

GENERAL DESCRIPTION
— Epilepsy is a disorder of the nervous system, marked by recurrent acute episodes of loss of consciousness, staring upward, convulsions, spitting of foam or crying like an animal. Between episodes, the patient's condition appears normal. Epileptic seizures are usually brief and may occur at any hour of the day.
— This disease is difficult to treat. It is linked to emotional stress and brain injury. Strong emotions such as fear, depression and anger inhibit the circulation of Heart and Liver Qi, which in turn leads to the production of Phlegm. Brain injury leads to stagnation of Qi, Blood and Phlegm in the Interior. Although the Heart, Liver, Spleen and Kidneys are all involved, Phlegm is the root cause.
— The initial stage of the disease is of the Excess type and is treated by eliminating Phlegm, calming Wind and opening the orifices. Chronic cases are of the Deficiency type; the primary treatment method is to tonify the Kidneys, Heart and Spleen while secondarily resolving Phlegm.

DIFFERENTIATION AND TREATMENT

a. Blockage by Wind-Phlegm

— Rebellion of Qi allows Wind and Phlegm to move upward to mist the clear cavity, transversely to invade the channels and collaterals and inward to disturb the Mind. Clinical manifestations include sudden loss of consciousness, staring upward, convulsion, clenched teeth, drooling, crying like an animal, a sticky white tongue coating and a rolling pulse. When the patient regains consciousness he appears normal except for drowsiness and dizziness.
— If there is concurrent Qi Stagnation with production of Phlegm, there will be stuffiness of the chest and mental depression. This

pattern is often induced by emotional stress and includes warning symptoms such as dizziness and rebellion of Qi before a seizure.

— If the pattern is one of Phlegm-Fire, clinical manifestations will include headache, red eyes, flushed face, restlessness and a sticky yellow tongue coating.
— If the pattern is one of stirring of Wind with Phlegm moving upward, clinical manifestations include dizziness and vertigo, muscular twitching, convulsions, rigidity of the limbs and deviation of the mouth and eye.
— The treatment principle is to eliminate Phlegm, open the orifices and calm Wind.
— The recommended formula is a variation of **Arrest Seizures Pill**:

Rhizoma Pinelliae	10 g
Rhizoma Arisaematis	10 g
Bulbus Fritillariae Cirrhosae	10 g
Rhizoma Acori Graminei	2-5 g
Radix Polygalae	10 g
Poria cum Ligno Hospite	10 g
Concha Margaritifera Usta	10 g
Scorpio	3 g
Bombyx Batryticatus	10 g

— Modifications:

  – For frequent episodes with incessant convulsion, add Cornu Antelopis (1-3 g) (to be taken separately), Ramulus Uncariae cum Uncis (12 g) and Concha Haliotidis (15 g) (decocted first).
  – For Phlegm-Fire, add Rhizoma Coptidis (3 g) and Radix Gentianae (3 g), and administer **Chorite-Schist Pill for Chronic Phlegm Syndromes**.

b. Heart and Kidney Deficiency

— Long-term epilepsy damages the Heart and Kidneys. Clinical manifestations include recurrent seizures of varying severity, listlessness, dizziness, palpitations, reduced appetite, sore and weak lumbar region and knees, pallor, a pale tongue with thin, white coating, and a thready and possibly rolling pulse. In severe cases, intelligence may be impaired.
— The treatment principle is to tonify the Kidneys, soothe the Heart, invigorate the Spleen and resolve Phlegm.
— The recommended formula is a variation of *Da Bu Yuan Jian* (**Great Tonify the Source Decoction**) and **Six Gentlemen Decoction**:

Radix Codonopsis Pilosulae	10 g
or Radix Ginseng	6 g
Rhizoma Dioscoreae	15 g
Radix Rehmanniae Praeparata	15 g
Fructus Lycii	12 g
Radix Angelicae Sinensis	10 g
Radix Salviae Miltiorrhizae	12 g
Rhizoma Pinelliae *(treated)*	10 g
Pericarpium Citri Reticulatae	5 g
Radix Polygalae	10 g
Poria cum Ligno Hispite	10 g

— Modifications:

  – For mental dullness, add alum-water-treated Radix Curcumae (12 g) and Rhizoma Acori Graminei (2–5 g) (*decocted later*).
  – For listlessness, administer Placenta Hominis frequently.
  – If the condition is due to brain injury, add Rhizoma Ligustici Chuanxiong (10 g), Eupolyphaga seu Steleophaga (10 g), Radix Achyranthis (10 g) and Flos Carthami (5 g) to activate the Blood and resolve Stasis.

7. EMOTIONALLY-RELATED PATTERNS

GENERAL DESCRIPTION

— Emotionally related patterns correspond to neurasthenia, hysteria and climacteric syndromes in Western medicine. They are caused by stagnation of Liver Qi, deficiency of the Zang and Phlegm-Fire.
— The treatment principles are to relieve stagnation of Liver Qi, to clear Fire and resolve Phlegm, and to nourish the Zang and calm the Mind.

Differentiation and treatment

a. Stagnation of Liver Qi

— Emotional irritation impairs the function of the Liver in promoting the free flow of Qi, thus resulting in Liver Qi Stagnation. Clinical manifestations include mental depression, restlessness, stuffiness of the chest, sighing, wandering distending pains in the costal and hypochondriac regions and a wiry pulse.
— The treatment principle is to soothe the Liver, regulate Qi and relieve depression.
— The recommended formula is a variation of **Bupleurum Soothing the Liver Decoction** and **Free and Relaxed Powder**:

Radix Bupleuri *(vinegar-treated)*	5 g
Radix Paeoniae Alba	10 g

Rhizoma Cyperi *(treated)*	10 g
Fructus Aurantii	5 g
Radix Curcumae	10 g
Flos Mume Albus	10 g
Cortex Albiziae	15 g

— Modifications:

- If stagnant Qi turns to Fire, add Cortex Moutan Radicis (10 g) and Fructus Gardeniae (10 g).
- For Liver and Heart Fire and Phlegm-Fire manifesting as irritability, mania and restlessness, add Arisaema cum Bile (10g), Bulbus Fritillariae Cirrhosae (10 g), Rhizoma Anemarrhenae (10 g), Radix Gentianae (2-5 g) and Rhizoma Coptidis (3 g).
- For stagnation of Qi and Blood with irregular menstruation, scanty flow or amenorrhoea, add Rhizoma Ligustici Chuanxiong (6 g), Flos Carthami (5 g) and Radix Salviae Miltiorrhizae (12 g).

b. Combination of Phlegm and Qi

— Heart and Spleen Qi Stagnation produces Phlegm, which combines with the stagnant Qi to cause the sensation of a foreign body in the throat which cannot be relieved by swallowing or spitting. Other symptoms include stuffiness of the chest and a wiry rolling pulse.
— The treatment principle is to regulate Qi, relieve Stagnation and resolve Phlegm.
— The recommended formula is a variation of **Pinellia and Magnolia Bark Decoction**:

Rhizoma Pinelliae	10 g
Cortex Magnoliae Officinalis	2 g
Folium Perillae	3 g
Rhizoma Cyperi *(treated)*	10 g
Fructus Aurantii	10 g
Radix Platycodi	6 g
Poria	10 g
Cortex Albiziae	15 g

— Modifications:

- If stagnant Qi turns to Fire and damages the Yin, remove Cortex Magnoliae Officinalis and Folium Perillae from the prescription and add Cortex Moutan Radicis (10g), Fructus Gardeniae (10 g), Radix Adenophorae (10 g), Radix Ophiopogonis (10 g) and Radix Paeoniae Alba (10 g).

c. Long-term stagnation of Qi deprives the Zang of nourishment

— Prolonged stagnation of Liver Qi leads to deficiency of Qi and Yin and deprives the Heart and Mind of nourishment. Clinical manifestations include absent-mindedness and restlessness.
— The treatment principle is to soothe the Heart, nourish Yin and relieve stagnation.
— The recommended formula is a variation of *Gan Mai Da Zao Tang* (**Licorice, Wheat and Jujube Decoction**):

Radix Glycyrrhizae	5-10 g
Wheat	15-30 g
Radix Rehmanniae	15 g
Radix Ophiopogonis	15 g
Fructus Schisandrae	5 g
Bulbus Lilii	15 g
Rhizoma Anemarrhenae	12 g
Radix Curcumae	10 g
Semen Ziziphi Spinosae	10 g
Poria cum Ligno Hospite	10 g
Cortex Albiziae	15 g

CASE STUDY 40.25
MELANCHOLIA

Female, age 40

This patient presented with depression, grief, weeping, suspiciousness, fear, poor memory, a thin, sticky tongue coating and a rapid, thready pulse. She had a history of depression for 5 years.

Pathogenesis: Deficiency of the Heart, disturbed by Phlegm-Damp.

Western diagnosis: Neurasthenia

Treatment principle: Nourish the Heart, calm the Mind, eliminate Phlegm and open the orifices.

The formula used was a variation of **Licorice, Wheat and Jujube Decoction**:

Radix Glycyrrhizae *(treated)*	9 g
Wheat	30 g
Fructus Ziziphi Jujubae	5 pieces
Herba Ecliptae	15 g
Rhizoma Acori Graminei	9 g
Iron cinder *(Sheng Tie Luo)*	30 g
Radix Curcumae	9 g
Rhizoma Arisaematis *(prepared)*	4.5 g
Semen Ziziphi Spinosae *(stir-baked)*	15 g

After five doses, the depression, grief and weeping improved, as did the insomnia. Because Qi and Blood were both deficient following a prolonged illness, Qi and Blood tonics such as Radix Angelicae Sinensis, Fructus Lycii and Radix

Codonopsis Pilosulae were then added to the formula.

The treatment was continued for a month, by which time all symptoms had disappeared.

d. Disharmony between the Heart and Kidneys

— In this pattern, stagnant Qi turns to Fire while Kidney Yin Deficiency leads to Empty Heart Fire. Clinical manifestations include dizziness and vertigo, palpitations, restlessness, insomnia, lumbar soreness, spermatorrhoea, irregular menstruation, a red tongue with scanty coating, and a thready pulse.
— The treatment principle is to nourish Yin, reduce Fire and harmonize the Heart and Kidneys.
— The recommended formula is a variation of **Heavenly Emperor Tonifying the Heart Pill** and **Six-Flavour Rehmannia Pill**:

Radix Rehmanniae	10–15 g
Radix Scrophulariae	10 g
Radix Ophiopogonis	10–15 g
Fructus Lycii	10 g
Fructus Schisandrae	2–5 g
Fructus Ligustri Lucidi	15 g
Rhizoma Coptidis	1.5–3 g
Semen Nelumbinis	10 g
Poria cum Ligno Hospite	
(Cinnabaris coated)	12 g
Os Draconis	15 g
(decocted first)	
Magnetitum	20 g
(decocted first)	

F. Miscellaneous other diseases

1. CHYLURIA

GENERAL DESCRIPTION
— Chyluria is a condition of chyle in the urine, which gives the urine a milky appearance. It is categorized in TCM as turbid urine and urinary disturbance and is caused by the downward movement of Damp-Heat and Essences and deficiency of the Spleen and Kidney.
— The treatment principle is to clear Damp-Heat and tonify the Spleen and Kidney.

DIFFERENTIATION AND TREATMENT

a. Downward movement of Damp-Heat

— Filariasis produces Dampness and Heat, which move downward and impair the Kidneys' function of dividing the clear from the turbid. The key sign is turbid urine, or urine with fatty clots and oil floating on the surface, or with streaks of blood and blood clots. Other clinical manifestations include hesitant painful urine accompanied by a burning sensation, and a sticky yellow tongue coating.
— The treatment principle is to clear Damp-Heat and separate the clear from the turbid.
— The recommended formula is a variation of **Dioscoreae Hypoglauca Decoction to Separate the Clear**:

Rhizoma Dioscoreae Septemlobae	10–15 g
Folium Pyrrosiae	10 g
Poria	10 g
Semen Plantaginis	10 g
(decocted wrapped)	
Rhizoma Acori Graminei	2–5 g
(added at end of decoction)	
Cortex Phellodendri	10 g
Talcum	10–15 g
(decocted wrapped)	

— Modifications:

  – For urinary obstruction, add Radix Linderae.
  – For scanty, deep-yellow urine, with pain and a burning sensation during urination, add Fructus Gardeniae and Caulis Akebiae.
  – For haematuria, add Herba Cephalanoploris and Radix Rubiae.
  – For Yin Deficiency, remove Rhizoma Acori Graminei from the prescription and add Rhizoma Anemarrhenae, Radix Rehmanniae and Radix Ophiopogonis.

CASE STUDY 40.26
CHYLURIA

Male, age 31

This patient had a history of recurrent attacks of turbid urine over 5 years. Upon admission to hospital, urinalysis showed positive ether test, pus cells ++ and a small quantity of red blood cells. Other clinical manifestations included turbid urine like rice water and milk with decaying, sticky, flesh-like clots in it, lumbar soreness, burning pain in the urethra, hesitant urination, dizziness, lassitude, a slightly red tongue with a sticky yellow coating, and a weak-floating pulse.

Pathogenesis: Spleen and Kidney Deficiency complicated with downward movement of Damp-Heat, the signs of Excess being more pronounced than the signs of Deficiency.

Western diagnosis: Chyluria

Treatment principle: Clear Damp-Heat and promote the Bladder's function of dividing the clear from the turbid.

The formula used was a variation of **Dioscorea Hypoglauca Decoction to Separate the Clear** and **Eight-Herb Powder for Rectification:**

Rhizoma Dioscoreae Hypoglauca	12 g
Folium Pyrrosiae	12 g
Cortex Phellodendri	10 g
Rhizoma Anemarrhenae	10 g
Semen Coicis *(raw)*	15 g
Excrementum Bombycis	10 g
Poria	10 g
Semen Plantaginis	10 g
(decocted wrapped)	
Medulla Junci	3 g

After three doses, the flesh-like clots disappeared and the urine became less turbid. After a further three doses, the urine became clear and the ether test was negative. At this point Radix Angelicae Pubescentis (10 g), Ramulus Loranthi (12 g) and Semen Cuscutae (12 g) were added to the prescription.

A month after admission to hospital, the patient had a mild relapse. Although the urine was not visibly turbid, he had lumbar soreness, dizziness, lassitude and hesitant urination. Radix Angelicae Pubescentis was removed from the prescription and Fructus Lycii, Semen Astragali Complanati and Fructus Tribuli were added to nourish the Kidneys and subdue the Liver.

After urinalysis showed negative three times, the treatment method was altered, primarily to invigorate the Spleen and Kidneys and secondarily to clear Heat, in order to consolidate the therapeutic results. The patient's urine remained clear following exercise or eating oily food, although he still felt slightly tired and sore in the lumbar region on exertion, and he was discharged from the hospital.

b. Deficiency and Sinking of Spleen Qi

— Sinking of Spleen Qi results in a downward flowing of Essences. The key symptom is recurrent episodes of turbid urine, often induced by stress or overwork or an excessive intake of oily foods; other clinical manifestations include a bearing-down sensation in the lower abdomen, lassitude, a pale tongue with a white coating, and a soft, thready pulse.

— The treatment principle is to tonify and raise Qi.

— The recommended formula is a variation of **Tonifying the Middle and Benefiting Qi Decoction:**

Radix Codonopsis Pilosulae	10 g
Radix Astragali seu Hedysari	10 g
Rhizoma Atractylodis	
Macrocephalae	10 g
Rhizoma Dioscoreae	15 g
Rhizoma Cimicifugae	3 g
Radix Bupleuri	3 g
Rhizoma Dioscoreae Septemlobae	10 g
Semen Euryales	10 g
Poria	10 g

— Modifications:

  – If Spleen Deficiency affects the Kidneys, leading to lumbar soreness and cold limbs, add Fructus Alpiniae Oxyphyllae (10 g) and Radix Aconiti Praeparata (10 g).

  – For turbid urine mixed with blood, add Herba Cephalanoploris (10 g) and Colla Corii Asini (10g, stir-baked in Pollen Typhae).

  – For Damp-Heat, add Cortex Phellodendri (10 g) and Rhizoma Alismatis (10 g).

c. Kidney Deficiency with impairment of the storing of Essence

— Impairment of the Kidneys' function of storing Essence allows the downward discharge of Essential substances. Clinical manifestations include long-term turbidity of urine, listlessness, sore and weak lumbar region and knees, dizziness and tinnitus.

— The treatment principle is to tonify the Kidneys and strengthen the function of storing the Essence.

— If there is underlying Yin Deficiency, the recommended formula is **Six-Flavour Rehmannia Pill with Anemarrhena and Phellodendri;** for underlying Yang Deficiency, the recommended formula is **Kidney Qi Pill**. In either case, the core formula consists of:

Radix Rehmanniae Praeparata	10–15 g
Fructus Corni	10 g
Rhizoma Dioscoreae	10 g

Semen Cuscutae	15 g
Fructus Rosae Laevigatae	15 g
Semen Euryales	10 g
Poria	10 g
Rhizoma Alismatis	10 g

— Modifications:

- For Yin Deficiency complicated with Damp-Heat, add Rhizoma Anemarrhenae (10 g) and Cortex Phellodendri (10 g).
- For Yang Deficiency, add Radix Aconiti Praeparata (2–5 g), Cortex Cinnamomi (2–5 g) and Cornu Cervi (2–5 g).
- For Sinking of Spleen Qi, add Radix Codonopsis Pilosulae (10 g), Radix Astragali seu Hedysari (10 g) and Rhizoma Cimicifugae (3 g).
- For haematuria, add Plastrum Testudinis (15 g), Herba Ecliptae (15 g) and Colla Corii Asini (10 g) (melted and taken separately).

2. LEUCOCYTOPENIA AND THROMBOCYTOPENIA

GENERAL DESCRIPTION

— Leucocytopenia and thrombocytopenia are both categorized in TCM as consumption and haemorrhagic patterns. Their causes are very complicated and are linked to deficiency of Qi and Blood of the Spleen and Heart, Liver and Kidney Yin Deficiency, general Yin Deficiency with Blood Heat, and Spleen and Kidney Yang Deficiency. Leucocytopenia usually presents with Qi and Yang Deficiency while thrombocytopenia usually exhibits Qi and Yin Deficiency with Empty Fire.

DIFFERENTIATION AND TREATMENT

a. Heart and Spleen Deficiency

— Spleen Deficiency implies insufficiency of the source of Qi and Blood and impairment of the Spleen's function of controlling Blood. Clinical manifestations include dizziness, lassitude, reduced appetite, susceptibility to the common cold, bleeding gums, epistaxis, petechiae, a profuse pinkish menstrual flow, pallor, a pale tongue with thin coating, and a soft, thready pulse.
— The treatment principle is to tonify the Heart and Spleen, nourish Qi and Blood, and control Blood.

The recommended formula is **Tonifying the Spleen Decoction**:

Radix Astragali seu Hedysari	10–20 g
Radix Codonopsis Pilosulae	10 g
Rhizoma Atractylodis Macrocephalae	10 g
Radix Angelicae Sinensis	10 g
Fructus Psoraleae	10 g
Arillus Longan	10 g
Caulis Spatholobae	15 g
Radix Glycyrrhizae (treated)	3 g
Ganoderma Lucidum	10 g

— Modifications:

- For haemorrhage, add stir-baked Rhizoma Zingiberis (2 – 5 g), Colla Corii Asini (10 g, melted and taken separately) and Herba Agrimoniae (15 g).

b. Liver and Kidney Yin Deficiency

— Liver and Kidney Yin Deficiency produces Fire, which impairs the Liver's function of storing Blood. Clinical manifestations include dizziness, blurred vision, tinnitus, lumbar soreness, five-palm Heat, night sweats, bleeding gums, epistaxis, petechiae, a shortened menstrual cycle, profuse red menstrual flow, a red tongue with scanty coating, and a rapid, thready pulse.
— The treatment principle is to nourish Yin, reduce Fire and tonify the Liver and Kidneys.
— The recommended formula is a variation of **Six-Flavour Rehmanniae Pill**:

Radix Rehmanniae Praeparata	15 g
Radix Rehmanniae	15 g
Fructus Corni	10 g
Fructus Ligustici Lucidi	15 g
Herba Ecliptae	15 g
Cortex Moutan Radicis	10 g
Plastrum Testudinis	15 g
Semen Cuscutae	15 g

— Modifications:

- For pronounced Empty Fire, add Rhizoma Anemarrhenae (10 g) and Cortex Phellodendri (10 g).
- For pronounced bleeding, add Colla Corii Asini (10g, melted and taken separately), Radix Rubiae (10–15 g) and Radix Notoginseng (1.5–3 g, ground to powder and taken separately).

c. Spleen and Kidney Yang Deficiency

— Yang Deficiency can be a consequence of Qi Deficiency or of Yin Deficiency. Spleen and Kidney Yang Deficiency implies insufficiency of Essence and Blood. Clinical manifestations include dizziness and vertigo, lumbar soreness, tinnitus, listlessness, cold limbs, impotence, spermatorrhoea, a pale tongue and a deep, thready pulse.

— The treatment principle is to warm and tonify the Spleen and Kidneys and replenish Essence and Blood.

— The recommended formula is:

Radix Rehmanniae Praeparata	15 g
Fructus Corni	12 g
Semen Cuscutae	15 g
Fructus Psoraleae	10 g
Cornu Cervi Pantotrichum	2 g
or Cornu Cervi	5 g
(*powdered and taken separately*)	
Herba Epimedii	10–15 g
Herba Cistanchis	10 g
Radix Ginseng	5–10 g
Radix Astragali seu Hedysari	10–20 g

CASE STUDY 40.27
THROMBOCYTOPENIC PURPURA

Male, age 3

This patient had had purpura for a month, his lower limbs being completely covered by purpura or pointed haemorrhagic spots. He had a pale tongue tinged with purple. Blood test showed platelets 20 000 – 40 000/mm³. Myelogram revealed decreased hyperplasia of granulocyte series, and absence of hyperplasia of megakaryocytic series.

Pathogenesis: Spleen and Kidney Yang Deficiency and failure of Qi to control Blood.

Western diagnosis: Primary thrombocytopenic purpura

Treatment principle: Warm the Kidneys, nourish Blood, tonify Qi and control Blood.

The formula used consisted of:

Radix Rehmanniae Praeparata	12 g
Cornu Cervi	10 g
(*decocted first*)	
Fructus Lycii	10 g
Fructus Psoraleae	12 g
Rhizoma Drynariae	10 g
Semen Cuscutae	15 g
Radix Astragali seu Hedysari	15 g
Rhizoma Atractylodis	
Macrocephalae	10 g

Radix Angelica Sinensis	10 g
Herba Agrimoniae	15 g
Radix Glycyrrhizae (*treated*)	3 g

After administration of seven doses, the purpura has disappeared except from two lesions the size of a broad bean. There were no new haemorrhagic spots. Because the boy suffered from night sweats, herbs that nourish Yin and stop sweating were added to the prescription, such as Radix Paeoniae Alba and Fructus Mume.

Seven further doses were given, by which time a blood test showed platelets increased to 100 000/mm³.

---

3. DIABETES

GENERAL DESCRIPTION

— Diabetes is marked by thirst with excessive drinking, hunger with excessive eating and profuse production of urine which has a sweet taste. It is categorized as upper, middle and lower types of diabetes.

— This disease is caused by Yin Deficiency with Dryness and Heat. The treatment principle is thus to nourish Yin, promote Body Fluids and clear Fire.

— The late stage of the disease presents with Qi and Yin Deficiency. If Yin Deficiency affects Yang, herbs that tonify Qi and warm the Kidneys are included in the treatment.

DIFFERENTIATION AND TREATMENT

a. Upper diabetes

— Dryness and Heat consume Body Fluids, causing Lung Yin Deficiency. Clinical manifestations include restlessness, thirst with excessive drinking, frequent and profuse urination, a dry tongue with a red tip and border and a thin, yellow coating.

— The treatment principle is to clear Lung Heat, moisten Dryness, promote Body Fluids and relieve thirst.

— The recommended formula is a variation of *Xiao Ke Fang* (**Prescription to Treat Diabetes**) in combination with **White Tiger plus Ginseng Decoction**:

Radix Adenophorae	10–15 g
Radix Ophiopogonis	10–15 g
Herba Dendrobii	15 g
Rhizoma Coptidis	2–5 g
Radix Rehmanniae	15 g

Rhizoma Anemarrhenae	10 g
Cortex Lycii Radicis	10–15 g
Rhizoma Phragmitis	15 g

— Modifications:

- For severe Heat with restlessness and a desire to drink large quantities of fluid, add raw Gypsum Fibrosum (15–30 g) (decocted first).
- For Qi and Yin Deficiency with shortness of breath, spontaneous sweating and lassitude, add Radix Astragali seu Hedysari (10 g), Radix Codonopsis Pilosulae (10 g) and Fructus Schisandrae (2–5 g).

b. Middle diabetes

— Retention of Heat in the Stomach causes constant hunger and consumes Body Fluid. Clinical manifestations include constant hunger with excessive eating, an empty and uncomfortable sensation in the stomach, restlessness, thirst, profuse sweating, constipation with dry stool, emaciation, a dry yellow tongue coating and a rolling, rapid pulse.
— The treatment principle is to clear Stomach Heat, nourish Yin and promote Body Fluids.
— The recommended formula is a variation of **Jade Woman Decoction**:

Radix Rehmanniae	15 g
Radix Ophiopogonis	15 g
Rhizoma Anemarrhenae	12 g
Gypsum Fibrosum *(raw)*	15 g
Rhizoma Coptidis	3 g
Radix Trichosanthis	15 g
Herba Dendrobii	12 g

— Modifications:

- For Stomach Fire with constipation, add raw Radix et Rhizoma Rhei (10 g) at the end of the decoction to reduce Fire in the Large Intestine.

c. Lower diabetes

— Deficiency of Kidney Essence impairs the storing function of the Kidneys. Clinical manifestations include frequent passing of profuse thick, sticky urine, a dry mouth and tongue, thirst with excessive drinking, dizziness, blurred vision, sore and weak lumbar region and knees, a red tongue and a thready, rapid pulse.
— The treatment principle is to nourish the

Kidneys and strengthen their storing function.
— The recommended formula is a variation of **Six-Flavour Rehmannia Pill**:

Radix Rehmanniae or Radix Rehmanniae Praeparata	15–30 g
Fructus Corni	10 g
Rhizoma Dioscoreae	15–30 g
Cortex Moutan Radicis	10 g
Fructus Lycii	15 g
Rhizoma Alismatis	15 g

— Modifications:

- If the urine is profuse and turbid, add Fructus Rubi (10 g), Semen Cuscutae (15 g) and Ootheca Mantidis (10 g).
- For Qi Deficiency, add Radix Ginseng (5–10 g), Radix Astragali seu Hedysari (10 g) and Rhizoma Polygonati (15 g).
- For Spleen Deficiency with Dampness, remove Radix Rehmanniae, Cortex Moutan Radicis and Fructus Corni from the prescription and add Radix Codonopsis Pilosulae (10 g), Rhizoma Atractylodis Macrocephalae (12g), Semen Dolichoris (15 g), Radix Puerariae (15 g) and Endothelium Corneum Gigeriae Galli (10 g).
- If Yin Deficiency affects Yang, producing symptoms of urination equal to the amount drunk, lumbar soreness and cold limbs, add Radix Aconiti Praeparata (2–5 g), Cortex Cinnamomi (2–5 g), Semen Cuscutae (15 g) and Cornu Cervi (3–5 g) (*decocted separately*).

CASE STUDY 40.28
DIABETES

Male, age 21

This patient presented with loss of body weight, thirst with a desire to drink large quantities, excessive hunger, profuse urine, irritability, a sensation of heat in the chest, a bitter taste and sticky sensation in the mouth, lumbar soreness, a scaly skin, a dark purple tongue with a sticky white coating, and a thready pulse. Examinations showed sugar in his urine ++++, ketone bodies positive and blood sugar 603mg/100ml.

Western diagnosis: Diabetes

Treatment principle: Clear Heat, nourish the Stomach, relieve thirst and promote Body Fluids.

The first formula used was a variation of *Xiao Ke Fang* (**Prescription for Diabetes**) and *Er Dong Tang* (**Two-Tuber Decoction**). After administration of five doses, the results were not satisfactory and the case was reviewed. Because the diabetes had developed to a severe stage, both the Yin and Yang of the body were damaged; upper, middle and lower forms of diabetes were all present, the lower form being the most severe.

The treatment principle was therefore modified, primarily to warm the Kidneys and secondarily to nourish Lung and Stomach Yin. The following formula was prescribed:

Radix Rehmanniae Praeparata	12 g
Fructus Corni	10 g
Radix Aconiti Praeparata	3 g
Cortex Cinnamomi	2 g
Herba Cistanchis	10 g
Fructus Schisandrae	5 g
Radix Adenophorae	10 g
Radix Asparagi	10 g
Radix Ophiopogonis	10 g
Rhizoma Anemarrhenae	10 g
Radix Trichosanthis	12 g
Radix Paeoniae Alba	10 g
Herba Dendrobii	10 g

After administration of 50 doses of this formula, all signs and symptoms had disappeared except for a sensation of five-palm Heat. The patient was not excessively thirsty and the volume of urine decreased, while his body weight increased. Ketone bodies were negative and sugar in the urine decreased to ++.

4. URTICARIA

GENERAL DESCRIPTION

— Urticaria is an allergic skin disease marked by weals of varying shape and size and intolerable itching; the weals appear and disappear from time to time.
— The causes of urticaria include deficiency of Lung and Defensive Qi complicated with invasion of External Wind, disharmony between the Spleen and Stomach with improper diet, and Blood Heat complicated with External Wind. The primary treatment method is to eliminate Wind while the secondary treatment methods include clearing Heat, cooling Blood, dispersing Cold, resolving Dampness and, in chronic cases, tonifying Blood and Qi.

DIFFERENTIATION

a. Wind-Heat

— Wind and Heat combine to invade the muscles and skin. Clinical manifestations include red or purple-red skin eruptions with a burning sensation and severe itching, restlessness, a red tongue with thin coating, and a superficial, rapid pulse. The symptoms are aggravated by exposure to heat.
— The treatment principle is to eliminate Wind and clear Heat.
— The recommended formula is:

Herba Schizonepetae	10 g
Radix Ledebouriellae	10 g
Fructus Arctii	10–15 g
Periostracum Cicadae	2–5 g
Herba Menthae *(decocted later)*	2–3 g
Flos Lonicerae	10 g
Fructus Forsythiae	10 g
Radix Rehmanniae	10–15 g
Radix Paeoniae Rubra	10 g

— Modifications:

  – For Heat in the Blood, with red overlapping skin eruptions, add Cortex Moutan Radicis (10 g), Radix Scrophulariae (15 g) and Radix Lithospermi seu Arnebiae (*Zi Cao*) (10–20 g).
  – For retention of Damp-Heat on the body surface with a sticky yellow tongue coating, add Radix Sophorae Flavescentis (10 g) and Fructus Kochiae (12 g).
  – For abdominal pain and constipation, add Radix et Rhizoma Rhei (5–10 g).
  – For fever and restlessness, add Gypsum Fibrosum (15 g) (decocted first) and Rhizoma Anemarrhenae (10 g).

b. Wind-Cold

— Invasion by Wind-Cold causes disharmony between the Nutrient and Defensive Qi. Clinical manifestations include pale red skin eruptions which are induced or aggravated by exposure to Wind and alleviated by warmth, a thin, white tongue coating and a superficial, tense pulse.
— The treatment principle is to eliminate Wind and disperse Cold.
— The recommended formula is a variation of *Ma Huang Gui Zhi Ge Ban Tang* (**Half-Decoction of Ephedra and Cinnamon Twig**) and *Jing Fang Bai Du San* (**Schizonepeta and Ledebouriella Powder to Overcome Pathogenic Influences**):

Herba Ephedrae	2–3 g
Ramulus Cinnamomi	2–5 g
Radix Paeoniae Alba	10 g

Herba Schizonepetae	10 g
Radix Ledebouriellae	10 g
Folium Perillae	2–3 g
Rhizoma Zingiberis Recens	2–3 slices

— Modifications:

- For Dampness, add Rhizoma seu Radix Notopterygii (5 –10 g) and Radix Angelicae Pubescentis (5–10 g).
- If Wind-Damp predominates, add Fructus Xanthii (10–15 g) and raw Semen Coicis (15 g).
- For Qi Deficiency and weakness of Defensive Qi, with susceptibility to the common cold which may induce new attacks of urticaria, add Radix Astragali seu Hedysari (10 g) and Rhizoma Atractylodis Macrocephalae (10 g).

CASE STUDY 40.29
URTICARIA

Female, age 24

This patient had a history of urticaria and chronic diarrhoea for 2 years. The day before she was seen at the hospital, she noted new skin eruptions all over her body, accompanied by aversion to cold, and fever (39.4˚C). The skin eruptions were papular and caused intolerable itching. Other signs and symptoms included thirst, scanty deep-yellow urine, loose stools with four motions daily, a red tongue border with a sticky white coating, and a rapid pulse.

Pathogenesis: Spleen Deficiency with excess Dampness, complicated with invasion by pathogenic Wind-Cold, causing stagnation of Nutritive and Defensive Qi.

Treatment principle: Eliminate Wind, disperse Cold and resolve Dampness.

The formula consisted of:

Herba Schizonepetae	5 g
Radix Ledebouriellae	5 g
Rhizoma seu Radix Notopterygii	5 g
Herba Spirodelae *(Fu Ping)*	5 g
Cortex Magnoliae Officinalis	5 g
Herba Agastachis	10 g
Fructus Arctii	10 g
Radix Paeoniae Rubra	10 g
Red Poria *(Chi Fu Ling)*	10 g
Periostracum Cicadae	3 g

After two doses, her temperature dropped to 37.8˚C, the diarrhoea stopped, the itching improved and there were signs of Dampness turning to Heat. Herba Agastachis, Rhizoma seu Radix Notopterygii and Cortex Magnoliae Officinalis were therefore removed from the

prescription and replaced by Bombyx Batryticatus (10 g), Fructus Kochiae (10 g), Cortex Moutan Radicis (10 g) and Cortex Dictamni Radicis (10 g) to strengthen the action of eliminating Wind and to relieve itching.

After one dose of this new formula, the fever subsided and the skin eruptions disappeared.

---

c. **Blood Deficiency**

— Blood Deficiency produces Wind which stays in the muscles and skin. Clinical manifestations include recurrent episodes of pale red skin eruptions which are more itchy at night, pallor, a slightly red tongue and a thready pulse. Women may experience more frequent attacks during the pre- and postmenstrual periods.

— The treatment principle is to nourish Blood and eliminate Wind.

— The recommended formula is a variation of **Four-Substance Decoction:**

Radix Angelicae Sinensis	10 g
Radix Rehmanniae	10 g
Radix Paeoniae Alba	10 g
Rhizoma Ligustici Chuanxiong	5 g
Radix Polygoni Multiflori	15–30 g
Herba Schizonepetae	10 g
Radix Ledebouriellae	10 g
Bombyx Batryticatus	10 g

— Modifications:

- For red skin eruptions which are aggravated by heat, add Cortex Moutan Radicis (10 g), Radix Paeoniae Rubra (10g) and Radix Scrophulariae (10–15 g).
- For sweating and aversion to Wind, add Radix Astragali seu Hedysari (10 g) and Rhizoma Atractylodis Macrocephalae (10 g).
- If urticaria is induced by food, or abdominal pain and diarrhoea are present in any of the patterns described above, add Fructus Crataegi, Massa Fermentata Medicinalis and Radix Aucklandiae.
- If urticaria is caused by roundworms, add Fructus Quisqualis *(Shi Jun Zi)* (10 g) and Cortex Meliae *(Ku Lian Gen Pi)* (15 g).
- For stubborn chronic urticaria, add insects that eliminate Wind such as Bombyx Batryticatus (10g), Scorpio (2–5 g), Periostracum Cicadae (2–5g) and Zaocys (10–15 g).

Gynaecological disorders **41**

A. Important points in the differentiation of gynaecological disorders

— The key signs and symptoms in diagnosing gynaecological disorders are those relating to menstruation, leucorrhoea, pregnancy and labour. Systemic signs and symptoms are secondary in importance and should be disregarded if they conflict with the key symptoms.

a. Deficiency-type patterns

i. Qi Deficiency
— Clinical manifestations include a shortened menstrual cycle with profuse thin, pinkish flow, uterine bleeding, uterine prolapse, persistent pale lochia following childbirth and spontaneous secretion of milk after delivery.

ii. Blood Deficiency
— Clinical manifestations include a prolonged menstrual cycle with scanty thin, pinkish flow, amenorrhoea, postmenstrual abdominal pain, miscarriage and insufficient lactation.

iii. Spleen Deficiency
— Clinical manifestations include persistent uterine bleeding, a profuse thin, odourless , white vaginal discharge, pernicious vomiting and oedema during pregnancy.

iv. Kidney Deficiency
— The manifestation of Kidney Yin Deficiency include a scanty red or dark menstrual flow, irregular menstruation, uterine bleeding, amenorrhoea, miscarriage and eclampsia or threatened eclampsia.
— The manifestations of Kidney Yang Deficiency include a thin, pinkish menstrual flow, irregular menstruation, uterine bleeding, a profuse thin vaginal discharge and infertility or miscarriage.

b. Excess-type patterns

i. Qi Stagnation
— Clinical manifestations include an irregular menstrual cycle, hesitant and painful menstruation, pelvic inflammation, pernicious vomiting, palpable abdominal masses and retarded secretion of milk.

ii. Blood Stagnation
— Clinical manifestations include a prolonged menstrual cycle, dysmenorrhoea, uterine bleeding, amenorrhoea, pelvic inflammation, palpable abdominal masses, persistent purple lochia with clots and boring abdominal pain which is aggravated by pressure.

iii. Phlegm-Damp
— Clinical manifestations include a profuse vaginal discharge, amenorrhoea, infertility, pernicious vomiting and oedema during pregnancy.

c. Heat patterns

i. Excess-type Heat patterns
— Clinical manifestations include a shortened menstrual cycle with profuse deep-red flow, epistaxis during menstruation, uterine bleeding, vaginal bleeding during pregnancy and thick, deep-yellow leucorrhoea.

ii. Deficiency-type Heat patterns
— Clinical manifestations include a shortened menstrual cycle with bright-red flow, or a prolonged dribbling flow, hypertension during pregnancy and threatened eclampsia.

d. Cold patterns

i. Deficiency-type Cold patterns
— Clinical manifestations include a prolonged menstrual cycle with scanty pinkish flow, dysmenorrhoea, amenorrhoea, a watery vaginal discharge, pernicious vomiting, infertility, palpable abdominal masses and lingering abdominal pain which is alleviated by warmth and pressure.

ii. Excess-type Cold patterns
— Clinical manifestations include a prolonged menstrual cycle with scanty dark-red flow, infertility, palpable abdominal masses, dysmenorrhoea, amenorrhoea and abdominal colic which is alleviated by warmth.

B. Menstrual disorders

1. IRREGULAR MENSTRUATION

GENERAL DESCRIPTION
— Irregular menstruation refers to abnormal changes in the frequency or duration of the menstrual period or in the amount, colour and quality of the flow. It includes shortened cycle, prolonged cycle, irregular cycle, excessive amount of menstrual flow, scanty flow, etc.
— In differentiating menstrual patterns, the cycle and amount of flow determine whether the pattern is Hot or Cold; the colour and quality of the flow determine whether the pattern is one of Excess or Deficiency. A shortened cycle with profuse flow suggests a Heat pattern; a prolonged cycle with scanty flow suggests a Cold pattern; a deep-red thick flow suggests a pattern of the Excess type; and a thin pinkish flow suggests a pattern of the Deficiency type.

a. Shortened menstrual cycle

i. Heat in the Blood
— This pattern may result from retention of Heat, Yin Deficiency with Empty Fire, or Fire originating from Liver Qi Stagnation, all of which act on the Chong and Ren channels, forcing the menses to flow ahead of schedule. Clinical manifestations include a shortened menstrual cycle with a profuse thick, deep-red or purple flow, restlessness, a

red tongue with yellow coating and a rapid, forceful pulse.
— The treatment principle is to clear Heat and cool Blood.
— The recommended formula is a variation of **Four-Substance Decoction:**

Radix Rehmanniae	15–30 g
Cortex Moutan Radicis	10 g
Radix Paeoniae Rubra	10 g
Radix Paeoniae Alba	10 g
Radix Scutellariae	10 g
Fructus Gardeniae	10 g
Herba Schizonepetae (*charred*)	10 g
Radix Rubiae	10 g

— Modifications:

– For Stagnant Liver Qi turning to Fire, with symptoms of a bitter taste in the mouth, stuffiness of the chest and distending breast pain, add Radix Bupleuri (5 g), Fructus Meliae Toosendan (10 g) and Rhizoma Cyperi (10 g).
– For Yin Deficiency, add Fructus Ligustri Lucidi (15 g), Herba Ecliptae (15 g) and Radix Ophiopogonis (10–15 g).

ii. Qi Deficiency
— Spleen Qi Deficiency implies impairment of the Spleen's function of controlling Blood, thus leading to a shortened menstrual cycle. Clinical manifestations include a shortened menstrual cycle with profuse thin, pinkish flow, lassitude, a pale tongue and a weak, thready pulse.
— The treatment principle is to tonify Qi and control Blood.
— The recommended formula is a variation of **Tonifying the Spleen Decoction** and **Tonifying the Middle and Benefiting Qi Decoction**:

Radix Astragali seu Hedysari	15–20 g
Radix Codonopsis Pilosulae	10 g
Rhizoma Atractylodis Macrocephalae	10 g
Radix Glycyrrhizae	3 g
Radix Angelicae Sinensis	10 g
Arillus Longan	10 g
Poria	10 g
Semen Ziziphi Spinosae	10 g
Rhizoma Cimicifugae	3 g
Radix Bupleuri	3 g
Fructus Ziziphi Jujubae	3–5 pieces

— Modifications:

– For excessive bleeding, add charred Cortex Trachycarpi (10 g), stir-baked

Rhizoma Zingiberis (5 g), Colla Corii Asini (10g) (melted and taken separately) and Os Sepiellae seu Sepiae (15 g).

b. Prolonged menstrual cycle

i. Cold in the Blood

— This pattern may be due to exposure to cold during menstruation or retention of Cold in the uterus which coagulates the Blood. Clinical manifestations include a prolonged menstrual cycle with scanty dark-red flow, lower abdominal pain, aversion to cold, cold limbs, pallor, a pale tongue with white coating, and a deep and tense or wiry pulse.

— The treatment principle is to warm the channels and disperse Cold.

— The recommended formula is a variation of **Warm the Menses Decoction**:

Fructus Evodiae	3 g
Ramulus Cinnamomi	2–5 g
Radix Angelicae Sinensis	10 g
Rhizoma Ligustici Chuanxiong	5–10 g
Folium Artemisiae Argyi	10 g
Rhizoma Zingiberis	3–5 g
Colla Corii Asini	10 g
(melted and taken separately)	

— Modifications:

  – For Blood Stagnation with a clotted purple flow, add Semen Persicae (10 g), Flos Carthami (5–10 g) and Faeces Trogopterorum (10 g).

ii. Blood Deficiency

— Blood Deficiency implies weakness of the Chong and Ren channels which does not allow the timely flow of menses. Clinical manifestations include a prolonged menstrual cycle with scanty pinkish flow, sallow complexion, dizziness and vertigo, palpitations, a pale tongue and a thready pulse.

— The treatment principle is to benefit Qi and Blood and regulate menstruation.

— The recommended formula is a variation of **Four-Substance Decoction** and *Ren Shen Yang Rong Tang* (**Ginseng Decoction to Nourish the Nutritive Qi**):

Radix Angelicae Sinensis	10 g
Radix Rehmanniae Praeparata	15–20 g
Radix Paeoniae Alba	10 g
Rhizoma Ligustici Chuanxiong	5–10 g
Radix Codonopsis Pilosulae	10 g
Radix Astragali seu Hedysari	10 g
Cortex Cinnamomi *(treated)*	2–5 g

Folium Artemisiae Argyi	10 g
Rhizoma Cyperi *(treated)*	10 g

iii. Qi Stagnation

— Liver Qi Stagnation leads to stagnation of Blood, which blocks the Chong and Ren channels and causes a prolonged menstrual cycle. Clinical manifestations include a prolonged menstrual cycle with scanty, normal or dark-red flow, distending abdominal pain, stuffiness of the chest, breast distension, hypochondriac pain and a wiry pulse.

— The treatment principle is to activate Qi and resolve Stagnation.

— The recommended formula is a variation of *Si Zhi Xiang Fu Wan* (**Four-Preparation Cyperi Pill**):

Rhizoma Cyperi	10 g
Radix Linderae	5–10 g
Radix Bupleuri	5 g
Rhizoma Ligustici Chuanxiong	5–10 g
Radix Angelicae Sinensis	10 g
Herba Lycopi *(Ze Lan)*	10 g
Radix Aucklandiae	5 g
Caulis Perillae *(Su Geng)*	5–10 g

— Modifications:

  – For Stagnation of Qi and Blood, add Semen Persicae (10 g) and Flos Carthami (5–10 g).

c. Irregular menstrual cycle

i. Liver Qi Stagnation

— In cases of Liver Qi Stagnation, stagnation of Qi leads to disorders of Blood, thus causing irregular menstruation. Clinical manifestations include irregular menstrual cycle with hesitant flow, stuffiness of the chest, distending pain in the breasts, hypochondrium and flanks and a wiry pulse.

— The treatment principle is to soothe the Liver, resolve Stagnation, harmonize the Blood and regulate menstruation.

— The recommended formula is a variation of **Free and Relaxed Powder**:

Radix Bupleuri *(vinegar treated)*	5 g
Rhizoma Cyperi	10 g
Radix Angelicae Sinensis	10 g
Rhizoma Ligustici Chuanxiong	6 g
Pericarpium Citri Reticulatae Viride	5 g
Pericarpium Citri Reticulatae	5 g
Flos Mume Albus	5 g
Radix Paeoniae Rubra	10 g
Radix Paeoniae Alba	10 g

— Modifications:

- For abdominal pain during menstruation with hesitant flow, add Semen Persicae (10 g) and Herba Lycopi (10 g).
- For Stagnant Liver Qi turning to Fire, add Cortex Moutan Radicis (10g) and Fructus Gardeniae (10 g).

CASE STUDY 41.1
IRREGULAR MENSTRUATION

Female, age 32

This patient complained of a shortened menstrual cycle (two periods per month, each lasting 3–7 days). The flow was scanty and purplish-red with clots and she experienced abdominal distension and occasional pain. During the premenstrual period, she often experienced stuffiness of the chest, irritability and distending pain in the breasts. Her tongue was red with a yellow coating and her pulse was wiry, rapid and thready.

Pathogenesis: Stagnant Liver Qi turning to Fire.

Treatment principle: Clear Liver Heat and soothe the Liver.

The formula used was a variation of **Free and Relaxed Powder with Moutan and Gardenia**:

Cortex Moutan Radicis	10 g
Fructus Gardeniae	10 g
Radix Bupleuri (*vinegar-treated*)	5 g
Radix Angelicae Sinensis	10 g
Radix Paeoniae Rubra	10 g
Rhizoma Cyperi (*prepared*)	10 g
Radix Curcumae	10 g
Cortex Albiziae	15 g
Herba Leonuri	10 g
Rhizoma Atractylodis Macrocephalae	10 g
Poria	10 g
Radix Glycyrrhizae	3 g

This prescription was taken during the premenstrual and menstrual periods, and the patient was advised to take the patent medicine **Free and Relaxed Powder with Moutan and Gardenia** during the rest of the month. After 2 months, her menstrual cycle became normal.

ii. Kidney Deficiency

— Kidney Deficiency implies irregularity of the Chong and Ren channels. Clinical manifestations include irregular menstrual cycle with scanty pinkish flow, dizziness, tinnitus, lumbar soreness, dull pain and a bearing-down sensation in the lower abdomen, a pale tongue and a deep, thready pulse.
— For Kidney Yin Deficiency, the recommended formula is a variation of *Zhi Bai Di Huang Wan* (**Six-Flavour Rehmannia Pill with Anemarrhena and Phellodendri**); for Kidney Yang Deficiency, it is a variation of *Ai Fu Nuan Gong Wan* (**Mugwort and Prepared Aconite Pill for Warming the Womb**):
— In either case, the core formula consists of:

Radix Rehmanniae Praeparata	15–30 g
Fructus Corni	10 g
Rhizoma Dioscoreae	15 g
Semen Cuscutae	15 g
Radix Angelicae Sinensis	10 g
Radix Paeoniae Alba	10 g
Rhizoma Ligustici Chuanxiong	6 g

— Modifications:

- For Yin Deficiency with Empty Fire, add Rhizoma Anemarrhenae (10 g), Cortex Phellodendri (5–10 g) and Cortex Moutan Radicis (10 g).
- For Yang Deficiency, add Cortex Cinnamomi (2–3 g), Radix Dipsaci (10 g) and Folium Artemisiae Argyi (10 g).
- For Qi Deficiency, add Radix Astragali seu Hedysari (10–15 g) and Radix Codonopsis Pilosulae (10 g).

---

2. FUNCTIONAL UTERINE BLEEDING

GENERAL DESCRIPTION

— Functional uterine bleeding is treated in three stages. First, the method of astringing and stopping bleeding is used to stop the bleeding. Then the causes are established and treated. Finally, if there has been a substantial loss of blood, Qi and Blood are tonified.

DIFFERENTIATION AND TREATMENT

a. Heat in the Blood

— This pattern may arise from retention of Heat in the Interior, stagnant Qi turning to Fire, or Yin Deficiency producing Internal Heat. The Heat causes the Blood to move recklessly, thus weakening the Chong and Ren channels. Clinical manifestations include haemorrhage of thick, sticky red-purple or dark purple blood with clots,

restlessness, a red tongue and a rapid, forceful pulse.
— The treatment principle is to clear Heat, cool Blood, strengthen the Chong channel and stop bleeding.
— The recommended formula is a variation of **Stabilize the Menses Pill**:

Radix Rehmanniae	15–30 g
Plastrum Testudinis	15 g
(*decocted first*)	
Radix Scutellariae	10 g
Fructus Gardeniae	10 g
Cortex Phellodendri	10 g
Cortex Moutan Radicis	10 g
Cortex Lycii Radicis	10 g
Cortex Trachycarpi (*charred*)	10 g
Radix Rubiae	10–15 g
Radix Sanguisorbae	10–20 g

— Modifications:
  – For persistent bleeding, add Colla Corii Asini (10 g, stir-baked in Pollen Typhae) and powder of Radix Notoginseng (1.5–3 g, taken separately).
  – If the bleeding stops gradually, and there is deficiency of Yin and Blood, remove Radix Sanguisorbae and Cortex Trachycarpi from the prescription and add Colla Corii Asini (10 g, melted and taken separately) and Radix Ophiopogonis (15 g).

b. Blood Stagnation

— Stagnation of Blood prevents the return of the Blood to its channels. Clinical manifestations include prolonged dribbling flow of dark purple blood with clots, lower abdominal pain which is aggravated by pressure but alleviated by discharge of clots, a purple tongue and a deep and wiry, or hesitant pulse.
— The treatment principle is to resolve Blood Stasis and stop bleeding.
— The recommended formula is **Sudden Smile Powder** with additions:

Pollen Typhae	10 g
Faeces Trogopterorum	10 g
Radix Notoginseng (*powdered*)	1.5–3 g
(*taken separately*)	
Radix Rubiae	15 g
Radix Angelicae Sinensis	10 g
Radix Salviae Miltiorrhizae	15 g
Rhizoma Ligustici Chuanxiong	10 g
Cortex Moutan Radicis	10 g
Radix Paeoniae Rubra	10 g
Herba Leonuri	10–20 g

— Modifications:
  – For Heat in the Blood, add Radix Rehmanniae (15–30 g), Fructus Gardeniae (10 g) and Radix Scutellariae (10 g).

CASE STUDY 41.2
FUNCTIONAL UTERINE BLEEDING

Female, age 22

This patient complained of excessive uterine bleeding for the past 3 years, worsening during the most recent months. Severe bleeding with abdominal pain and large clots lasted for 7 days, the total duration of each menstrual period being more than 10 days. During the premenstrual period she experienced stuffiness of the chest and irritability. Before the severe bleeding began she had had amenorrhoea for 3 months. Her tongue was red with a thin yellow coating and her pulse was wiry and thready.

Pathogenesis: Uterine bleeding due to stagnation of Blood.

Western diagnosis: Functional uterine bleeding

Treatment principle: Primarily to resolve Blood Stasis and stop bleeding; secondarily to provide tonification.

The formula used consisted of:

Radix Angelicae Sinensis	10 g
Radix Paeoniae Rubra	10 g
Cortex Moutan Radicis	10 g
Radix Salviae Miltiorrhizae	15 g
Sudden Smile Powder	12 g
(*decocted wrapped*)	
Herba Leonuri	15 g
Rhizoma Cyperi (*prepared*)	10 g
Rhizoma Corydalis	10 g
Radix Dipsaci	12 g
Ramulus Loranthi	12 g
Cortex Cinnamomi	1.5 g
(*added at end of decoction*)	
Fructus Crataegi	15 g

After three doses, uterine bleeding substantially decreased and abdominal pain disappeared.

This prescription was taken during the premenstrual and menstrual periods; herbs that regulate the menstrual cycle were prescribed for the rest of the month. After 6 months of treatment, the patient fully recovered.

---

c. Qi Deficiency

— Spleen Qi Deficiency implies inability of the Spleen to control the Blood and weakness of

the Chong and Ren channels. Clinical manifestations include uterine haemorrhage or prolonged dribbling flow of thin pinkish blood, pallor or facial puffiness, a pale tongue and a soft, thready pulse.
— The treatment principle is to tonify Qi and control Blood.
— The recommended formula is a variation of **Tonifying the Spleen Decoction**:

Radix Astragali seu Hedysari	15–30 g
Radix Codonopsis Pilosulae	10 g
Rhizoma Atractylodis Macrocephalae	10 g
Rhizoma Zingiberis (*stir-baked*)	2–5 g
Radix Rehmanniae	15 g
Radix Polygoni Multiflori (*treated*)	15 g
Os Sepiellae seu Sepiae	15 g

— Modifications:

– For severe haemorrhage resulting in Collapse of Qi, decoct 15–30 g of Radix Ginseng and administer with 1 g of Yunnan Baiyao powder or 3 g of powdered Radix Notoginseng. Blood transfusion should also be given as first aid.

CASE STUDY 41.3
FUNCTIONAL UTERINE BLEEDING

Female, age 44

This patient's most recent period had continued for 20 days. Initially, the flow was purplish-red with clots, then it turned to a pinkish dribble without clots. She was now presenting with a pinkish watery flow, lassitude, dull pain on the left side of her abdomen, a pale tongue with no coating, and a weak, thready pulse.

Pathogenesis: Deficiency of Qi not allowing the Spleen to control Blood.

Treatment principle: Tonify Qi and control Blood.

The formula used was a variation of **Tonifying the Spleen Decoction**:

Radix Astragalus seu Hedysari (*treated*)	15 g
Radix Codonopsis Pilosulae	10 g
Rhizoma Atractylodis Macrocephalae	10 g
Radix Angelicae Sinensis	10 g
Colla Corii Asini (*melted*)	10 g
Rhizoma Zingiberis (*charred*)	3 g
Os Sepiellae seu Sepiae	12 g
Cortex Phellodendri	6 g
Cortex Ailanthi	12 g

After three doses, the flow stopped. The patient returned to work a few days later and gynaecological examination 20 days later was negative.

---

3. DYSMENORRHOEA

GENERAL DESCRIPTION

— Premenstrual abdominal pain often results from stagnation of Qi, pain during menstruation results from stagnation of Blood and postmenstrual pain results from deficiency of Blood.
— If distension is more pronounced than pain, Qi Stagnation is suggested. If pain is more pronounced than distension, Blood Stagnation is suggested. If pain is accompanied by a sensation of cold, Cold is suggested. Burning pain suggests Heat. Violent, colicky or stabbing pain which is aggravated by pressure suggests an Excess-type pattern. Lingering, dull pain that is alleviated by pressure suggests a Deficiency-type pattern.
— The treatment principles are to regulate Qi during the premenstrual period, to activate Blood and resolve Stasis during the menstrual period and to tonify Deficiency during the postmenstrual period.

DIFFERENTIATION AND TREATMENT

a. Stagnation of Qi and Blood

— Stagnation of Liver Qi due to emotional stress leads to stagnation of Qi and Blood, allowing Blood to be retained in the uterus. Clinical manifestations include distending lower abdominal pain in the premenstrual and menstrual periods and a scanty and hesitant flow of dark purple blood.
— If Qi Stagnation predominates, there may be distending pain in the breasts and the costal and hypochondriac regions, with distension more pronounced than pain. If Blood Stagnation predominates, pain will be more pronounced than distension; it will be aggravated by pressure and alleviated by the discharge of clots. There may also be a dark-purple tongue and a wiry pulse. If Cold predominates, pain is accompanied by a sensation of cold and is alleviated by warmth.
— The treatment principle is to activate Qi and Blood, resolve Stasis and relieve pain.
— The recommended formula is a variation of

Blood Mansion Eliminating Stasis Decoction:

Radix Angelicae Sinensis	10 g
Rhizoma Ligustici Chuanxiong	10 g
Radix Salviae Miltiorrhizae	15 g
Semen Persicae	10 g
Flos Carthami	10 g
Radix Bupleuri	5 g
Rhizoma Cyperi	10 g
Pericarpium Citri Reticulatae Viride	5 g
Pericarpium Citri Reticulatae	5 g
Rhizoma Corydalis	10g

— Modifications:

- For Qi Stagnation, add Radix Linderae (5–10 g) and Caulis Perillae (5–10 g).
- For Blood Stagnation, add Rhizoma Sparganii (5–10 g), Rhizoma Zedoariae (5–10 g) and 12 g of **Sudden Smile Powder**.
- For stagnation of Cold, add Cortex Cinnamomi (2–5 g), Fructus Evodiae (2 g) and Folium Artemisiae (10 g).

CASE STUDY 41.4
DYSMENORRHOEA

Female, age 29

This patient complained of dysmenorrhoea for over 10 years, becoming worse in recent years. She did not conceive for 4 years after her marriage. Gynaecological examination showed retroversion of the uterus with poor motion, thickened and tender appendix and a moderate degree of erosion and congestion of the cervix. She had violent lower abdominal pain on the first 2 days of her period and a profuse flow of purplish blood with clots. During the premenstrual period she experienced stuffiness of the chest, irritability and distending breast pain. When the period was over she experienced dizziness, lumbar soreness, tinnitus and palpitations. She had a sticky yellow tongue coating and a wiry, thready pulse.

Pathogenesis: Stagnation of Qi and Blood, and Liver and Kidney Deficiency.

Treatment principle: Regulate Qi and resolve Blood Stasis during the premenstrual and menstrual periods and regulate the Liver and Kidneys when the period is over.

During the premenstrual and menstrual periods, a variation of *Ge Xia Zhu Yu Tang* (**Drive Out Blood Stasis Below the Diaphragm Decoction**) was prescribed:

Rhizoma Cyperi (*prepared*)	12 g
Radix Angelicae Sinensis	10 g

Radix Paeoniae Rubra	10 g
Fructus Aurantii	5 g
Radix Aucklandiae	3 g
Semen Persicae	10 g
Flos Carthami	6 g
Faeces Trogopterorum	12 g
Resina Olibani	2 g
Resina Myrrhae	2 g

For the rest of the month, a combination of *Gui Shao Di Huang Tang* (**Angelica, Peony and Rehmannia Decoction**) and **Free and Relaxed Powder** was prescribed.

After 3 months of treatment, the dysmenorrhoea disappeared. After another 2 months, the patient became pregnant.

---

b. Deficiency of Qi and Blood

— Deficiency of Qi and Blood deprives the vessels of the uterus of nourishment. Qi Deficiency also leads to Blood Stagnation. Clinical manifestations include a lingering, dull pain during or after the menstrual period which is alleviated by pressure; a scanty thin, pinkish menstrual flow, pallor, lassitude, a pale tongue and a weak, thready pulse.

— The treatment principle is to tonify Qi and Blood and harmonize the collaterals.

— The recommended formula is a variation of *Dang Gui Shao Yao San* (**Angelica and Peony Powder**):

Radix Angelicae Sinensis	10 g
Radix Rehmanniae Praeparata	15 g
Radix Paeoniae Alba	10 g
Rhizoma Ligustici Chuanxiong	5–10 g
Radix Codonopsis Pilosulae	10 g
Radix Astragali seu Hedysari	15 g
Ramulus Cinnamomi	5 g
Radix Glycyrrhizae	3 g

— Modifications:

- For Cold, add Folium Artemisiae (10 g) and Fructus Evodiae (2–3 g).
- For Qi Stagnation, add Rhizoma Cyperi (10g), Radix Linderae (5–10g) and Radix Aucklandiae (3–5g).

CASE STUDY 41.5
DYSMENORRHOEA

Female, age 40

Since her marriage, this patient had given birth to four children and had had two abortions. During the past year, she had had a dull lower abdominal pain before and during her menstrual periods. The pain is alleviated by warmth and pressure. Her menstrual flow was profuse and pinkish in colour. Other symptoms and signs included pallor, dizziness, blurred vision, sore and weak lumbar region and knees, lassitude and loose stool. Her tongue was pale and flabby with a thin, white coating and her pulse was weak and thready. Gynaecological examination revealed no abnormality.

Pathogenesis: Qi and Blood Deficiency and Spleen and Kidney Deficiency.

Treatment principle: Tonify Qi and Blood, warm and invigorate the Spleen and Kidneys.

The formula used consisted of:

Radix Astragali seu Hedysari (*treated*)	15 g
Radix Codonopsis Pilosulae	10 g
Rhizoma Atractylodis Macrocephalae	10 g
Poria	10 g
Radix Angelicae Sinensis	10 g
Radix Paeoniae Alba	10 g
Radix Rehmanniae Praeparata	12 g
Rhizoma Ligustici Chuanxiong	6 g
Fructus Amomi	3 g
(*added at end of decoction*)	
Rhizoma Cyperi (*prepared*)	10 g
Rhizoma Zingiberis (*baked*)	5 g
Fructus Psoraleae	10 g
Rhizoma Corydalis	10 g

After 2 months of treatment, the volume of menstrual flow decreased and dysmenorrhoea disappeared.

4. AMENORRHOEA

GENERAL DESCRIPTION

— Primary amenorrhoea is diagnosed when menarche has not occurred by the age of 18. Secondary amenorrhoea is the cessation of menstruation for 3 months in succession.
— The condition is differentiated into Excess and Deficiency types. The Deficiency type is the result of Liver and Kidney Deficiency while the Excess type is caused by Qi and Blood Stagnation and retention of Phlegm-Damp in the Interior.

DIFFERENTIATION AND TREATMENT

a. Liver and Kidney Deficiency

— Liver and Kidney Deficiency can result from developmental insufficiency or from excessive childbearing or sexual activity. Clinical manifestations include primary or secondary amenorrhoea, hypoplasia of the uterus, sallow complexion, sore and weak lumbar region and knees, dizziness, tinnitus, pain in the heels, lassitude, a dark-pale tongue and a thready and weak or deep and hesitant pulse.
— The treatment principle is to tonify the Liver and Kidneys, nourish Blood and regulate menstruation.
— In cases of Kidney Yin Deficiency, the recommended formula is a variation of **Six-Flavour Rehmannia Pill**; in cases of Kidney Yang Deficiency, it is a variation of **Restoring the Right Pill**. In either case, the core formula consists of:

Radix Rehmanniae Praeparata	15–30 g
Fructus Corni	10–15 g
Fructus Lycii	15 g
Semen Cuscutae	15 g
Radix Paeoniae Alba	10 g
Rhizoma Dioscoreae	15 g
Radix Angelicae Sinensis	10 g
Radix Bidentatae	10–15 g

— Modifications:

  – For Yin Deficiency with Empty Fire, add Rhizoma Anemarrhenae (10 g), Cortex Moutan Radicis (10 g) and Cortex Lycii Radicis (10 g).
  – For Yang Deficiency, add Herba Epimedii (10g), Radix Aconiti Praeparata (2–5 g) and Cortex Cinnamomi (2–5 g).

CASE STUDY 41.6
AMENORRHOEA

Female, age 24

This patient's periods had begun at the age of 15, with a period once every 2 or 3 months. 6 years later, her periods stopped, but returned after treatment with Chinese herbal medicine. She had now had no period for 10 months, but did not present with any other significant symptoms. Her tongue was red with a thin coating and her pulse was thready and wiry. She was unmarried.

Pathogenesis: Deficiency of the Kidneys and of Liver Blood.

Treatment principle: Primarily to tonify the Kidneys and nourish Blood; secondarily to induce menstruation.

The formula used consisted of:

Radix Rehmanniae Praeparata	15 g
Radix Dipsaci	10 g
Herba Epimedii	10 g
Semen Cuscutae	15 g

Radix Angelicae Sinensis	10 g
Radix Paeoniae Alba	10 g
Rhizoma Ligustici Chuanxiong	6 g
Semen Biotae	10 g
Herba Lycopi	12 g
Fructus Leonuri	12 g
Radix Achyranthis Bidentatae	10 g

After 15 doses of this prescription, the patient's menstrual period returned with a normal colour and quality of flow. The period lasted for 6 days, after which she took **Six-Flavour Rehmannia Pill** plus *Wu Zi Bu Shen Wan* (**Five-Seed Pill to Tonify the Kidneys**) and *Tiao Jing Pian* (**Regulate the Menses Pill**). 40 days later, her second period arrived, with a normal colour and quality of flow. She continued treatment to consolidate the therapeutic results.

b. Qi and Blood Deficiency

— Qi and Blood Deficiency implies emptiness of the Sea of Blood, which deprives the Chong and Ren channels of nourishment. Clinical manifestations include amenorrhoea following a history of scanty and pinkish menstrual flow, pallor, lassitude, dizziness and vertigo, palpitation, a pale tongue and a thready, weak pulse.
— The treatment principle is to benefit Qi, nourish Blood and promote menstruation.
— The recommended formula is a variation of *Ba Zhen Tang* (**Eight-Precious Decoction**):

Radix Angelicae Sinensis	10 g
Radix Rehmanniae Praeparata	15 g
Radix Paeoniae Alba	10 g
Rhizoma Ligustici Chuanxiong	5–10 g
Radix Codonopsis Pilosulae	10 g
Radix Astragali seu Hedysari	10–15 g
Rhizoma Atractylodis Macrocephalae	10 g
Radix Glycyrrhizae (*treated*)	3 g
Radix Salviae Miltiorrhizae	15 g
Herba Leonuri	15 g

— Modifications:
  – For Spleen Deficiency with reduced appetite and loose stools, remove Radix Rehmanniae Praeparata from the prescription and add Radix Aucklandiae (3–5 g), Pericarpium Citri Reticulatae (5 g), Massa Fermentata Medicinalis (10 g) and Fructus Crataegi (15 g).

c. Qi and Blood Stagnation

— Stagnation of Qi and Blood results from Liver Qi Stagnation or retention of Cold. Blockage of the Chong and Ren channels by stagnation Qi and Blood leads to amenorrhoea. Clinical manifestations include secondary amenorrhoea, lower abdominal distending pain, depression, a purple tongue or purple spots on the tongue and a deep and wiry or hesitant pulse.
— The treatment principle is to activate the circulation of Qi and Blood, resolve Blood Stasis and promote menstruation.
— The recommended formula is a variation of **Blood Mansion Eliminating Stasis Decoction**:

Radix Angelicae Sinensis	10 g
Rhizoma Ligustici Chuanxiong	10 g
Radix Paeoniae Alba	10 g
Radix Salviae Miltiorrhizae	10 g
Radix Bupleuri	5 g
Fructus Aurantii	5–10 g
Rhizoma Cyperi	10 g
Radix Achyranthis Bidentatae	10–15 g
Semen Persicae	10 g
Flos Carthami	5–15 g

— Modifications:
  – For Cold patterns marked by lower abdominal pain and distension accompanied by a feeling of cold and cold limbs, add Cortex Cinnamomi (2–3 g), Fructus Evodiae (2–3 g) and Radix Linderae (5–10).
  – If Stagnant Qi turns to Fire which combines with Blood Stasis, giving rise to restlessness, irritability, thirst and a bitter taste in the mouth, add Cortex Moutan Radicis (10 g), Fructus Gardeniae (10 g) and Radix Rubiae (10–15 g).

d. Retention of Phlegm-Damp in the Interior

— Phlegm-Damp in the Interior blocks the collaterals, including those of the uterus. Clinical manifestations include amenorrhoea, obesity, profuse vaginal discharge, lassitude, a sticky white tongue coating and a rolling pulse.
— The treatment principle is to activate Qi, resolve Phlegm, dry Dampness and invigorate the Spleen.
— The recommended formula is *Cang Fu Dao Tan Wan* (**Atractylodis and Cyperi Pill to Eliminate Phlegm**):

Rhizoma Pinelliae	10 g
Pericarpium Citri Reticulatae	5–10 g
Poria	10 g
Rhizoma Atractylodis	10 g
Rhizoma Cyperi	10 g

Rhizoma Arisaematis	10 g
Fructus Aurantii	5–10 g
Cortex Magnoliae Officinalis	2–3 g
Radix Achyranthis Bidentatae	10–15 g

— Modifications:

- For Blood Stagnation, add Rhizoma Ligustici Chuanxiong (10 g) and Herba Leonuri (15 g).

C. Leucorrhoea

1. SIMPLE LEUCORRHOEA

GENERAL DESCRIPTION

— Disorders of vaginal discharge are marked by a persistent discharge of abnormal fluid from the vagina, accompanied by lumbar soreness, dizziness and lassitude. The colour of the discharge may be white, yellow or red-white.
— Leucorrhoea is a symptom of various gynaecological disorders, including vaginitis, cervicitis, pelvic inflammation and cervical cancer. The causes of these disorders include downward movement of Damp-Heat, stagnant Liver Qi turning to Fire that moves down with Dampness, Spleen Deficiency with downward movement of Turbid Damp and constitutional Kidney Deficiency which impairs the function of the Dai channel and allows the downward movement of Turbid Damp.
— Patterns of Excess are marked by downward movement of Damp-Heat, while Deficiency conditions are caused by impaired function of the Dai channel due to Spleen and Kidney Deficiency.

DIFFERENTIATION AND TREATMENT

a. **Spleen Deficiency with downward movement of Turbid Damp**

— Spleen Deficiency produces Dampness, which then moves downward. Clinical manifestations include a thin, odourless, white or slightly yellow vaginal discharge, pallor, lassitude, reduced appetite, loose stools, a pale tongue with a sticky white coating, and a soft or thready and soft pulse.
— The treatment principle is to benefit Qi, invigorate the Spleen, lift Yang and resolve Dampness.

— The recommended formula is a variation of **End Discharge Decoction**:

Rhizoma Atractylodis Macrocephalae	10–12 g
Rhizoma Atractylodis	5–10 g
Radix Codonopsis Pilosulae	10 g
Rhizoma Dioscoreae	15 g
Radix Astragali seu Hedysari	10 g
Poria	12 g
Semen Coicis	15 g
Semen Dolichoris	15 g
Radix Bupleuri	2–5 g
Rhizoma Cimicifugae	2–5 g

— Modifications:

- If Cold-Damp is severe, giving rise to profuse, watery leucorrhoea and lower abdominal pain accompanied by a sensation of cold, add Cortex Cinnamomi (2-5 g), Radix Angelicae Dahuricae (10 g) and Os Sepiellae seu Sepiae (15 g).
- For Damp-Heat, giving rise to a yellow, foul-smelling vaginal discharge, remove Radix Codonopsis Pilosulae and Radix Astragali seu Hedysari from the prescription and add Cortex Phellodendri (10 g), Cortex Ailanthi (10-15 g) and Rhizoma Dioscoreae Septemlobae (10g).

b. **Damp-Heat in the Liver channel**

— This pattern is due to Heat in the Liver channel, which combines with Dampness and moves downward. Clinical manifestations include a yellow-green, sticky and smelly vaginal discharge, pruritus vulvae, scanty and deep-red urine, a red tongue with a sticky yellow coating, and a wiry, rolling pulse.
— The treatment principle is to clear Liver Heat and expel Dampness.
— The recommended formula is a variation of **Gentiana Draining the Liver Decoction**:

Radix Gentianae	2–5 g
Cortex Phellodendri	10 g
Fructus Gardeniae	10 g
Cortex Moutan Radicis	10 g
Radix Bupleuri	5 g
Caulis Akebiae	2 g
Semen Plantaginis (*decocted wrapped*)	10 g
Semen Coicis	15 g
Rhizoma Alismatis	10 g

— Modifications:

- For red vaginal discharge, add Herba

Cephalanoploris (10 g), Cortex Ailanthi (15 g) and Radix Paeoniae Rubra (10 g).

- For pruritus vulvae, steam and wash the diseased area with a decoction made up of Fructus Cnidii (15-30 g), Cortex Phellodendri (10–15 g), Radix Sophorae Flavescentis (15 g) and Alum (10 g).
- For trichomonal vaginitis, grind Fructus Cnidii and dried alum into a powder (3:1) and mix with melted gelatine to make an ointment for external application. Apply once per day in the evening for 5 consecutive days.
- Or steam and wash the diseased area with a decoction of Radix Stemonae (15 g), Radix Sophorae Flavescentis (15 g), dried alum (10 g) and Folium Persicae (15 g) once daily for 5–7 consecutive days.

CASE STUDY 41.7
LEUCORRHOEA

Female, age 40

This patient complained of a profuse, thick, yellow vaginal discharge with pruritus. Her menstrual cycle was normal, with a profuse, red flow. She also had lumbar soreness, poor appetite, yellow urine and a red tongue with a thick, sticky yellow coating. A smear of vaginal secretion showed fungus +.

Pathogenesis: Leucorrhoea due to downward movement of Damp-Heat.

Western diagnosis: Colpomycosis

Treatment principle: Clear Heat, eliminate Damp, kill fungus and relieve pruritus.

The formula used consisted of:

Radix Gentianae	9 g
Radix Rehmanniae	12 g
Rhizoma Smilacis Glabrae	15 g
Semen Arecae	9 g
Polyporus Umbellatus	9 g
Poria	9 g
Rhizoma Alismatis	9 g

After three doses the leucorrhoea decreased and the pruritus disappeared. After a further three doses, the vaginal discharge and urine were normal and a smear of vaginal secretion showed negative.

---

c. **Kidney Deficiency**

— Kidney Deficiency implies impairment of

the function of the Dai channel in controlling leucorrhoea, resulting in the downward movement of Turbid Damp. Clinical manifestations include a profuse, odourless vaginal discharge that looks like egg white, sore and weak lumbar region and knees, a dark complexion and a deep thready pulse.

— The treatment principle is to benefit the Kidneys and astringe the discharge.

— The recommended formula is:

Semen Cuscutae	15 g
Fructus Rubi	10–15 g
Radix Dipsaci	10 g
Semen Euryales	10 g
Fructus Rosae Laevigatae	10 g
Fructus Corni	10 g
Os Sepiellae seu Sepiae	15 g

— Modifications:

- For Yin Deficiency, remove Radix Dipsaci from the prescription and add Radix Rehmanniae (15 g), Cortex Moutan Radicis (10 g), Rhizoma Anemarrhenae (10 g) and Cortex Phellodendri (5–10 g).
- For Yang Deficiency, add Fructus Alpiniae Oxyphyllae (10 g) and Cortex Eucommiae (10 g).
- For cancer with a red-white vaginal discharge, add Radix Sophorae Subprostatae (15 g), Radix Sophorae Flavescentis (15 g), Herba Solani Nigri (*Long Kui*) and Rhizoma Paris Polyphyllae (*Zao Xiu*)

  or

- prepare a paste of Arsenolitum (Pi Shi), alum, realgar and Resina Olibani for external application.

---

2. CHRONIC PELVIC INFLAMMATION

GENERAL DESCRIPTION

— Chronic pelvic inflammation may or may not arise out of acute pelvic inflammation. It involves the fallopian tubes, ovaries and connective tissues of the pelvic cavity. In TCM, it falls into the categories of palpable abdominal masses, leucorrhoea, dysmenorrhoea, irregular menstruation and infertility. It may be caused by retention of Damp-Heat and stagnant Blood, or by stagnation of Cold and Qi.

DIFFERENTIATION AND TREATMENT

a. **Retention of Damp-Heat and stagnant Blood in the uterus**

— This pattern results from contact with pathogens during menstruation or after childbirth when the collaterals of the uterus are empty, or through sexual activity. Clinical manifestations include low-grade fever, soreness in the lumbo-sacral region and lower abdominal pain or a bearing-down sensation, all of which are aggravated during menstruation or on exertion. Other signs and symptoms include a foul yellow vaginal discharge, irregular menstruation, shortened menstrual cycle, infertility, a dark-purple tongue with a sticky yellow coating, and a soft, hesitant or wiry pulse.
— The treatment principle is to clear Heat, expel Dampness, activate the Blood and resolve Stasis.
— The recommended formula is a variation of *Hong Teng Jian* (**Sargentodoxa Decoction**) plus **Four-Marvel Pill**:

Caulis Sargentodoxae	15–30 g
Herba Patriniae	15–30 g
Cortex Moutan Radicis	10g
Flos Lonicerae	15g
Rhizoma Atractylodis	10g
Cortex Phellodendri	10g
Semen Coicis	10g
Semen Persicae	10g
Rhizoma Corydalis	10g
Rhizoma Zedoariae	5–10g
Rhizoma Cyperi	10g
Resina Olibani	2–5g
Resina Myrrhae	2–5g
Faeces Trogopterorum	10g

— Modifications:

– For low-grade fever, add Carapax Trionycis (15 g) (decocted first) and Cortex Lycii Radicis (10 g).
– For palpable masses, add Squama Manitis (15 g) (decocted first) and Rhizoma Sparganii (10 g).
– For constipation and distending abdominal pain, add raw Radix et Rhizoma Rhei (5 –10 g) and Cortex Magnoliae Officinalis (2–5 g).

CASE STUDY 41.8
OVARIAN CYST

Female, age 28

This patient complained of distending pain in the right lower abdomen and low-grade fever (37.5 – 38°C) for 2 months. Gynaecological examination showed a cyst 5×6 cm on the right ovary. Her tongue was slightly purple, with a slightly yellow sticky coating, and her pulse was wiry and rolling.

Pathogenesis: Stagnation of Qi and Blood, complicated by retention of Heat.

Western diagnosis: Ovarian cyst

Treatment principle: Circulate Qi, resolve Blood Stasis and disperse palpable masses.

The formula used consisted of:

Radix Angelicae Sinensis	10 g
Radix Paeoniae Rubra	10 g
Semen Persicae	10 g
Flos Carthami	6 g
Rhizoma Sparganii	6 g
Rhizoma Zedoariae	6 g
Rhizoma Cyperi (*prepared*)	10 g

After six doses, the cyst apparently decreased in size and the patient had a painful sensation in the right lower abdomen. Herba Salviae Sinensis (*Shi Jian Chuan*) (12 g) was then added to the prescription to clear Heat, eliminate Dampness and resolve Stasis.

After a further five doses, the cyst disappeared, but the patient still had fever (37.6°C) and distension and dull pain in the lower right abdomen, suggesting retention of residual Heat. Flos Lonicerae (10 g), Caulis Sargentodoxae (15 g) and baked Squama Manitis (12 g, decocted first) were then added to the prescription to clear Heat and Toxins, activate Blood circulation and remove obstruction from the channels.

After five doses of this new formula, the patient had fully recovered.

---

b. **Stagnation of Cold and Qi**

— Exposure to Cold during menstruation or after childbirth leads to stagnation of Cold, Qi and Blood in the uterus. Clinical manifestations include soreness of the lumbo-sacral region, lower abdominal pain, a bearing-down sensation, aversion to cold, irregular menstruation, prolonged menstrual cycle, dysmenorrhoea, purple menstrual discharge with clots, a profuse thin, white vaginal discharge, a pale tongue or purple spots on the tongue and a sticky white coating.
— The treatment principle is to warm the channels, disperse Cold and activate Qi and Blood.
— The recommended formula is a variation of

Shao Fu Zhu Yu Tang (**Drive Out Blood Stasis in the Lower Abdomen Decoction**):

Cortex Cinnamomi	2–5 g
Fructus Evodiae	1.5–3 g
Radix Angelicae Sinensis	10 g
Rhizoma Ligustici Chuanxiong	10 g
Fructus Foeniculi	2–3 g
(*added at end of decoction*)	
Radix Linderae	5–10 g
Lignum Aquilariae Resinatum	2–3 g
(*added at end of decoction*)	
Resina Myrrhae	2–5 g
Faeces Trogopterorum	10 g
Rhizoma Corydalis	10 g

— Modifications:

- For Liver Qi Stagnation with distending hypochondriac and breast pain, add Radix Bupleuri (5 g), Pericarpium Citri Reticulatae Viride (5 g) and Semen Citri Reticulatae (10 g).
- For Qi Deficiency following a prolonged illness, add Radix Astragali seu Hedysari (10 –15 g) and Radix Codonopsis Pilosulae (10 g).
- For low-grade fever and a profuse yellow discharge, add Cortex Phellodendri (10 g), Caulis Sargentodoxae (15 g) and Cortex Ailanthi (10–15g).
- For Kidney Yang Deficiency with lower abdominal pain and a sensation of cold, add Radix Aconiti Praeparata (2–5g) and Semen Litchi (*Li Zhi He*) (10–15g).

D. Disorders of pregnancy and delivery

1. THREATENED AND HABITUAL MISCARRIAGE

GENERAL DESCRIPTION

— TCM terms for threatened miscarriage include abdominal pain during pregnancy, restlessness of the fetus and uterine bleeding during pregnancy. The TCM term for habitual miscarriage is 'slippery fetus'. Both types of miscarriage can be caused by deficiency of Qi and Blood, or of the Kidneys, which deprives the fetus of nourishment. Another cause is Yin Deficiency giving rise to Heat in the Blood which disturbs the Chong and Ren channels.
— The treatment principles are variously to

benefit the Kidneys, tonify Qi and Blood, clear Heat, cool Blood and protect the fetus.

DIFFERENTIATION AND TREATMENT

a. Qi and Blood Deficiency

— Qi Deficiency implies an inability to carry the fetus and Blood Deficiency implies an inability to nourish the fetus. Both conditions result in uterine bleeding during pregnancy. Clinical manifestations include slight bleeding from the vagina in the early stage of pregnancy, a bearing-down sensation in the lower abdomen, listlessness, pallor, a pale tongue and a deficient, rolling pulse.
— The treatment principle is to tonify Qi, nourish Blood and protect the fetus.
— The recommended formula is a variation of *Ju Yuan Jian* (**Lift the Source Decoction**):

Radix Codonopsis Pilosulae	10 g
Radix Astragali seu Hedysari	10–15 g
Rhizoma Atractylodis Macrocephalae	12 g
Colla Corii Asini	10 g
(*melted and taken separately*)	
Ramulus Loranthi	15 g
Radix Boehmeriae	15 g
Rhizoma Cimicifugae	3 g

— Modifications:

- For Spleen Deficiency with reduced appetite and loose stool, remove Colla Corii Asini from the prescription and add Fructus Amomi (2–3 g) (added at end of decoction), Radix Aucklandiae (3 g) and stir-baked Rhizoma Zingiberis (2–5 g).
- For pronounced Blood Deficiency, add Radix Rehmanniae Praeparata (15 g) and Radix Angelicae Sinensis (10 g).

b. Kidney Qi Deficiency

— Kidney Deficiency implies weakness of the Chong and Ren channels. This deprives the fetus of nourishment and results in threatened or habitual miscarriage. Clinical manifestations include bleeding from the vagina in the early stage of pregnancy, a bearing-down sensation in the lower abdomen, lumbar soreness, weakness of the knees, dizziness, tinnitus, frequent urination, a pale tongue and a deep and weak pulse.
— The treatment principle is to tonify the Kidneys and protect the fetus.

— The recommended formula is a variation of *Shou Tai Wan* (**Fetus Longevity Pill**):

Radix Dipsaci	15 g
Cortex Eucommiae	10–12 g
Ramulus Loranthi	15 g
Semen Cuscutae	15 g
Rhizoma Atractylodis Macrocephalae	12 g
Folium Artemisiae Argyi	10 g
Colla Corii Asini	10 g
(*melted and taken separately*)	

— Modifications:

– For Qi Deficiency, add Radix Codonopsis Pilosulae (10 g) and Radix Astragali seu Hedysari (10–15 g).
– For excessive bleeding, add Radix Boehmeriae (15 g).

CASE STUDY 41.9
THREATENED MISCARRIAGE

Female, age 30

In the 5 years since her marriage, this patient had had three miscarriages, each occurring at approximately 40 days of pregnancy. She had a delayed menstrual cycle with dysmenorrhoea and a moderate amount of flow. Premenstrually, she had stuffiness of the chest, irritability and distending breast pain. She also had lumbar soreness and a cold sensation in the lower abdomen. She was 1 month pregnant and had been resting in bed. Her tongue was red and her pulse was deep and thready.

Pathogenesis: Kidney Deficiency complicated with retention of Fire in the Liver channel.

Treatment principle: Tonify the Kidneys, reduce Liver Fire and prevent miscarriage.

The formula used consisted of:

Radix Rehmanniae	8 g
Radix Rehmanniae Praeparata	8 g
Radix Dipsaci	12 g
Colla Corii Asini (*melted*)	10 g
Ramulus Loranthi	15 g
Semen Cuscutae	15 g
Radix Paeoniae Alba	10 g
Radix Boehmeriae	30 g
Folium Artemisiae Argyi (*charred*)	10 g

Later, Ramulus Uncariae cum Uncis (12 g), Caulis Bambusae in Taeniam (10 g) and Pericarpium Citri Reticulatae (5 g) were added to the prescription to treat headache, irritability, thirst and retching.

The patient took these herbs for over 5 months, and finally gave birth to a boy at full term.

---

c. **Yin Deficiency and Heat in the Blood**

— Yin Deficiency produces internal Heat. Heat in the Blood disturbs the Chong and Ren channels, causing uterine bleeding during pregnancy. Clinical manifestations include loss of thick red blood during early pregnancy, restlessness, thirst with desire to drink, scanty and yellow urine, a red tongue with thin yellow coating, and a thready, rolling and rapid pulse.
— The treatment principle is to clear Heat, nourish Yin, cool Blood and protect the fetus.
— The recommended formula is *Bao Yin Jian* (**Protect the Yin Decoction**) with additions:

Radix Rehmanniae	15 g
Radix Rehmanniae Praeparata	15 g
Radix Paeoniae Alba	10 g
Colla Corii Asini	10 g
(*melted and taken separately*)	
Herba Ecliptae	15 g
Radix Dipsaci	12 g
Radix Scutellariae	10–15 g
Cortex Phellodendri	10 g
Radix Boehmeriae	15 g
Radix Sanguisorbae	10 g

---

2. PERSISTENT LOCHIA

GENERAL DESCRIPTION

— Lochia continuing for more than 2 or 3 weeks after labour is persistent. Its main causes are weakness of the Chong and Ren channels after childbirth, deficient Qi failing to control Blood and stagnation of Blood in the Interior. Other causes include deficiency of Yin and Blood, Empty Fire, Stagnant Liver Qi turning to Fire and invasion by Heat Toxins.

DIFFERENTIATION AND TREATMENT

a. **Qi Deficiency**

— Weakness of the Chong and Ren channels after childbirth makes Qi unable to control Blood. Clinical manifestations include profuse, pinkish, odourless lochia, a bearing-down sensation, lassitude, dislike of speaking, a swollen pale tongue and a thready, weak pulse.
— The treatment principle is to tonify Qi and control Blood.
— The recommended formula is a variation of **Tonifying the Middle and Benefiting Qi Decoction**:

Radix Codonopsis Pilosulae	10 g
Radix Astragali seu Hedysari	10–15 g
Rhizoma Atractylodis Macrocephalae	10 g
Rhizoma Cimicifugae	3 g
Radix Bupleuri	3 g
Radix Angelicae Sinensis	10 g
Radix Paeoniae Rubra	10 g
Radix Paeoniae Alba	10 g
Arillus Longan	10 g
Cornu Cervi Degelatinatium	10 g
Folium Artemisiae Argyi	10 g

— Modifications:

- For Blood Stagnation, add Herba Leonuri (15 g) and 12 g of **Sudden Smile Powder**.

CASE STUDY 41.10
PERSISTENT LOCHIA

Female, age 29

Lochia ceased 10 days after this patient's labour, but she then carried heavy objects which caused her to begin bleeding again. She had been bleeding for 2 months, with a red flow and clots but little abdominal pain. Her tongue was slightly purple with a thin coating and her pulse was thready.

Pathogenesis: Physical strain caused damage to the vessels, leading to stagnation of Blood in the Interior.

Treatment principle: Primarily to tonify Qi and control Blood; secondarily to resolve Blood Stasis and stop bleeding.

The formula used consisted of:

Radix Astragali seu Hedysari (*treated*)	12 g
Rhizoma Atractylodis Macrocephalae	10 g
Radix Angelicae Sinensis	10 g
Radix Paeoniae Rubra	6 g
Rhizoma Ligustici Chuanxiong	5 g
Rhizoma Zingiberis (*baked*)	3 g
Sudden Smile Powder (*decocted wrapped*)	15 g
Radix Rubiae (charred)	10 g
Herba Leonuri	15 g

After three doses, bleeding stopped.

---

b. **Blood Stagnation**

— Stagnation of Blood in the uterus prevents the circulation of Blood in the vessels. Clinical manifestations include scanty dark-purple lochia with clots, lower abdominal pain which is aggravated by pressure, a purple tongue or purple spots on the tongue and a wiry or deep and forceful pulse.

— The treatment principle is to activate the Blood, resolve Stasis and stop bleeding.
— The recommended formula is a variation of *Sheng Hua Tang* (**Generation and Transformation Decoction**):

Radix Angelicae Sinensis	10 g
Rhizoma Ligustici Chuanxiong	10 g
Radix Salviae Miltiorrhizae	15 g
Radix Paeoniae Rubra	10 g
Herba Leonuri	15 g
Herba Lycopi	10–15 g
Fructus Crataegi	15 g
Rhizoma Zingiberis (*stir-baked*)	2–5 g
Herba Taraxaci	10 g
Faeces Trogopterorum	10 g

— Modifications:

- For invasion by pathogenic Cold, giving rise to lower abdominal pain with a cold sensation and a general aversion to cold, add Cortex Cinnamomi or Ramulus Cinnamomi (2–5 g) (*decocted later*) or Ramulus Cinnamomi (5–10 g) and Folium Artemisiae Argyi (10 g).
- For stagnation of Qi with stuffiness of the chest and abdominal distension, add Rhizoma Cyperi (10 g) and Radix Linderae (5–10 g).

CASE STUDY 41.11
PERSISTENT LOCHIA

Female, age 30

This patient complained of persistent uterine bleeding for 13 days following abortion. The blood flow was dribbling and purplish-red in colour with clots. Other symptoms and signs included dull lower abdominal pain, a slightly yellow tongue coating and a thready, wiry pulse. Her appetite and energy level remained good.

Pathogenesis: Retention of residual Blood Stasis following abortion.

Treatment principle: Resolve Blood Stasis.

The formula used was a variation of **Generation and Transformation Decoction**:

Radix Angelicae Sinensis	10g
Rhizoma Ligustici Chuanxiong	10g
Semen Persicae	10g
Fructus Crataegi (*raw*)	15g
Herba Leonuri	15g
Rhizoma Zingiberis (*baked*)	2g
Herba Lycopi	10g
Radix Salviae Miltiorrhizae	10g

After two doses, the bleeding stopped.

c. Heat in the Blood

— In this pattern, the Blood becomes reckless due to Yin Deficiency with Empty Fire, or due to pathogenic factors turning to Heat. Clinical manifestations include persistent thick red or foul lochia, fever, flushed face, thirst, a red tongue and a thready, rapid pulse.
— The treatment principle is to nourish Yin, clear Heat and Fire and stop bleeding.
— The recommended formula is a variation of **Protect the Yin Decoction**:

Radix Rehmanniae	15–30 g
Radix Paeoniae Rubra *or* Radix Paeoniae Alba	10 g
Radix Scutellariae	10 g
Cortex Moutan Radicis	10 g
Cortex Phellodendri	10 g
Herba Ecliptae	15 g
Radix Rubiae	15 g
Os Sepiellae seu Sepiae	12 g

— Modifications:

- For pronounced Yin Deficiency, add Fructus Lycii (10–15 g) and Colla Corii Asini (10g).
- For pronounced Heat and Fire, add Flos Lonicerae (10 –15 g), Fructus Forsythiae (10 g) and Herba Patriniae (10–15 g).
- In any of the above conditions, if there is infection with foul lochia or fever, reduce the dosage of the tonics and add Radix Bupleuri (10 g), Radix Scutellariae (10 g), Flos Lonicerae (15 g) and Fructus Forsythiae (10 g) to clear Heat and Fire Poison.

---

3. POSTPARTUM URINARY DISORDERS

GENERAL DESCRIPTION
— Retention of urine, frequent urination and urinary incontinence may occur during the postpartum period due to deficiency of Upright Qi, damage to the collaterals of the uterus and deficiency of Kidney Qi following childbirth, all of which impair the function of the Bladder in controlling urine.

DIFFERENTIATION AND TREATMENT

a. Kidney Deficiency

— This may be the result of a constitutional Kidney Qi deficiency or of excessive child-bearing, both of which impair the function of the Bladder in controlling urination. Clinical manifestations include postpartum retention of urine with distension, fullness and pain in the lower abdomen, or urinary frequency or incontinence; soreness and a cold sensation in the lumbar region and knees, lassitude, dizziness, tinnitus, a pale tongue and a deep, thready pulse.
— The treatment principle is to tonify the Kidneys and produce Qi.
— The recommended formula is **Kidney Qi Pill**:

Radix Rehmanniae Praeparata	10–15 g
Fructus Corni	10 g
Rhizoma Dioscoreae	15 g
Cortex Cinnamomi or Ramulus Cinnamomi	25 g
Radix Aconiti Praeparata	2–5 g
Poria	10 g
Rhizoma Alismatis	10 g

— Modifications:

- For severe urinary incontinence, remove Rhizoma Alismatis from the prescription and add Fructus Schisandrae (5 g), Fructus Alpiniae Oxyphyllae (10 g) and Ootheca Mantidis (10–15 g).
- For lumbar pain, add Cortex Eucommiae (10 g), Radix Dipsaci (10 g) and Fructus Alpiniae Oxyphyllae (10 g).
- For retention of urine with abdominal distension and fullness, add Radix Linderae (5 g), Polyporus Umbellatus (12 g) and Semen Plantaginis (12 g) (decocted wrapped).

b. Qi Deficiency

— Deficiency of Lung Qi implies impairment of the Lungs' function of regulating the water passages. Deficiency of Spleen Qi implies impairment of the Spleen's function of transformation and transportation of Water and Dampness. Clinical manifestations include postpartum retention of urine, lower abdominal distension and fullness, dislike of speaking, lassitude, pallor and a soft, weak pulse.
— The treatment principle is to tonify Qi and move Water.
— The recommended formula is:

Radix Astragali seu Hedysari	10–15 g
Rhizoma Atractylodis Macrocephalae	12 g

Radix Ophiopogonis	10–15 g
Poria	10 g
Medulla Tetrapanacis	5 g
Rhizoma Alismatis	10–15 g

— Modifications:

- If Qi Deficiency is complicated with Blood Stagnation, giving rise to painful and hesitant urination with haematuria, add Pollen Typhae (10 g), Rhizoma Imperatae (15 g) and 1 g of powdered Succinum (to be taken separately).
- For abdominal distension and fullness, add Radix Linderae (5–10 g) and Fructus Aurantii (5–10 g).
- For urinary frequency or incontinence, remove Medulla Tetrapanacis and Rhizoma Alismatis from the prescription and add Fructus Alpiniae Oxyphyllae (10 g), Fructus Corni (10 g), Semen Cuscutae (10 –15 g), Rhizoma Cimicifugae (3 g) and Radix Bupleuri (3 g).
- For postpartum retention of urine, fill the umbilicus with salt and place ten slices of Chinese green onion on the salt. Apply moxibustion on top of the onion.

4. DISORDERS OF LACTATION

GENERAL DESCRIPTION

— Insufficiency or lack of milk, and spontaneous secretion of milk may be caused by deficiency of Qi and Blood, or by Liver Qi Stagnation or Liver Fire.

DIFFERENTIATION AND TREATMENT

a. Deficient lactation

i. Deficiency of Qi and Blood
— Qi and Blood Deficiency implies insufficiency of the source of milk. Clinical manifestations include scanty and thin milk, or a complete absence of milk, soft breasts without distension or pain, pallor, palpitation, shortness of breath, spontaneous sweating, a pale tongue and a weak, thready pulse.
— The treatment principle is primarily to tonify Qi and Blood and secondarily to promote the secretion of milk.
— The recommended formula is a variation of

Tong Ru Dan (**Special Pill to Promote Lactation**):

Radix Astragali seu Hedysari (*raw*)	10–20 g
Radix Codonopsis Pilosulae	10 g
Radix Angelicae Sinensis	10 g
Radix Paeoniae Alba	10 g
Radix Rehmanniae Praeparata	15–20 g
Radix Ophiopogonis	15 g
Medulla Tetrapanacis	2–5 g
Radix Platycodi	5 g
Semen Vaccariae	10–15 g

— Modifications:

- For Spleen and Stomach Deficiency with impairment of transformation and transportation, remove Radix Rehmanniae Praeparata from the prescription and add Radix Atractylodis Macrocephalae (10 g) and Massa Fermentata Medicinalis (10 g).

ii. Liver Qi Stagnation
— Stagnation of Liver Qi blocks the channels and collaterals, preventing the secretion of milk. Clinical manifestations include stagnation of milk, breast distension and pain, distension and fullness of the chest and hypochondrium, depression, a thin tongue coating and a wiry pulse.
— The treatment principle is to soothe the Liver, relieve stagnation and promote the secretion of milk.
— The recommended formula is a variation of *Xia Ru Yong Quan San* (**Yong Quan Powder to Promote Lactation**):

Radix Bupleuri	5 g
Pericarpium Citri Reticulatae Viride	5 g
Radix Angelicae Sinensis	10 g
Rhizoma Ligustici Chuanxiong	6 g
Radix Trichosanthis	15 g
Squama Manitis	10–15 g
Semen Vaccariae	10 g
Radix Platycodi	5 g
Medulla Tetrapanacis or Caulis Akebiae	2–3 g

— Modifications:

- If there is pronounced distension, hardness and pain of the breasts, add Radix Angelicae Dahuricae (10 g) and Herba Taraxaci (15 g) and apply externally a decoction of Pericarpium Citri Reticulatae or minced fresh Herba Taraxaci or Folium Hibisci (*Fu Rong Ye*).

b. Spontaneous secretion of milk

i. *Qi Deficiency*

— In this pattern, Qi is deficient and fails to control the secretion of milk. Clinical manifestations include the spontaneous secretion of small amounts of thin milk, absence of breast distension, lassitude, a pale tongue and a thready, weak pulse.
— The treatment principle is primarily to tonify Qi and Blood and secondarily to astringe milk.
— The recommended formula is a variation of **Eight-Precious Decoction**:

Radix Astragali seu Hedysari	10–20 g
Radix Codonopsis Pilosulae	10 g
Rhizoma Atractylodis Macrocephalae	10 g
Radix Angelicae Sinensis	10 g
Radix Rehmanniae Praeparata	15 g
Radix Paeoniae Alba	10 g
Fructus Schisandrae	5 g
Semen Euryales	10 g
Os Draconis	15 g
(decocted first)	

ii. *Liver Heat*

— In this pattern, Liver Fire forces milk to flow out. Clinical manifestations include spontaneous secretion of milk, breast distension, a bitter taste in the mouth, restlessness, irritability, a red tongue with yellow coating, and a wiry, rapid pulse.
— The treatment principle is to soothe the Liver, relieve Stagnation and clear Heat.
— The recommended formula is a variation of *Dan Zhi Xiao Yao San* (**Free and Relaxed Powder with Moutan and Gardenia**):

Radix Bupleuri *(vinegar-treated)*	5 g
Radix Paeoniae Alba	10 g
Cortex Moutan Radicis	10 g
Fructus Gardeniae	10 g
Radix Scutellariae	10 g
Radix Rehmanniae	10–15 g
Fructus Meliae Toosendan	10 g
Fructus Aurantii Immaturus	5 g
Radix Ophiopogonis	10 g
Radix Paeoniae Rubra	10 g
Radix Glycyrrhizae *(raw)*	3 g

— To stop the secretion of milk, administer a decoction of 60 g of Fructus Hordei Germinatus, and/or wrap 250 g of Natrii Sulfas in cloth and apply to the breasts.

E. Miscellaneous disorders

1. MENOPAUSAL SYNDROMES

GENERAL DESCRIPTION

— Menopausal syndrome refers to a series of signs and symptoms due to the decline of ovarian function before and after the cessation of menstruation. These include irregular menstruation, dizziness, palpitation, restlessness, insomnia, irritability, tinnitus and hypertension.
— The cause of menopausal syndrome is linked to Kidney Deficiency leading to deficiency of the Chong and Ren channels, giving rise to functional disturbance of the Zang Fu and irregularity of the Yin and Yang of the body.
— The treatment principle is primarily to tonify the Kidneys and regulate Yin and Yang and secondarily to soothe the Liver and Heart.

DIFFERENTIATION AND TREATMENT

a. Kidney Deficiency and hyperactivity of the Liver

— Deficiency of the Kidneys leads to Liver Yang Rising and disharmony between the Heart and Kidneys. Clinical manifestations include hot flushes, restlessness, irritability, mental and emotional tension, dizziness, blurred vision, palpitation, insomnia, five-palm Heat, irregular menstruation, night sweats, tidal fever, abnormal sensations of the skin, a red tongue and a thready, wiry and rapid pulse.
— The treatment principle is to nourish Yin, suppress Yang, clear Fire and tonify the Liver and Kidneys.
— The recommended formula is a variation of **Six-Flavour Rehmannia Pill with Anemarrhena and Phellodendron**:

Radix Rehmanniae	15–30 g
Fructus Corni	10 g
Fructus Lycii	10–15 g
Rhizoma Anemarrhenae	10 g
Cortex Phellodendri	10 g
Os Draconis	15 g
(decocted first)	
Concha Ostreae	15–20 g
(decocted first)	
Plastrum Testudinis	10–15 g
(decocted first)	
Radix Polygoni Multiflori	15 g
Cortex Moutan Radicis	10 g

Rhizoma Dioscoreae	15 g
Poria	10 g

— Modifications:

- For emotional fluctuations such as laughing and crying without reason, restlessness, insomnia and yawning, add Radix Glycyrrhizae (5 g), wheat (15–30 g), Fructus Ziziphi Jujubae (15–10 pieces) and Radix Stemonae (15–30 g).

b. Spleen and Kidney Deficiency

— Kidney Deficiency implies a decline of Ming Men Fire and weakness of the Chong and Ren channels. Spleen Deficiency implies insufficiency of the source of Qi and Blood. Clinical manifestations include irregular menstruation, cold limbs, aversion to cold, lumbar soreness, urgent urination, loose stools, lassitude, sallow complexion, a pale or dark tongue and a deep, thready and weak pulse.
— The treatment principle is to tonify the Kidneys, strengthen Yang and invigorate the Spleen.
— The recommended formula is a variation of **Restoring the Right Pill:**

Radix Rehmanniae Praeparata	15–30 g
Fructus Corni	10 g
Rhizoma Dioscoreae	15 g
Fructus Lycii	10 g
Radix Aconiti Praeparata	2–5 g
Cortex Cinnamomi	2–5 g
Cornu Cervi	5–10 g
Semen Cuscutae	15 g
Radix Angelicae Sinensis	10 g
Radix Codonopsis Pilosulae	10 g
Rhizoma Atractylodis Macrocephalae	10 g

— Modifications:

- For Kidney Yang Deficiency and Heart Fire as a result of disharmony between the Heart and Kidneys, add Rhizoma Coptidis (2–5 g), which combines with Cortex Cinnamomi to harmonize the Heart and Kidneys.
- For oedema of the face and feet, remove Radix Rehmanniae Praeparata from the prescription and add Poria (12 g), Radix Astragali seu Hedysari (12 g) and Radix Stephaniae Tetrandrae (10 g).
- For irregularity between Yin and Yang with hypertension, prescribe Rhizoma Curculiginis (10 g), Herba Epimedii (10 g), Radix Morindae Officinalis (10 g), Rhizoma Anemarrhenae (10 g), Cortex Phellodendri (10 g) and Radix Angelicae Sinensis (10 g).

CASE STUDY 41.12
MENOPAUSAL SYNDROME

Female, age 48

This patient complained of irregular menstruation for 3 years. 6 months previously, she had developed dizziness, insomnia, irritability, stuffiness of the chest, palpitation, mental tension and weeping without obvious reason following a conflict. She was currently presenting with loss of body weight, lassitude, depression, sighing, talking to herself, dream-disturbed sleep, anxiety, a red tongue with scanty coating, and a wiry, thready pulse.

Pathogenesis: Loss of balance of Yin and Yang, stagnation of Liver Qi, Deficiency of Yin and Blood and dysfunction of the Heart in housing the Mind.

Treatment principle: Nourish Yin and Blood, soothe the Liver and relieve Stagnant Liver Qi, nourish the Heart and calm the Mind.

The formula used was a variation of **Licorice, Wheat and Jujube Decoction**, with herbs that soothe the Heart and calm the Mind:

Radix Rehmanniae Praeparata	30 g
Radix Angelicae Sinensis	10 g
Radix Paeoniae Alba	10 g
Radix Bupleuri (*vinegar-treated*)	6 g
Rhizoma Cyperi (*prepared*)	10 g
Wheat	30 g
Radix Glycyrrhizae	10 g
Fructus Ziziphi Jujubae	5 pieces
Semen Ziziphi Spinosae	10 g
Semen Biotae	10 g
Os Draconis	150 g
(*decocted first*)	
Poria cum Ligno Hospite	10 g
Concha Margaritifera Usta	20 g
(*decocted first*)	

After 20 doses, all symptoms had disappeared. A follow-up visit 6 months later showed no relapse.

Appendix 1:
Pin Yin names of herbs
with Latin equivalents

Ai Ye	Folium Artemisiae Argyi
Ba Ji Tian	Radix Morindae Officinalis
Bai Bu	Radix Stemonae
Bai Dou Kou	Semen Amomi Cardomomi
Bai Fu Zi	Rhizoma Typhonii
Bai Guo	Semen Ginkgo
Bai Hua She	Agkistrodon Acutus (also Bungarus Parvus)
Bai Hua She She Cao	Herba Hedyotis Diffusae
Bai Ji	Rhizoma Bletilla
Bai Jiang Cao	Herba Patriniae
Bai Jie Zi	Semen Sinapis Albae
Bai Shao	Radix Paeoniae Alba
Bai Tou Weng	Radix Pulsatillae
Bai Qian	Rhizoma Cynanchi Stauntonii
Bai Wei	Radix Ampelopsis
Bai Zhi	Radix Angelicae Dahuricae
Bai Zhu	Rhizoma Atractylodis Macrocephalae
Bai Zi Ren	Semen Biotae
Bei Mu	Bulbus Fritillariae
Ban Lan Gen	Radix Isatidis
Ban Xia	Rhizoma Pinelliae
Ban Zhi Lian	Herba Scutellariae Barbatae
Bei Sha Shen	Radix Glehniae
Bi Xie	Rhizoma Dioscoreae Septemlobae
Bian Dou	Semen Dolichoris
Bie Jia	Carapax Trionycis
Bing Long	Semen Arecae
Bo He	Herba Menthae
Bu Gu Zhi	Fructus Psoraleae
Can Sha	Excrementum Bombycis Mori
Cang Er Zi	Fructus Xanthii
Cang Zhu	Rhizoma Atractylodis
Cao Wu	Radix Aconiti Kusnezoffii
Ce Bai Ye	Cacumen Biotae
Chai Hu	Radix Bupleuri
Chan Tui	Periostracum Cicadae
Che Qian Zi	Semen Plantaginis
Chen Pi	Pericarpium Citri Reticulatae
Chen Xiang	Lignum Aquilariae Resinatum
Cheng Liu	Ramulus Tamarix Chinensis
Chi Fu Ling	Red Poria
Chi Shi Zhi	Halloysitum Rubrum
Chi Shao	Radix Paeoniae Rubra
Chou Wu Tong	Folium Clerodendri
Chuan Lian Zi	Fructus Meliae Toosendan
Chuan Mu Tong	Caulis Clematidis Armandii
Chuan Po Hua	Flos Magnoliae Officinalis
Chuan Shan Jia	Squama Manitis
Chuan Xin Lian	Herba Andrographitis
Chuan Xiong	Rhizoma Ligustici Chuanxiong
Chun Gen Pi	Cortex Ailanthi
Ci Ji Li	Fructus Tribuli
Ci Shi	Magnetitum
Da Ji	Herba seu Radix Cirsii Japonici
Da Huang	Radix et Rhizoma Rhei
Da Qing Ye	Folium Isatidis
Da Zao	Fructus Ziziphi Jujubae
Dai Mao	Carapax Eretmochaelydis
Dai Zhe Shi	Haematitum
Dan Shen	Radix Salviae Miltiorrhizae
Dan Zhu Ye	Herba Lophatheri
Dang Gui	Radix Angelicae Sinensis
Dang Shen	Radix Codonopsis Pilosulae
Deng Xin Cao	Medulla Junci Effusi
Di Bie Chong	Eupolyphaga seu Steleophaga
Di Gu Pi	Cortex Lycii Radicis
Di Long	Lumbricus
Di Yu	Radix Sanguisorbae
Ding Xiang	Flos Caryophylli
Dong Chong Xie Cao	Cordyceps
Dong Gua Zi	Semen Benincasae
Du Huo	Radix Angelicae Pubescentis
Du Zhong	Cortex Eucommiae
E Jiao	Colla Corii Asini
E Zhu	Rhizoma Zedoariae
Fan Xie Ye	Folium Cassiae
Fang Feng	Radix Ledebouriellae
Fang Ji	Radix Stephaniae Tetrandrae
Feng Mi	Mel
Fo Shou	Fructus Citri Sarcodactylis
Fu Ling	Poria
Fu Pen Zi	Fructus Rubi
Fu Ping	Herba Spirodelae
Fu Rong Ye	Herba Hibisci
Fu Xiao Mai	Fructus Tritici Levis
Fu Zi	Radix Aconiti Praeparata
Gan Cao	Radix Glycyrrhizae
Gan Jiang	Rhizoma Zingiberis
Gao Liang Jiang	Rhizoma Alpiniae Officinalis
Ge Gen	Radix Puerariae
Ge Jie	Gecko
Ge Ke	Concha Meretricis seu Cyclinae
Gou Ji	Rhizoma Cibotii
Gou Teng	Ramulus Uncariae cum Uncis
Gou Qi Zi	Fructus Lycii

Gu Sui Bu	Rhizoma Drynariae	*Luo Shi Teng*	Caulis Trachelospermi
Gu Ya	Fructus Oryzae Germinatus	*Ma Bo*	Lasiosphaera seu Calvatia
Gua Lou	Fructus Trichosanthis	*Ma Chi Xian*	Herba Portulacae
Gui Ban	Plastrum Testudinis	*Ma Dou Ling*	Fructus Aristolochiae
Gui Zhi	Ramulus Cinnamomi	*Ma Huang*	Herba Ephedrae
Hai Feng Teng	Caulis Piperis Futokadsurae	*Ma Huang Gen*	Radix Ephedrae
Hai Gou Shen	Peniet Testes Callorhini	*Mai Dong*	Radix Ophiopogonis
Hai Jin Sha	Spora Lygodii	*Mai Ya*	Fructus Hordei Germinatus
Hai Ma	Hippocampus	*Man Jing Qi*	Fructus Viticis
Hai Zao	Sargassum	*Mang Xiao*	Natrii Sulfas
He Huan Pi	Cortex Albizziae	*Mei Gui Hua*	Flos Rosae Rugosae
He Shou Wu	Radix Polygoni Multiflori	*Mo Han Lian*	Herba Ecliptae
He Zi	Fructus Chebulae	*Mo Yao*	Resina Myrrhae
Hong Hua	Flos Carthami	*Mu Dan Pi*	Cortex Moudan Radicis
Hong Shen	Radix Ginseng Rubra	*Mu Gua*	Fructus Chaenomelis
Hong Teng	Caulis Sargentodoxae	*Mu Hu Die*	Semen Oroxyli
Hou Po	Cortex Magnoliae Officinalis	*Mu Li*	Concha Ostreae
Hu Po	Succinum	*Mu Xiang*	Radix Aucklandiae
Hu Tao Rou	Semen Juglandis	*Nan Sha Shen*	Radix Adenophorae
Hu Zhang	Rhizoma Polygoni Cuspidati	*Niu Bang Zi*	Fructus Arctii
Hua Jiao	Pericarpium Zanthoxyli	*Niu Huang*	Calculus Bovis
Hua Shi	Talcum	*Niu Xi*	Radix Achyranthis Bidentatae
Huai Hua	Flos Sophorae	*Nu Zhen Zi*	Fructus Ligustri Lucidi
Huang Bai	Cortex Phellodendri	*Ou Jie*	Nodus Nelumbinis Rhizomatis
Huang Jing	Rhizoma Polygonati	*Pang Da Hai*	Semen Sterculiae Scaphigerae
Huang Lian	Rhizoma Coptidis	*Pao Jiang*	Baked ginger
Huang Qi	Radix Astragali seu Hedysari	*Pei Lan*	Herba Eupatorii
Huang Qin	Radix Scutellariae	*Pi Pa Ye*	Folium Eriobotryae
Huo Ma Ren	Fructus Cannabis	*Pi Shi*	Arsenolitum
Huo Xiang	Herba Agastachis	*Pu Huang*	Pollen Typhae
Ji Nei Jin	Endothelium Corneum Gigeriae Galli	*Qi Dai*	Umbilical cord
Ji Xue Teng	Caulis Spatholobi	*Qian Cao*	Radix Rubiae
Jiang Can	Bombyx Batryticatus	*Qian Hu*	Radix Peucedani
Jiang Huang	Rhizoma Curcumae Longae	*Qian Niu Zi*	Semen Pharbitides
Jie Geng	Radix Platycodi	*Qian Shi*	Semen Euryales
Jin Qian Cao	Herba Lysimachiae	*Qiang Huo*	Rhizoma seu Radix Notopterygii
Jin Yin Hua	Flos Lonicerae	*Qin Jiu*	Radix Gentianae Macrophyllae
Jin Ying Zi	Fructus Rosae Laevigatae	*Qin Pi*	Cortex Fraxini
Jing Jie	Herba Schizonepetae	*Qing Dai*	Indigo Naturalis
Ju Hua	Flos Chrysanthemi	*Qing Pi*	Pericarpium Citri Reticulatae Viride
Jue Ming Zi	Semen Cassiae	*Qing Hao*	Herba Artemisiae Chinghao
Ku Lian Gen Pi	Cortex Meliae	*Quan Xie*	Scorpio
Kuan Dong Hua	Flos Farfarae	*Ren Dong Teng*	Caulis Lonicerae
Kun Bu	Thallus Laminariae	*Ren Shen*	Radix Ginseng
Lai Fu Zi	Semen Raphani	*Rou Cong Rong*	Herba Cistanchis
Lei Gong Teng	Herba Tripterygii	*Rou Dou Kou*	Semen Myristicae
Li Zhi He	Semen Litchi	*Rou Gui*	Cortex Cinnamomi
Lian Qiao	Fructus Forsythiae	*Ru Xiang*	Resina Olibani
Lian Zi	Semen Nelumbinis	*San Leng*	Rhizoma Sparganii
Ling Yang Jiao	Cornu Antelopis	*San Qi*	Radix Notoginseng
Long Dan Cao	Radix Gentianae	*Sang Bai Pi*	Cortex Mori Radicis
Long Gu	Os Draconis	*Sang Ji Sheng*	Ramulus Loranthi
Long Kui	Herba Solani Nigri	*Sang Piao Xiao*	Ootheca Mantidis
Lu E Mei	Flos Mume	*Sang Ye*	Folium Mori
Lu Gen	Rhizoma Phragmitis	*Sang Zhi*	Ramulus Mori
Lu Jiao	Cornu Cervi	*Sha Ren*	Fructus Amomi
Lu Jiao Jiao	Colla Cornus Cervi	*Shan Dou Gen*	Radix Sophorae Subprostratae
Lu Jiao Shuang	Cornu Cervi Degelatinatium	*Shan Yao*	Rhizoma Dioscoreae
Lu Rong	Cornu Cervi Pantotrichum	*Shan Zha*	Fructus Crataegi
Luo Bu Ma	Folium Apocyni Veneti	*Shan Zhu Yu*	Fructus Corni

She Gan	Rhizoma Belamcandae	*Xuan Shen*	Radix Scrophulariae
Shen Qu	Massa Fermentata	*Xue Yu Tan*	Crinis Carbonisatus
Sheng Di Huang	Radix Rehmanniae	*Yan Hu Suo*	Rhizoma Corydalis
Sheng Jiang	Rhizoma Zingiberis Recens	*Yi Mu Cao*	Herba Leonuri
Sheng Ma	Rhizoma Cimicifugae	*Yi Tang*	Saccharum Granorum
Sheng Tie Luo	Iron cinder	*Yi Yi Ren*	Semen Coicis
Shi Gao	Gypsum Fibrosum	*Yi Zhi Ren*	Fructus Alpiniae Oxyphyllae
Shi Hu	Herba Dendrobii	*Yin Chai Hu*	Radix Stellariae
Shi Jian Chuan	Herba Salviae Sinensis	*Yin Chen Hao*	Herba Artemisiae Capillaris (also
Shi Jue Ming	Concha Haliotidis		Herba Artemisiae Scopariae)
Shi Jun Zi	Fructus Quisqualis	*Yin Yang Huo*	Herba Epimedii
Shi Liu Pi	Pericarpium Granati	*Ying Su Ke*	Pericarpium Papaveris
Shi Wei	Folium Pyrrosiae	*Yu Jin*	Radix Curcumae
Shu Di Huang	Radix Rehmanniae Praeparata	*Yu Li Ren*	Semen Pruni
Shui Zhi	Hirudo	*Yu Xing Cao*	Herba Houttuyniae
Su Geng	Caulis Perillae	*Yu Zhu*	Rhizoma Polygonati Odorati
Su Zi	Fructus Perillae	*Yuan Zhi*	Radix Polygalae
Suan Zao Ren	Semen Ziziphi Spinosae	*Zao Xin Tu*	Baked yellow earth
Suo Yang	Herba Cynomorii	*Zao Xiu*	Rhizoma Paradis
Tai Zi Shen	Radix Pseudostellariae	*Ze Lan*	Herba Lycopi
Tao Ren	Semen Persicae	*Ze Xie*	Rhizoma Alismatis
Tian Dong	Radix Asparagi	*Zhen Zhu*	Margarita
Tian Hua Fen	Radix Trichosanthis	*Zhen Zhu Mu*	Concha Margaritifera Usta
Tian Ma	Rhizoma Gastrodiae	*Zhi Mu*	Rhizoma Anemarrhenae
Tian Nan Xing	Rhizoma Arisaematis	*Zhi Qiao*	Fructus Aurantii
Ting Li Zi	Semen Lepidii seu Descurainiae	*Zhi Shi*	Fructus Aurantii Immaturus
Tong Ji Li	Semen Astragali Complanati	*Zhi Zi*	Fructus Gardeniae
Tu Fu Ling	Rhizoma Smilacis Glabrae	*Zhu Li*	Succus Bambusae
Tu Si Zi	Semen Cuscutae	*Zhu Ling*	Polyporus Umbellatus
Wa Leng Zi	Concha Arcae	*Zhu Me Gen*	Radix Boehmeriae
Wang Bu Liu Xing	Semen Vaccariae	*Zhu Ru*	Caulis Bambusae
Wei Ling Xian	Radix Clematis	*Zhu Sha*	Cinnabaris
Wu Bei Zi	Galla Chinensis	*Zhu Ye*	Folium Phyllostachyos
Wu Gong	Scolopendra	*Zi Cao*	Radix Lithospermum seu Arnebiae
Wu Jia Pi	Cortex Acanthopanacis Radicis	*Zi He Che*	Placenta Hominis
Wu Ling Zhi	Faeces Trogopterorum	*Zi Su Ye*	Folium Perillae
Wu Mei	Fructus Mume	*Zi Wan*	Radix Asteris
Wu Shao She	Zaocys	*Zi Zhu*	Folium Callicarpae
Wu Tou	Radix Aconiti	*Zong Lu Tan*	Petiolus Trachycarpi Carbonisatus
Wu Wei Zi	Fructus Schisandrae		
Wu Yao	Radix Linderae		
Wu Zei Gu	Os Sepiae		
Wu Zhu Yu	Fructus Evodiae		
Xi Jiao	Cornu Rhinoceri Asiatici		
Xi Xian Cao	Herba Siegesbeckiae		
Xi Xin	Herba Asari		
Xi Yang Shen	Panacis Quinquefolii Radix		
Xia Ku Cao	Spica Prunellae		
Xian He Cao	Herba Agrimoniae		
Xian Mao	Rhizoma Curculiginis		
Xiang Fu	Rhizoma Cyperi		
Xiang Ru	Herba Elsholtzia		
Xiang Yuan	Fructus Citri		
Xiao Hui Xiang	Fructus Foeniculi		
Xiao Ji	Herba Cephalanoploris		
Xie Bai	Bulbus Allii Macrostemi		
Xin Yi Hua	Flos Magnoliae		
Xing Ren	Semen Armeniacae		
Xu Duan	Radix Dipsaci		
Xuan Fu Hua	Flos Inulae		

Appendix 2:
Latin names of herbs
with Pin Yin equivalents

Latin	Pin Yin
Acanthopanacis Radicis, Cortex	*Wu Jia Pi*
Achyranthis Bidentatae, Radix	*Niu Xi*
Aconiti, Radix	*Wu Tou*
Aconiti Kusnezoffii, Radix	*Cao Wu*
Aconiti Praeparata, Radix	*Fu Zi*
Adenophorae, Radix	*Nan Sha Shen*
Agastachis, Herba	*Huo Xiang*
Agkistrodon Acutus	*Bai Hua She*
Agrimoniae, Herba	*Xian He Cao*
Ailanthi, Cortex	*Chun Gen Pi*
Albizziae, Cortex	*He Huan Pi*
Alismatis, Rhizoma	*Ze Xie*
Allii Macrostemi, Bulbus	*Xie Bai*
Alpiniae Officinalis, Rhizoma	*Gao Liang Jiang*
Alpiniae Oxyphyllae, Fructus	*Yi Zhi Ren*
Amomi Cardomomi, Semen	*Bai Dou Kou*
Amomi, Fructus	*Sha Ren*
Ampelopsis, Radix	*Bai Wei*
Anemarrhenae, Rhizoma	*Zhi Mu*
Andrographitis, Herba	*Chuan Xin Lian*
Angelicae Dahuricae, Radix	*Bai Zhi*
Angelicae Pubescentis, Radix	*Du Huo*
Angelicae Sinensis, Radix	*Dang Gui*
Antelopis, Cornu	*Ling Yang Jiao*
Apocyni Veneti, Folium	*Luo Bu Ma*
Aquilariae Resinatum, Lignum	*Chen Xiang*
Arctii, Fructus	*Niu Bang Zi*
Arecae, Semen	*Bing Long*
Arisaematis, Rhizoma	*Tian Nan Xing*
Aristolochiae, Fructus	*Ma Dou Ling*
Armeniacae, Semen	*Xing Ren*
Arsenolitum	*Pi Shi*
Artemisiae Argyi, Folium	*Ai Ye*
Artemisiae Capillaris, Herba	*Yin Chen Hao*
Artemisiae Chinghao, Herba	*Qing Hao*
Asari, Herba	*Xi Xin*
Asparagi, Radix	*Tian Dong*
Asteris, Radix	*Zi Wan*
Astragali Complanati, Semen	*Tong Ji Li*
Astragali seu Hedysari, Radix	*Huang Qi*
Atractylodis, Rhizoma	*Cang Zhu*
Atractylodis Macrocephalae, Rhizoma	*Bai Zhu*
Aucklandiae, Radix	*Mu Xiang*
Aurantii, Fructus	*Zhi Qiao*
Aurantii Immaturus, Fructus	*Zhi Shi*
Bambusae, Caulis	*Zhu Ru*
Bambusae, Succus	*Zhu Li*
Batryticatus, Bombyx	*Jiang Can*
Belamcandae, Rhizoma	*She Gan*
Benincasae, Semen	*Dong Gua Zi*
Biotae, Cacumen	*Ce Bai Ye*
Biotae, Semen	*Bai Zi Ren*
Bletillae, Rhizoma	*Bai Ji*
Boehmeriae, Radix	*Zhu Me Gen*
Bombycis Mori, Excrementum	*Can Sha*
Bovis, Calculus	*Niu Huang*
Bupleuri, Radix	*Chai Hu*
Callicarpae, Folium	*Zi Zhu*
Callorhini, Peni et Testes	*Hai Gou Shen*
Cannabis, Fructus	*Huo Ma Ren*
Carthami, Flos	*Hong Hua*
Caryophylli, Flos	*Ding Xiang*
Cassiae, Folium	*Fan Xie Ye*
Cassiae, Semen	*Jue Ming Zi*
Cephalanoploris, Herba	*Xiao Ji*
Cervi, Cornu	*Lu Jiao*
Cervi, Colla Cornus	*Lu Jiao Jiao*
Cervi Degelatinatium, Cornu	*Lu Jiao Shuang*
Cervi Pantotrichum, Cornu	*Lu Rong*
Chaenomelis, Fructus	*Mu Gua*
Chebulae, Fructus	*He Zi*
Chinensis, Galla	*Wu Bei Zi*
Chrysanthemi, Flos	*Ju Hua*
Cibotii, Rhizoma	*Gou Ji*
Cicadae, Periostracum	*Chan Tui*
Cimicifugae, Rhizoma	*Sheng Ma*
Cinnabaris	*Zhu Sha*
Cinnamomi, Cortex	*Rou Gui*
Cinnamomi, Ramulus	*Gui Zhi*
Cirsii Japonici, Herba seu Radix	*Da Ji*
Cistanchis, Herba	*Rou Cong Rong*
Citri, Fructus	*Xiang Yuan*
Citri Reticulatae, Pericarpium	*Chen Pi*
Citri Reticulatae Viride, Pericarpium	*Qing Pi*
Citri Sarcodactylis, Fructus	*Fo Shou*
Clematidis, Radix	*Wei Ling Xian*
Clematidis Armandii, Caulis	*Chuan Mu Tong*
Clerodendri, Folium	*Chou Wu Tong*
Codonopsis Pilosulae, Radix	*Dang Shen*
Coicis, Semen	*Yi Yi Ren*
Concha Arcae	*Wa Leng Zi*
Coptidis, Rhizoma	*Huang Lian*
Cordyceps	*Dong Chong Xie Cao*
Corydalis, Rhizoma	*Yan Hu Suo*
Corii Asini, Colla	*E Jiao*
Corneum Gigeriae Galli, Endothelium	*Ji Nei Jin*

Corni, Fructus	*Shan Zhu Yu*	Isatidis, Folium	*Da Qing Ye*
Crataegi, Fructus	*Shan Zha*	Isatidis, Radix	*Ban Lan Gen*
Crinis Carbonatus	*Xue Yu Tan*	Juglandis, Semen	*Hu Tao Rou*
Curculiginis, Rhizoma	*Xian Mao*	Junci Effusi, Medulla	*Deng Xin Cao*
Curcumae, Radix	*Yu Jin*	Laminariae, Thallus	*Kun Bu*
Curcumae Longae, Rhizoma	*Jiang Huang*	Lasiosphera seu Calvatia	*MaBo*
Cuscutae, Semen	*Tu Si Zi*	Ledebouriellae, Radix	*Fang Feng*
Cynanchi Stauntonii, Rhizoma	*Bai Qian*	Leonuri, Herba	*Yi Mu Cao*
Cynomorii, Herba	*Suo Yang*	Lepidii seu Descurainiae, Semen	*Ting Li Zi*
Cyperi, Rhizoma	*Xiang Fu*	Ligustici Chuanxiong, Rhizoma	*Chuan Xiong*
Dendrobii, Herba	*Shi Hu*	Ligustri Lucidi, Fructus	*Nu Zhen Zi*
Dioscoreae, Rhizoma	*Shan Yao*	Linderae, Radix	*Wu Yao*
Dioscoreae Septemlobae, Rhizoma	*Bi Xie*	Litchi, Semen	*Li Zhi He*
Dipsaci, Radix	*Xu Duan*	Lithospermum seu Arnebiae, Radix	*Zi Cao*
Dolichoris, Semen	*Bian Dou*	Lophatheri, Herba	*Dan Zhu Ye*
Draconis, Os	*Long Gu*	Lonicerae, Caulis	*Ren Dong Teng*
Drynariae, Rhizoma	*Gu Sui Bu*	Lonicerae, Flos	*Jin Yin Hua*
Ecliptae, Herba	*Mo Han Lian*	Loranthi, Ramulus	*Sang Ji Sheng*
Elsholtzia, Herba	*Xiang Ru*	Lumbricus	*Di Long*
Ephedrae, Herba	*Ma Huang*	Lycii, Fructus	*Gou Qi Zi*
Ephedrae, Radix	*Ma Huang Gen*	Lycii Radicis, Cortex	*Di Gu Pi*
Epimedii, Herba	*Yin Yang Huo*	Lycopi, Herba	*Ze Lan*
Eretmochaelydis, Carapax	*Dai Mao*	Lygodii, Spora	*Hai Jin Sha*
Eriobotryae, Folium	*Pi Pa Ye*	Lysimachiae, Herba	*Jin Qian Cao*
Eucommiae, Cortex	*Du Zhong*	Magnetitum	*Ci Shi*
Eupatorii, Herba	*Pei Lan*	Magnoliae, Flos	*Xin Yi Hua*
Eupolyphaga seu Steleophaga	*Di Bie Chong*	Magnoliae Officinalis, Cortex	*Hou Po*
Euryales, Semen	*Qian Shi*	Magnoliae Officinalis, Flos	*Chuan Po Hua*
Evodiae, Fructus	*Wu Zhu Yu*	Manitis, Squama	*Chuan Shan Jia*
Farfarae, Flos	*Kuan Dong Hua*	Mantidis, Ootheca	*Sang Piao Xiao*
Foeniculi, Fructus	*Xiao Hui Xiang*	Margarita	*Zhen Zhu*
Forsythiae, Fructus	*Lian Qiao*	Margaritifera Usta, Concha	*Zhen Zhu Mu*
Fraxini, Cortex	*Qin Pi*	Massa Fermentata	*Shen Qu*
Fritillariae, Bulbus	*Bei Mu*	Mel	*Feng Mi*
Gardeniae, Fructus	*Zhi Zi*	Meliae, Cortex	*Ku Lian Gen Pi*
Gastrodiae, Rhizoma	*Tian Ma*	Meliae Toosendan, Fructus	*Chuan Lian Zi*
Gecko	*Ge Jie*	Menthae, Herba	*Bo He*
Gentianae, Radix	*Long Dan Cao*	Meretricis seu Cyclinae, Concha	*Ge Ke*
Gentianae Macrophyllae, Radix	*Qin Jiu*	Mori, Folium	*Sang Ye*
Ginkgo, Semen	*Bai Guo*	Mori, Ramulus	*Sang Zhi*
Ginseng, Radix	*Ren Shen*	Mori Radicis, Cortex	*Sang Bai Pi*
Ginseng Rubra, Radix	*Hong Shen*	Morindae Officinalis, Radix	*Ba Ji Tian*
Glehniae, Radix	*Bei Sha Shen*	Moutan Radicis, Cortex	*Mu Dan Pi*
Glycyrrhizae, Radix	*Gan Cao*	Mume, Flos	*Lu E Mei*
Granati, Pericarpium	*Shi Liu Pi*	Mume, Fructus	*Wu Mei*
Gypsum Fibrosum	*Shi Gao*	Myristicae, Semen	*Rou Dou Kou*
Haematitum	*Dai Zhe Shi*	Myrrhae, Resina	*Mo Yao*
Haliotidis, Concha	*Shi Jue Ming*	Natrii Sulfas	*Mang Xiao*
Halloysitum Rubrum	*Chi Shi Zhi*	Nelumbinis, Semen	*Lian Zi*
Hedyotis Diffusae, Herba	*Bai Hua She She Cao*	Nelumbinis Rhizomatis, Nodus	*Ou Jie*
Herba Salviae Sinensis	*Shi Jian Chuan*	Notoginseng, Radix	*San Qi*
Hibisci, Herba	*Fu Rong Ye*	Notopterygii, Rhizoma seu Radix	*Qiang Huo*
Hippocampus	*Hai Ma*	Olibani, Resina	*Ru Xiang*
Hirudo	*Shui Zhi*	Ophiopogonis, Radix	*Mai Dong*
Hominis, Placenta	*Zi He Che*	Oroxyli, Semen	*Mu Hu Die*
Houttuyniae, Herba	*Yu Xing Cao*	Oryzae Germinatus, Fructus	*Gu Ya*
Hordei Germinatus, Fructus	*Mai Ya*	Ostreae, Concha	*Mu Li*
Indigo Naturalis	*Qing Dai*	Paeoniae Alba, Radix	*Bai Shao*
Inulae, Flos	*Xuan Fu Hua*	Paeoniae Rubra, Radix	*Chi Shao*
Iron cinder	*Sheng Tie Luo*	Panacis Quinquefolii, Radix	*Xi Yang Shen*

Papaveris, Pericarpium	*Ying Su Ke*	Sophorae Subprostratae, Radix	*Shan Dou Gen*
Paradis, Rhizoma	*Zao Xiu*	Sparganii, Rhizoma	*San Leng*
Patriniae, Herba	*Bai Jiang Cao*	Spatholobae, Caulis	*Ji Xue Teng*
Perillae, Caulis	*Su Geng*	Spirodelae, Herba	*Fu Ping*
Perillae, Folium	*Zi Su Ye*	Stellariae, Radix	*Yin Chai Hu*
Perillae, Fructus	*Su Zi*	Stemonae, Radix	*Bai Bu*
Persicae, Semen	*Tao Ren*	Stephaniae Tetrandrae, Radix	*Fang Ji*
Peucedani, Radix	*Qian Hu*	Sterculiae Scaphigerae, Semen	*Pang Da Hai*
Pharbitides, Semen	*Qian Niu Zi*	Succinum	*Hu Po*
Phellodendri, Cortex	*Huang Bai*	Talcum	*Hua Shi*
Phragmitis, Rhizoma	*Lu Gen*	Testudinis, Plastrum	*Gui Ban*
Phyllostachyos, Folium	*Zhu Ye*	Trachelospermi, Caulis	*Luo Shi Teng*
Pinelliae, Rhizoma	*Ban Xia*	Trachycarpi Carbonisatus, Petiolus	*Zong Lu Tan*
Piperis Futokadsurae, Caulis	*Hai Feng Teng*	Tribuli, Fructus	*Ci Ji Li*
Plantaginis, Semen	*Che Qian Qi*	Trichosanthis, Fructus	*Gua Lou*
Platycodi, Radix	*Jie Geng*	Trichosanthis, Radix	*Tian Hua Fen*
Polygalae, Radix	*Yuan Zhi*	Trionycis, Carapax	*Bie Jia*
Polygonati Odorati, Rhizoma	*Yu Zhu*	Tripterygii, Herba	*Lei Gong Teng*
Polygoni Cuspidati, Rhizoma	*Hu Zhang*	Trogopterorum, Faeces	*Wu Ling Zhi*
Polygoni Multiflori, Radix	*He Shou Wu*	Typhae, Pollen	*Pu Huang*
Polygonati, Rhizoma	*Huang Jing*	Typhonii, Rhizoma	*Bai Fu Zi*
Poria	*Fu Ling*	Umbellatus, Polyporus	*Zhu Ling*
Poria (red)	*Chi Fu Ling*	Umbilical cord	*Qi Dai*
Portulacae, Herba	*Ma Chi Xian*	Uncariae cum Uncis, Ramulus	*Gou Teng*
Prunellae, Spica	*Xia Ku Cao*	Vaccariae, Semen	*Wang Bu Liu Xing*
Pruni, Semen	*Yu Li Ren*	Viticis, Fructus	*Man Jing Zi*
Pseudostellariae, Radix	*Tai Zi Shen*	Yellow earth (baked)	*Zao Xin Tu*
Psoraleae, Fructus	*Bu Gu Zhi*	Xanthii, Fructus	*Cang Er Zi*
Puerariae, Radix	*Ge Gen*	Zanthoxyli, Pericarpium	*Hua Jiao*
Pulsatilla, Radix	*Bai Tou Weng*	Zaocys	*Wu Shao She*
Pyrrosiae, Folium	*Shi Wei*	Zedoariae, Rhizoma	*E Zhu*
Quisqualis, Fructus	*Shi Jun Zi*	Zingiberis, Rhizoma (dried)	*Gan Jiang*
Ramulus Tamarix Chinensis	*Cheng Liu*	Zingiberis, Rhizoma (baked)	*Pao Jiang*
Raphani, Semen	*Lai Fu Zi*	Zingiberis Recens, Rhizoma	*Sheng Jiang*
Rehmanniae, Radix	*Sheng Di Huang*	Ziziphi Jujubae, Fructus	*Da Zao*
Rehmanniae Praeparata, Radix	*Shu Di Huang*	Ziziphi Spinosae, Semen	*Suan Zao Ren*
Rhei, Radix et Rhizoma	*Da Huang*		
Rhinoceri Asiatici, Cornu	*Xi Jiao*		
Rosae Laevigatae, Fructus	*Jin Ying Zi*		
Rosae Rugosae, Flos	*Mei Gui Hua*		
Rubi, Fructus	*Fu Pen Zi*		
Rubiae, Radix	*Qian Cao*		
Saccharum Granorum	*Yi Tang*		
Salviae Miltiorrhizae, Radix	*Dan Shen*		
Sanguisorbae, Radix	*Di Yu*		
Sargassum	*Hai Zao*		
Sargentodoxae, Caulis	*Hong Teng*		
Schisandrae, Fructus	*Wu Wei Zi*		
Schizonepetae, Herba	*Jing Jie*		
Scolopendra	*Wu Gong*		
Scorpio	*Quan Xie*		
Scrophulariae, Radix	*Xuan Shen*		
Scutellariae, Radix	*Huang Qin*		
Scutellariae Barbatae, Herba	*Ban Zhi Lian*		
Sepiae, Os	*Wu Zei Gu*		
Siegesbeckiae, Herba	*Xi Xian Cao*		
Sinapis Albae, Semen	*Bai Jie Zi*		
Smilacis Glabrae, Rhizoma	*Tu Fu Ling*		
Solani Nigri, Herba	*Long Kui*		
Sophorae, Flos	*Huai Hua*		

Appendix 3:
Pin Yin names of formulae
with English equivalents

An Gong Niu Huang Wan
Calm the Palace Pill with Cattle Gallstone

Ba Zhen Tang
Eight-Precious Decoction

Ba Zheng San
Eight-Herb Powder for Rectification

Bai He Gu Jin Tang
Lily Bulb Decoction to Preserve the Metal

Bai Hu Cheng Qi Tang
White Tiger Decoction for Ordering the Qi

Bai Hu Jia Cang Zhu Tang
White Tiger Decoction with Atractylodis

Bai Hu Jia Gui Zhi Tang
White Tiger Ramulus Cinnamomi Decoction

Bai Hu Jia Ren Shen Tang
White Tiger plus Ginseng Decoction

Bai Hu Tang
White Tiger Decoction

Bai Tou Weng Tang
Pulsatilla Decoction

Ban Xia Bai Zhu Tian Ma Tang
Pinellia-Atractylodes-Gastrodia Decoction

Ban Xia Hou Po Tang
Pinellia and Magnolia Bark Decoction

Bao He Wan
Preserving and Harmonizing Pill

Bao Yin Jian
Protect the Yin Decoction

Bei Mu Gua Lou San
Fritillaria-Trichosanthes Powder

Bei Xie Fen Qing Yin
Dioscorea Hypoglauca Decoction to Separate the Clear

Bie Jia Jian Wan
Turtle Shell Pill

Bu Fei E Jiao Tang
Tonifying the Lung Decoction with Ass-Hide Gelatin

Bu Huan Jin Zheng Qi San
Rectify the Qi Powder Worth More Than Gold

Bu Yang Huan Wu Tang
Tonify the Yang to Restore Five-tenths Decoction

Bu Zhong Yi Qi Tang
Tonifying the Middle and Benefitting Qi Decoction

Cang Fu Dao Tan Wan
Atractylodes and Cyperi Pill to Eliminate Phlegm

Chai Ge Jie Ji Tang
Bupleurum and Kudzu Decoction to Release the Muscle Layer

Chai Hu Shu Gan Tang
Bupleurum Soothing the Liver Decoction

Chuan Xiong Cha Tiao San
Ligusticum-Green Tea Regulating Powder

Ci Zhu Wan
Magnetite and Cinnabar Pill

Cong Bai Qi Wei Yin
Scallion Decoction with Seven Ingredients

Cong Chi Tang
Scallion and Prepared Soybean Decoction

Cong Chi Jie Geng Tang
Scallion and Prepared Soybean Decoction with Platycodon

Da An Wan
Great Tranquility Pill

Da Bu Yin Wan
Great Tonify the Yin Pill

Da Bu Yuan Jian
Great Tonify the Source Decoction

Da Cheng Qi Tang
Major Order the Qi Decoction

Da Ding Feng Zhu
Major Arrest Wind Pearl

Da Huang Mu Dan Tang
Rhubarb and Moutan Decoction

Da Huang Fu Zi Tang
Rhubarb and Prepared Aconite Decoction

Da Jian Zhong Tang
Major Strengthening the Middle Decoction

Da Qing Long Tang
  Major Bluegreen Dragon Decoction

Da Xian Xiong Tang
  Major Sinking into the Chest Decoction

Dai Ge San
  Indigo Naturalis-Concha Meretricis Powder

Dan Shen Yin
  Salvia Decoction

Dan Zhi Xiao Yao San
  Free and Relaxed Powder with Moutan and Gardenia

Dang Gui Bu Xue Tang
  Angelica Decoction to Tonify the Blood

Dang Gui Jian Zhong Tang
  Angelica Strengthening the Middle Decoction

Dang Gui Liu Huang Tang
  Dang Gui and Six-Yellow Decoction

Dang Gui Long Hui Wan
  Dang Gui, Gentiana and Aloe Pill

Dang Gui Shao Yao San
  Angelica and Peony Powder

Dang Gui Si Ni Tang
  Angelica Four Rebellious Decoction

Dang Gui Si Ni Jia Wu Zhu Yu Sheng Jiang Tang
  Angelica Four Rebellious Decoction with Evodia and
  Ginger

Dao Chi San
  Eliminating Redness Powder

Dao Tan Tang
  Eliminating Phlegm Decoction

Di Huang Yin Zi
  Rehmannia Decoction

Ding Chuan Tang
  Arrest Wheezing Decoction

Ding Xian Wan
  Arrest Seizures Pill

Ding Xiang Shi Di Tang
  Clove and Persimmon Calyx Decoction

Du Huo Ji Sheng Tang
  Angelica Pubescens-Loranthus Decoction

E Jiao Ji Zi Huang Tang
  Ass-Hide Gelatin and Egg Yolk Decoction

Er Miao San
  Two-Marvel Powder

Fang Ji Huang Qi Tang
  Stephania and Astragalus Decoction

Fu Fang Cheng Qi Tang
  Revised Major Order the Qi Decoction

Fu Yuan Huo Xue Tang
  Revive Health by Invigorating the Blood Decoction

Fu Zi Li Zhong Wan
  Prepared Aconite Pill to Regulate the Middle

Fu Zi Tang
  Prepared Aconite Decoction

Gan Lu Xiao Du Dan
  Sweet Dew Special Pill to Eliminate Toxin

Gan Mai Da Zao Tang
  Licorice, Wheat and Jujube Decoction

Ge Gen Qin Lian Tang
  Kudzu, Coptis and Scutellaria Decoction

Ge Xia Zhu Yu Tang
  Drive Out Blood Stasis Below the Diaphragm Decoction

Geng Yi Wan
  Pill Requiring a Change of Clothes

Gu Chong Tang
  Stabilize Gushing Decoction

Gu Jing Wan
  Stabilize the Menses Pill

Gua Lou Xie Bai Ban Xia Tang
  Trichosanthis-Allium-Pinellia Decoction

Gui Pi Tang
  Tonifying the Spleen Decoction

Gui Shao Di Huang Tang
  Angelica, Peony and Rehmannia Decoction

Gui Zhi Fu Zi Tang
  Cinnamon Twig Decoction plus Prepared Aconite

Gui Zhi Tang
  Cinnamon Twig Decoction

Gui Zhi Jia Ge Gen Tang
  Cinnamon Twig Decoction plus Kudzu

Gui Zhi Jia Hou Po Xing Zi Tang
  Cinnamon Twig Decoction plus Magnolia Bark and
  Apricot Kernel

Gui Zhi Jia Ren Shen Tang
  Cinnamon Twig Decoction plus Ginseng

Hei Xiao Yao San
  Black Free and Relaxed Powder

Hong Teng Jian
  Sargentodoxa Decoction

Hou Po Wen Zhong Tang
  Magnolia Bark Decoction for Warming the Middle

Hu Qian Wan
  Hidden Tiger Pill

Hua Ban Tang
  Decoction for Relieving Feverish Rash

Huai Hua San
  Sophora Japonica Flower Powder

Huang Lian Jie Du Tang
  Coptis Decoction to Relieve Toxicity

Huang Long Tang
    Yellow Dragon Decoction

Huang Qi Jian Zhong Tang
    Astragalus Decoction to Construct the Middle

Huang Tu Tang
    Yellow Earth Decoction

Hui Yang Jiu Ji Tang
    Restore Collapsed Yang Decoction

Huo Xiang Zheng Qi San
    Agastache Upright Qi Powder

Ji Chuan Jian
    Benefit the River Decoction

Ji Ming San
    Powder to Take at Cock's Crow

Ji Sheng Shen Qi Wan
    Invigorate the Kidney Qi Pill

Jia Jian Wei Rui Tang
    Modified Polygonatum Oderatum Decoction

Jian Pi Wan
    Strengthen the Spleen Pill

Jiao Ai Tang
    Ass-Hide Gelatin and Mugwort Decoction

Jin Ling Zi San
    Melia Toosendan Powder

Jin Suo Gu Jing Wan
    Metal Lock Pill to Stabilize the Essence

Jing Fang Bai Du San
    Schizonepeta and Ledebouriella Powder to Overcome
    Pathogenic Influences

Jiu Wei Qiang Hu Tang
    Nine-Herb Decoction with Notopterygium

Ju Pi Zhu Ru Tang
    Tangerine Peel and Bamboo Shaving Decoction

Ju Yuan Jian
    Lift the Source Decoction

Li Zhong Wan
    Regulating the Middle Decoction

Liang Gu Wan
    Galangal and Cyperus Pill

Ling Gan Wu Wei Jiang Xin Tang
    Poria-Glycyrrhiza-Schisandra-Zingiber-Asarum
    Decoction

Ling Gui Zhu Gan Tang
    Poria-Ramulus Cinnamomi-Atractylodes-Glycyrrhiza
    Decoction

Ling Jiao Gou Teng Tang
    Antelope Horn and Uncaria Decoction

Ling Ma Bai Hu Tang
    White Tiger Decoction with Antelopis and Gastrodia

Liu Jun Zi Tang
    Six Gentlemen Decoction

Liu Wei Di Huang Wan
    Six-Flavour Rehmanniae Pill

Liu Yi San
    Six-to-One Powder

Long Dan Xie Gan Tang
    Gentiana Draining the Liver Decoction

Ma Huang Tang
    Ephedra Decoction

Ma Huang Fu Zi Xi Xin Tang
    Ephedra, Asarum and Prepared Aconite Decoction

Ma Huang Gui Zhi Ge Ban Tang
    Half-Decoction of Ephedra and Cinnamon Twig

Ma Xing Shi Gan Tang
    Ephedra-Prunus-Gypsum-Glycyrrhiza Decoction

Ma Zi Ren Wan
    Hemp Seed Pill

Mang Shi Gun Tan Wan
    Chlorite-Schist Pill for Chronic Phlegm Syndromes

Mu Li San
    Oyster Shell Powder

Niu Huang Qing Xin Wan
    Cattle Gallstone Pill to Clear the Heart

Nuan Gan Jian
    Warm the Liver Decoction

Ping Wei San
    Balancing the Stomach Powder

Pu Ji Xiao Du Yin
    Universal Benefit Decoction to Eliminate Toxin

Qi Ju Di Huang Wan
    Lycium Fruit, Chrysanthemum and Rehmannia Pill

Qian Zheng San
    Lead to Symmetry Powder

Qiang Huo Sheng Shi Tang
    Notopterygium Dispelling Dampness Decoction

Qing Hao Bie Jia Tang
    Artemisia Annua and Soft-shelled Turtle Shell Decoction

Qing Qi Hua Tan Wan
    Clearing Heat-Resolving Phlegm Decoction

Qing Shu Yi Qi Tang
    Clear Summerheat and Augment the Qi Decoction

Qing Wei San
    Clearing the Stomach Powder

Qing Wen Bai Du Yin
    Clear Epidemics and Overcome Toxin Decoction

Qing Ying Tang
    Clear the Nutritive Level Decoction

Ren Shen Bai Du San
Ginseng Powder to Overcome Pathogenic Influences

Ren Shen Ge Jie San
Ginseng and Gecko Powder

Ren Shen Hu Tao Tang
Ginseng and Walnut Decoction

Ren Shen Yang Rong Tang
Ginseng Decoction to Nourish the Nutritive Qi

Run Chang Wan
Moisten the Intestines Pill

San Ao Tang
Three-Unbinding Decoction

San Ren Tang
Three-Nut Decoction

San Wu Bei Ji Wan
Three Substance Pill for Emergencies

San Zi Yang Qin Tang
Three-Seed Nourishing Parents Decoction

Sang Ju Yin
Mulberry Leaf and Chrysanthemum Decoction

Sang Piao Xiao San
Mantis Egg-Case Powder

Sang Xing Tang
Mulberry Leaf and Apricot Kernel Decoction

Sha Shen Mai Dong Tang
Glehnia-Ophiopogonis Decoction

Shao Fu Zhu Yu Tang
Drive Out Blood Stasis in the Lower Abdomen Decoction

Shao Yao Tang
Peony Decoction

She Gan Ma Huang Tang
Belamcanda and Ephedra Decoction

Shen Fu Tang
Panax-Aconitum Decoction

Shen Fu Long Mu Tang
Panax-Aconitum Decoction with Long Gu and Mu Li

Shen Ling Bai Zhu San
Panax-Poria-Atractylodis Powder

Shen Qi Wan
Kidney Qi Pill

Sheng Fu Tang
Ginseng and Aconite Decoction

Sheng Hua Tang
Generation and Transformation Decoction

Sheng Ma Ge Gen Tang
Cimicifuga and Kudzu Decoction

Sheng Mai San
Generating the Pulse Powder

Sheng Tie Luo Yin
Iron Filings Decoction

Shi Hui San
Ten Partially-charred Substance Powder

Shi Pi San
Strengthening the Spleen Decoction

Shi Xiao San
Sudden Smile Powder

Shi Zao Tang
Ten-Jujube Decoction

Shou Tai Wan
Foetus Longevity Pill

Shui Lu Er Xian Dan
Water and Earth Immortals Special Pill

Si Jun Zi Tang
Four Gentlemen Decoction

Si Miao Wan
Four-Marvel Pill

Si Miao Yong An Tang
Four-Valiant Decoction for Well-Being

Si Ni Jia Ren Shen Tang
Four Rebellious Decoction with Ginseng

Si Ni Jiu Ji Tang
Four Rebellious Restore Collapsed Yang Decoction

Si Ni Tang
Four Rebellious Decoction

Si Shen Wan
Four-Miracle Pill

Si Wu Tang
Four Substance Decoction

Si Zhi Xiang Fu Wan
Four-Preparation Cyperi Pill

Su He Xiang Wan
Styrax Pill

Su Zi Jiang Qi Tang
Perilla Seed Lowering Qi Decoction

Suan Zao Ren Tang
Sour Jujube Decoction

Tao Ren Cheng Qi Tang
Peach Pit Decoction to Order the Qi

Tian Ma Gou Teng Yin
Gastrodia-Uncaria Decoction

Tian Tai Wu Yao San
Top-Quality Lindera Powder

Tian Wang Bu Xin Dan
Heavenly Emperor Tonifying the Heart Pill

Tiao Wei Cheng Qi Tang
Regulate the Stomach and Order the Qi Decoction

Ting Li Da Zao Xie Fei Tang
Descurainia and Jujube Decoction to Drain the Lungs

Tong Ru Dan
Special Pill to Promote Lactation

Tong Xie Yao Fang
Important Formula for Painful Diarrhoea

Tong Yang Si Ni Tang
Unblock the Yang Four Rebellious Decoction

Wan Dai Tang
End Discharge Decoction

Wei Jing Tang
Reed Decoction

Wei Ling San
Calm the Stomach with Poria Decoction

Wen Dan Tang
Warming the Gall Bladder Decoction

Wen Jing Tang
Warm the Menses Decoction

Wen Pi Tang
Warm the Spleen Decoction

Wu Ling San
Five Ingredient Powder with Poria

Wu Pi San
Five-Peel Powder

Wu Wei Xiao Du Yin
Five-Ingredient Decoction to Eliminate Toxin

Wu Zhi Yin
Five Juice Decoction

Wu Zhu Yu Tang
Evodia Decoction

Xi Jiao Di Huang Tang
Rhinoceros Horn and Rehmannia Decoction

Xia Ru Yong Quan San
Yong Quan Powder to Promote Lactation

Xian Fang Huo Ming Yin
Sublime Formula for Sustaining Life

Xiang Lian Wan
Aucklandia and Coptis Pill

Xiang Ru Yin
Elsholtzia Decoction

Xiang Sha Liu Jun Zi Tang
Six Gentlemen Decoction with Aucklandia and Amomum

Xiang Su San
Cyperus and Perilla Leaf Powder

Xiao Chai Hu Tang
Small Bupleurum Decoction

Xiao Cheng Qi Tang
Minor Order the Qi Decoction

Xiao Feng San
Eliminate Wind Powder

Xiao Huo Luo Dan
Minor Invigorate the Collaterals Special Pill

Xiao Ji Yin Zi
Cephalanoplos Decoction

Xiao Jian Zhong Tang
Minor Strengthening the Middle Decoction

Xiao Ke Fang
Prescription to Treat Diabetes

Xiao Qing Long Tang
Small Green Dragon Decoction

Xiao Xian Xiong Tang
Small Sinking Chest Decoction

Xiao Yao San
Free and Relaxed Powder

Xie Bai San
Expelling Whiteness Powder

Xie Xin Tang
Drain the Epigastrium Decoction

Xuan Fu Dai Zhe Tang
Inula and Haematite Decoction

Xue Fu Zhu Yu Tang
Blood Mansion Eliminating Stasis Decoction

Yang He Tang
Yang-Heartening Decoction

Yang Yin Qing Fei Tang
Nourish the Yin and Clear the Lungs Decoction

Yi Guan Tang
Linking Decoction

Yi Huang Tang
Change Yellow (Discharge) Decoction

Yi Wei Tang
Benefitting the Stomach Decoction

Yi Yi Ren Tang
Coix Decoction

Yin Chen Hao Tang
Artemisia Yinchenhao Decoction

Yin Qiao San
Honeysuckle and Forsythia Powder

You Gui Wan
Restoring the Right Pill

Yu Nu Jian
Jade Woman Decoction

Yu Ping Feng San
Jade Windscreen Powder

Yue Ju Wan
Gardenia-Ligusticum Pill

Zai Zao San
   Renewal Powder

Zeng Ye Cheng Qi Tang
   Increase the Fluids and Order the Qi Decoction

Zhen Gan Xi Feng Tang
   Pacifying the Liver and Subduing Wind Decoction

Zhen Ren Yang Zang Tang
   True Man's Decoction to Nourish the Organs

Zhen Wu Tang
   True Warrior Decoction

Zhi Bai Di Huang Wan
   Six-Flavour Rehmannia Pill with Anemarrhena and
   Phellodendri

Zhi Bao Dan
   Greatest Treasure Special Pill

Zhi Gan Cao Tang
   Glycyrrhiza Decoction

Zhi Shi Dao Zhi Wan
   Citrus Aurantius Eliminating Stagnation Pill

Zhi Shi Xiao Pi Wan
   Immature Bitter Orange Pill to Reduce Focal Distension

Zhi Zhu Wan
   Aurantia Immaturus-Atractylodis Macrocephalae Pill

Zhi Zi Dou Chi Tang
   Gardenia and Prepared Soybean Decoction

Zhou Che Wan
   Vessel and Vehicle Pill

Zhu Ling Tang
   Polyporus Decoction

Zhu Sha An Shen Wan
   Cinnabar Pill to Calm the Spirit

Zhu Ye Liu Bang Tang
   Lophatheri-Tamarix-Arctii Decoction

Zhu Ye Shi Gao Tang
   Lophatherus and Gypsum Decoction

Zi Xue Dan
   Purple Snow Special Pill

Zuo Gui Wan
   Restoring the Left Pill

Zuo Gui Yin
   Restoring the Left Decoction

Zuo Jin Wan
   Left Metal Pill

Appendix 4:
English names of formulae with Pin Yin equivalents

Agastache Upright Qi Powder
Huo Xiang Zheng Qi San

Angelica and Peony Powder
Dang Gui Shao Yao San

Angelica Decoction to Tonify the Blood
Dang Gui Bu Xue Tang

Angelica Four Rebellious Decoction
Dang Gui Si Ni Tang

Angelica Four Rebellious Decoction with Evodia and Ginger
Dang Gui Si Ni Wu Zhu Yu Sheng Jiang Tang

Angelica, Peony and Rehmannia Decoction
Gui Shao Di Huang Tang

Angelica Pubescens-Loranthus Decoction
Du Huo Ji Sheng Tang

Angelica Strengthening the Middle Decoction
Dang Gui Jian Zhong Tang

Antelope Horn and Uncaria Decoction
Ling Jiao Gou Teng Tang

Arrest Seizures Pill
Ding Xian Wan

Arrest Wheezing Decoction
Ding Chuan Tang

Artemisia Annua and Soft-shelled Turtle Shell Decoction
Qing Hao Bie Jia Tang

Artemisia Yinchenhao Decoction
Yin Chen Hao Tang

Ass-Hide Gelatin and Egg Yolk Decoction
E Jiao Ji Zi Huang Tang

Ass-Hide Gelatin and Mugwort Decoction
Jiao Ai Tang

Astragalus Decoction to Construct the Middle
Huang Qi Jian Zhong Tang

Atractylodes and Cyperi Pill to Eliminate Phlegm
Cang Fu Dao Tan Wan

Aucklandia and Coptis Pill
Xiang Lian Wan

Aurantia Immaturus-Atractylodis Macrocephalae Pill
Zhi Zhu Wan

Balancing the Stomach Powder
Ping Wei An

Belamcanda and Ephedrae Decoction
She Gan Ma Huang Tang

Benefit the River Decoction
Ji Chuan Jian

Benefitting the Stomach Decoction
Yi Wei Tang

Black Free and Relaxed Powder
Hei Xiao Yao San

Blood Mansion Eliminating Stasis Decoction
Xue Fu Zhu Yu Tang

Bupleurum and Kudzu Decoction to Release the Muscle Layer
Chai Ge Jie Ji Tang

Bupleurum Soothing the Liver Decoction
Chai Hu Shu Gan Tang

Calm the Palace Pill with Cattle Gallstone
An Gong Niu Huang Wan

Calm the Stomach with Poria Powder
Wei Ling San

Cattle Gallstone Pill to Clear the Heart
Niu Huang Qing Xin Wan

Cephalanoplos Decoction
Xiao Ji Yin Zi

Change Yellow (Discharge) Decoction
Yi Huang Tang

Chlorite-Schist Pill for Chronic Phlegm Syndromes
Mang Shi Gun Tan Wan

Cimicifuga and Kudzu Decoction
Sheng Ma Ge Gen Tang

Cinnabar Pill to Calm the Spirit
Zhu Sha An Shen Wan

Cinnamon Twig Decoctioin
Gui Zhi Tang

Cinnamon Twig Decoction plus Ginseng
Gui Zhi Jia Ren Shen Tang

Cinnamon Twig Decoction plus Kudzu
Gui Zhi Jia Ge Gen Tang

Cinnamon Twig Decoction plus Magnolia Bark and Apricot Kernel
Gui Zhi Jia Hou Po Xing Zi Tang

Cinnamon Twig Decoction plus Prepared Aconite
Gui Zhi Fu Zi Tang

Citrus Aurantius Eliminating Stagnation Pill
Zhi Shi Dao Zhi Wan

Clear Epidemics and Overcome Toxin Decoction
Qing Wen Bai Du Yin

Clear Summerheat and Augment the Qi Decoction
Qing Shu Yi Qi Tang

Clear the Nutritive Level Decoction
Qing Ying Tang

Clearing Heat-Resolving Phlegm Decoction
Qing Qi Hua Tan Wan

Clearing the Stomach Powder
Qing Wei San

Clove and Persimmon Calyx Decoction
Ding Xiang Shi Di Tang

Coix Decoction
Yi Yi Ren Tang

Coptis Decoction to Relieve Toxicity
Huang Lian Jie Du Tang

Cyperus and Perilla Leaf Powder
Xiang Su San

Dang Gui and Six-Yellow Decoction
Dang Gui Liu Huang Tang

Dang Gui, Gentiana and Aloe Pill
Dang Gui Long Hui Wan

Decoction for Relieving Feverish Rash
Hua Ban Tang

Descurainia and Jujube Decoction to Drain the Lungs
Ting Li Da Zao Xie Fei Tang

Dioscoreae Hypoglauca Decoction to Separate the Clear
Bei Xie Fen Qing Yin

Drain the Epigastrium Decoction
Xie Xin Tang

Drive Out Blood Stasis Below the Diaphragm Decoction
Ge Xia Zhu Yu Tang

Drive Out Blood Stasis in the Lower Abdomen Decoction
Shao Fu Zhu Yu Tang

Eight-Herb Powder for Rectification
Ba Zheng San

Eight-Precious Decoction
Ba Zhen Tang

Eliminate Wind Powder
Xiao Feng San

Eliminating Phlegm Decoction
Dao Tan Tang

Eliminating Redness Powder
Dao Chi San

Elsholtzia Decoction
Xiang Ru Yin

End Discharge Decoction
Wan Dai Tang

Ephedra Decoction
Ma Huang Tang

Ephedra, Asarum and Prepared Aconite Decoction
Ma Huang Fu Zi Xi Xin Tang

Ephedra-Prunus-Gypsum-Glycyrrhiza Decoction
Ma Xing Shi Gan Tang

Evodia Decoction
Wu Zhu Yu Tang

Expelling Whiteness Powder
Xie Bai San

Five-Ingredient Decoction to Eliminate Toxin
Wu Wei Xiao Du Yin

Five Juice Decoction
Wu Zhi Yin

Five Ingredient Powder with Poria
Wu Ling San

Five-Peel Powder
Wu Pi San

Foetus Longevity Pill
Shou Tai Wan

Four Gentlemen Decoction
Si Jun Zi Tang

Four-Marvel Pill
Si Miao Wan

Four-Miracle Pill
Si Shen Wan

Four-Preparation Cyperi Pill
Si Zhi Siang Fu Wan

Four Rebellious Decoction
Si Ni Tang

Four Rebellious Decoction with Ginseng
Si Ni Jia Ren Shen Tang

Four Rebellious Restore Collapsed Yang Decoction
Si Ni Jiu Ji Tang

Four Substance Decoction
Si Wu Tang

Four-Valiant Decoction for Well-Being
Si Miao Yong An Tang

Free and Relaxed Powder
Xiao Yao San

Free and Relaxed Powder with Moutan and Gardenia
Dan Zhi Xiao Yao San

Fritillaria-Trichosanthis Powder
Bei Mu Gua Lou San

Galangal and Cyperus Pill
Liang Gu Wan

Gardenia and Prepared Soybean Decoction
Zhi Zi Dou Chi Tang

Gardenia-Ligusticum Pill
Yue Ju Wan

Gastrodia-Uncaria Decoction
Tian Ma Gou Teng Yin

Generating the Pulse Powder
Sheng Mai San

Generation and Transformation Decoction
Sheng Hua Tang

Gentiana Draining the Liver Decoctionn
Long Dan Xie Gan Tang

Ginseng and Aconite Decoction
Sheng Fu Tang

Ginseng and Gecko Powder
Ren Shen Ge Jie San

Ginseng and Walnut Decoction
Ren Shen Hu Tao Tang

Ginseng Decoction to Nourish the Nutritive Qi
Ren Shen Yang Rong Tang

Ginseng Powder to Overcome Pathogenic Influences
Ren Shen Bai Du San

Glehnia-Ophiopogonis Decoction
Sha Shen Mai Dong Tang

Glycyrrhiza Decoction
Zhi Gan Cao Tang

Great Tonify the Source Decoction
Da Bu Yuan Jian

Great Tonify the Yin Pill
Da Bu Yin Wan

Great Tranquility Pill
Da An Wan

Greatest Treasure Special Pill
Zhi Bao Dan

Half-Decoction of Ephedra and Cinnamon Twig
Ma Huang Gui Zhi Ge Ban Tang

Heavenly Emperor Tonifying the Heart Pill
Tian Wan Bu Xin Dan

Hemp Seed Pill
Ma Zi Ren Wan

Hidden Tiger Pill
Hu Qian Wan

Honeysuckle and Forsythia Powder
Yin Qiao San

Immature Bitter Orange Pill to Reduce Focal Distension
Zhi Shi Xiao Pi Wan

Important Formula for Painful Diarrhoea
Tong Xie Yao Fang

Increase the Fluids and Order the Qi Decoction
Zeng Ye Cheng Qi Tang

Indigo Naturalis-Concha Meretricis Powder
Dai Ge San

Inula and Haematite Decoction
Xuan Fu Dai Zhe Tang

Invigorate the Kidney Qi Pill
Ji Sheng Shen Qi Wan

Iron Filings Decoction
Sheng Tie Luo Yin

Jade Windscreen Powder
Yu Ping Feng San

Jade Woman Decoction
Yu Nu Jian

Kidney Qi Pill
Shen Qi Wan

Kudzu, Coptis and Scutellaria Decoction
Ge Gen Qin Lian Tang

Lead to Symmetry Powder
Qian Zheng San

Left Metal Pill
Zuo Jin Wan

Licorice, Wheat and Jujube Decoction
Gan Mai Da Zao Tang

Lift the Source Decoction
Ju Yuan Jian

Ligusticum-Green Tea Regulating Powder
Chuan Xiong Cha Tiao San

Lily Bulb Decoction to Preserve the Metal
Bai He Gu Jin Tang

Linking Decoction
Yi Guan Tang

Lophatheri-Tamarix-Arctii Decoction
Zhu Ye Liu Bang Tang

Lophatherus and Gypsum Decoction
Zhu Ye Shi Gao Tang

Lycium Fruit, Chrysanthemum and Rehmannia Pill
Qi Ju Di Huang Wan

Magnetite and Cinnabar Pill
Ci Zhu Wan

Magnolia Bark Decoction for Warming the Middle
Hou Po Wen Zhong Tang

Major Arrest Wind Pearl
Da Ding Feng Zhu

Major Bluegreen Dragon Decoction
Da Qing Long Tang

Major Order the Qi Decoction
Da Cheng Qi Tang

Major Sinking into the Chest Decoction
Da Xian Xiong Tang

Major Strengthening the Middle Decoction
Da Jian Zhong Tang

Mantis Egg-Case Powder
Sang Piao Xiao San

Melia Toosendan Powder
Jin Ling Zi San

Metal Lock Pill to Stablilise the Essence
Jin Suo Gu Jing Wan

Minor Invigorate the Collaterals Special Pill
Xiao Huo Luo Dan

Minor Order the Qi Decoction
Xiao Cheng Qi Tang

Minor Strengthening the Middle Decoction
Xiao Jian Zhong Tang

Modified Polygonatum Odoratum Decoction
Jia Jian Wei Rui Tang

Moisten the Intestines Pill
Run Chang Wan

Mulberry Leaf and Apricot Kernel Decoction
Sang Xing Tang

Mulberry Leaf and Chrysanthemum Decoction
Sang Ju Yin

Nine-Herb Decoction with Notopterygii
Jiu Wei Qiang Hu Tang

Notopterygium Dispelling Dampness Decoction
Qiang Huo Sheng Shi Tang

Nourish the Yin and Clear the Lungs Decoction
Yang Yin Qing Fei Tang

Oyster Shell Powder
Mu Li San

Pacifying the Liver and Subduing Wind Decoction
Zhen Gan Xi Feng Tang

Panax-Aconitum Decoction
Shen Fu Tang

Panax-Aconitum Decoction with Long Gu and Mu Li
Shen Fu Long Mu Tang

Panax-Poria-Atractylodis Powder
Shen Ling Bai Zhu San

Peach Pit Decoction to Order the Qi
Tao Ren Cheng Qi Tang

Peony Decoction
Shao Yao Tang

Perilla Seed Lowering Qi Decoction
Su Zi Jiang Qi Tang

Pill Requiring a Change of Clothes
Geng Yi Wan

Pinellia and Magnolia Bark Decoction
Ban Xia Hou Po Tang

Pinellia-Atractylodes-Gastrodia Decoction
Ban Xia Bai Zhu Tian Ma Tang

Polyporus Decoction
Zhu Ling Tang

Poria-Glycyrrhiza-Schisandra-Zingiber-Asarum Decoction
Ling Gan Wu Wei Jiang Xin Tang

Poria-Ramulus Cinnamomi-Atractylodes-Glycyrrhiza Decoction
Ling Gui Zhu Gan Tang

Powder to Take at Cock's Crow
Ji Ming San

Prepared Aconite Decoction
Fu Zi Tang

Prepared Aconite Pill to Regulate the Middle
Fu Zi Li Zhong Wan

Prescription to Treat Diabetes
Xiao Ke Fang

Preserving and Harmonizing Pill
Bao He Wan

Protect the Yin Decoction
Bao Yin Jian

Pulsatilla Decoction
Bai Tou Weng Tang

Purple Snow Special Pill
Zi Xue Dan

Rectify the Qi Powder Worth More Than Gold
Bu Huan Jin Zheng Qi San

Reed Decoction
Wei Jing Tang

Regulate the Stomach and Order the Qi Decoction
Tiao Wei Cheng Qi Tang

Regulating the Middle Decoction
Li Zhong Wan

Rehmannia Decoction
Di Huang Yin Zi

Renewal Powder
Zai Zao San

Restore Collapsed Yang Decoction
Hui Yang Jiu Ji Tang

Restoring the Left Decoction
Zuo Gui Yin

Restoring the Left Pill
Zuo Gui Wan

Restoring the Right Pill
You Gui Wan

Revised Major Order the Qi Decoction
Fu Fang Cheng Qi Tang

Revive Health by Invigorating the Blood Decoction
Fu Yuan Huo Xue Tang

Rhinoceros Horn and Rehmannia Decoction
Xi Jiao Di Huang Tang

Rhubarb and Moutan Decoction
Da Huang Mu Dan Tang

Rhubarb and Prepared Aconite Decoction
Da Huang Fu Zi Tang

Salvia Decoction
Dan Shen Yin

Sargentodoxa Decoction
Hong Teng Jian

Scallion and Prepared Soybean Decoction
Cong Chi Tang

Schizonepeta and Ledebouriella Powder to Overcome
Pathogenic Influences
Jing Fang Bai Du San

Six-Flavour Rehmanniae Pill
Liu Wei Di Huang Wan

Six-Flavour Rehmannia Pill with Anemarrhena and
Phellodendri
Zhi Bai Di Huang Wan

Six Gentlemen Decoction
Liu Jun Zi Tang

Six Gentlemen Decoction with Aucklandia and
Amomum
Xiang Sha Liu Jun Zi Tang

Six-to-One Powder
Liu Yi San

Small Bupleurum Decoction
Xiao Chai Hu Tang

Small Green Dragon Decoction
Xiao Qing Long Tang

Small Sinking Chest Decoction
Xiao Xian Xiong Tang

Sophora Japonica Flower Powder
Huai Hua San

Sour Jujube Decoction
Suan Zao Ren Tang

Special Pill to Promote Lactation
Tong Ru Dan

Stabilize Gushing Decoction
Gu Chong Tang

Stabilize the Menses Pill
Gu Jing Wan

Stephania and Astragalus Decoction
Fang Ji Huang Qi Tang

Strengthen the Spleen Pill
Jian Pi Wan

Strengthening the Spleen Decoction
Shi Pi Yin

Styrax Pill
Su He Xiang Wan

Sublime Formula for Sustaining Life
Xian Fang Huo Ming Yin

Sudden Smile Powder
Shi Xiao San

Sweet Dew Special Pill to Eliminate Toxin
Gan Lu Xiao Du Dan

Tangerine Peel and Bamboo Shaving Decoction
Ju Pi Zhu Ru Tang

Ten-Jujube Decoction
Shi Zao Tang

Ten Partially-charred Substance Powder
Shi Hui San

Three-Nut Decoction
San Ren Tang

Three-Seed Nourishing Parents Decoction
San Zi Yang Qin Tang

Three Substance Pill for Emergencies
San Wu Bei Ji Wan

Three-Unbinding Decoction
San Ao Tang

Tonify the Yang to Restore Five-tenths Decoction
Bu Yang Huan Wu Tang

Tonifying the Lung Decoction with Ass-Hide Gelatin
Bu Fei E Jiao Tang

Tonifying the Middle and Benefitting Qi Decoction
Bu Zhong Yi Qi Tang

Tonifying the Spleen Decoction
Gui Pi Tang

Top-Quality Lindera Powder
Tian Tai Wu Yao San

Trichosanthis-Allium-Pinellia Decoction
Gua Lou Xie Bai Ban Xia Tang

True Man's Decoction to Nourish the Organs
Zhen Ren Yang Zang Tang.

True Warrior Decoction
Zhen Wu Tang

Two-Marvel Powder
Er Miao San

Turtle Shell Pill
Bie Jia Jian Wan

Universal Benefit Decoction to Eliminate Toxin
Pu Ji Xiao Du Yin

Unblock the Yang Four Rebellious Decoction
Tong Yang Si Ni Tang

Vessel and Vehicle Pill
Zhou Che Wan

Warm the Liver Decoction
Nuan Gan Jian

Warm the Menses Decoction
Wen Jing Tang

Warm the Spleen Decoction
Wen Pi Tang

Warming the Gall Bladder Decoction
Wen Dan Tang

Water and Earth Immortals Special Pill
Shui Lu Er Xian Dan

White Tiger Decoction
Bai Hu Tang

White Tiger Decoction for Ordering the Qi
Bai Hu Cheng Qi Tang

White Tiger Decoction with Antelopis and Gastrodia
Ling Ma Bai Hu Tang

White Tiger Decoction with Atractylodis
Bai Hu Jia Cang Zhu Tang

White Tiger plus Ginseng Decoction
Bai Hu Jia Ren Shen Tang

White Tiger Ramulus Cinnamomi Decoction
Bai Hu Jia Gui Zhi Tang

Yang-Heartening Decoction
Yang He Tang

Yellow Dragon Decoction
Huang Long Tang

Yellow Earth Decoction
Huang Tu Tang

Yong Quan Powder to Promote Lactation
Xia Ru Yong Quan San

Appendix 5:
Formulae and constituent herbs

Angelica and Peony Powder
Dang Gui Shao Yao San
    Radix Angelicae Sinensis
    Radix Paeoniae
    Poria
    Rhizoma Alismatis
    Rhizoma Ligustici Chuanxiong

Angelica and Six-Yellow Decoction
Dang Gui Liu Hang Tang
    Radix Angelicae Sinensis
    Radix Rehmanniae
    Radix Rehmanniae Praeparata
    Radix Scutellariae
    Cortex Phellodendri
    Rhizoma Coptidis
    Radix Astragali seu Hedysari

Angelica Decoction to Tonify the Blood
Dang Gui Bu Xue Tang
    Radix Astragali seu Hedysari
    Radix Angelicae Sinensis

Angelica, Gentian and Aloe Pill
Dang Gui Long Hui Wan
    Radix Angelicae Sinensis
    Radix Gentianae
    Fructus Gardeniae
    Rhizoma Coptidis
    Cortex Phellodendri
    Radix Scutellariae
    Aloe
    Radix et Rhizoma Rhei
    Radix Aucklandiae
    Moschus

Angelica Pubescens-Loranthus Decoction
Du Huo Ji Sheng Tang
    Radix Angelicae Pubescentis
    Ramulus Loranthi
    Cortex Eucommiae
    Radix Achyranthis Bidentatae
    Radix Asari
    Radix Gentianae Macrophyllae
    Poria
    Cortex Cinnamomi
    Radix Ledebouriellae
    Rhizoma Ligustici Chuanxiong

    Radix Ginseng
    Radix Glycyrrhizae
    Radix Angelicae Sinensis
    Radix Paeoniae Alba
    Radix Rehmanniae

Angelica Strengthening the Middle Decoction
Dang Gui Jian Zhong Tang
    Radix Paeoniae
    Ramulus Cinnamomi
    Radix Glycyrrhizae Praeparata
    Rhizoma Zingiberis Recens
    Fructus Ziziphi Jujubae
    Saccharum Granorum
    Radix Angelicae Sinensis

Antelope Horn and Uncaria Decoction
Ling Jiao Gou Teng Tang
    Cornu Antelopis
    Folium Mori
    Bulbus Fritillariae Cirrhosae
    Radix Rehmanniae
    Caulis Uncariae cum Uncis
    Flos Chrysanthemi
    Poria cum Ligno Hospite
    Radix Paeoniae Alba
    Radix Glycyrrhizae
    Caulis Bambusae in Taeniam

Arrest Wheezing Decoction
Ding Chuan Tang
    Semen Ginkgo
    Herba Ephedrae
    Fructus Perillae
    Radix Glycyrrhizae
    Flos Farfarae
    Semen Armeniacae Amarum
    Cortex Mori Radicis
    Radix Scutellariae
    Rhizoma Pinelliae

Artemisia Annua and Soft-shelled Turtle Shell Decoction
Qing Hao Bie Jia Tang
    Herba Artemisiae Chinghao
    Carapax Trionycis
    Radix Rehmanniae
    Rhizoma Anemarrhenae
    Cortex Moutan Radicis

Artemisia Yinchenhao Decoction
Yin Chen Hao Tang
    Herba Artemisiae Capillaris
    Fructus Gardeniae
    Radix et Rhizoma Rhei

Ass-Hide Gelatin and Egg Yolk Decoction
E Jiao Ji Zi Huang Tang
    Colla Corii Asini
    Radix Paeoniae Alba
    Concha Haliotidis
    Ramulus Uncariae cum Uncis
    Radix Rehmanniae
    Radix Glycyrrhizae Praeparata
    Concha Ostreae
    Caulis Trachelospermi
    Poria cum Ligno Hospite
    Egg yolk

Ass-Hide Gelatin and Mugwort Decoction
Jiao Ai Tang
    Rhizoma Ligustici Chuanxiong
    Colla Corii Asini
    Radix Glycyrrhizae
    Folium Artemisiae Argyi
    Radix Angelicae Sinensis
    Radix Paeoniae
    Radix Rehmanniae

Atractylodes and Cyperi Pill to Eliminate Phlegm
Cang Fu Dao Tan Wan
    Rhizoma Atractylodis
    Rhizoma Cyperi
    Pericarpium Citri Reticulatae
    Rhizoma Pinelliae
    Rhizoma Arisaematis
    Poria
    Fructus Aurantii Immaturus
    Radix Glycyrrhizae
    Rhizoma Zingiberis Recens

Astragalus Decoction to Construct the Middle
Huang Qi Jian Zhong Tang
    Radix Paeoniae
    Ramulus Cinnamomi
    Radix Glycyrrhizae Praeparata
    Rhizoma Zingiberis Recens
    Fructus Ziziphi Jujubae
    Saccharum Granorum
    Radix Astragali seu Hedysari

Aucklandia and Coptis Pill
Xiang Lian Wan
    Rhizoma Coptidis
    Radix Aucklandiae

Aurantia Immaturus-Atractylodis Macrocephalae Pill
Zhi Zhu Wan
    Fructus Aurantii Immaturus
    Rhizoma Atractylodis Macrocephalae

Balancing the Stomach Powder
Ping Wei San
    Rhizoma Atractylodis
    Cortex Magnoliae Officinalis
    Pericarpium Citri Reticulatae
    Radix Glycyrrhizae

Belamcanda and Ephedra Decoction
She Gan Ma Huang Tang
    Rhizoma Belamcandae
    Herba Ephedrae
    Rhizoma Zingiberis Recens
    Herba Asari
    Radix Asteris
    Flos Farfarae
    Fructus Ziziphi Jujubae
    Rhizoma Pinelliae
    Fructus Schisandrae

Benefit the River Decoction
Ji Chuan Jian
    Radix Angelicae Sinensis
    Radix Achyranthis Bidentatae
    Herba Cistanchis
    Rhizoma Alismatis
    Rhizoma Cimicifugae
    Fructus Aurantii

Benefiting the Stomach Decoction
Yi Wei Tang
    Radix Ophiopogonis
    Radix Rehmanniae
    Rhizoma Polygonati Odorati
    Radix Adenophorae
    Crystallized brown sugar (*Bing Tang*)

Black Free and Relaxed Powder
Hei Xiao Yao San
    Radix Bupleuri
    Radix Angelicae Sinensis
    Radix Paeoniae Alba
    Rhizoma Atractylodis Macrocephalae
    Poria
    Radix Glycyrrhizae
    Radix Rehmanniae or Radix Rehmanniae
        Praeparata

Blood Mansion Eliminating Stasis Decoction
Xue Fu Zhu Yu Tang
    Semen Persicae
    Flos Carthami
    Radix Angelicae Sinensis
    Radix Rehmanniae
    Rhizoma Ligustici Chuanxiong
    Radix Paeoniae Rubra
    Radix Achyranthis Bidentatae
    Radix Platycodi
    Radix Bupleuri
    Fructus Aurantii
    Radix Glycyrrhizae

Bupleurum and Kudzu Decoction to Release the Muscle Layer
Chai Ge Jie Ji Tang
    Radix Bupleuri
    Radix Puerariae
    Radix Glycyrrhizae
    Radix Scutellariae
    Rhizoma seu Radix Notopterygii
    Radix Angelicae Dahuricae
    Radix Paeoniae
    Radix Platycodi

Bupleurum Soothing the Liver Decoction
Chai Hu Shu Gan Tang
    Pericarpium Citri Reticulatae
    Radix Bupleuri
    Rhizoma Ligustici Chuanxiong
    Rhizoma Cyperi
    Fructus Aurantii
    Radix Paeoniae
    Radix Glycyrrhizae Praeparata

Calm the Palace Pill with Cattle Gallstone
An Gong Niu Hang Wan
    Folium Artemisiae
    Rhizoma Cyperi
    Fructus Evodiae
    Rhizoma Ligustici Chuanxiong
    Radix Paeoniae Alba
    Radix Astragali seu Hedysari
    Radix Dipsaci
    Radix Rehmanniae
    Cortex Cinnamomi
    Radix Angelicae Sinensis

Calm the Stomach with Poria Powder
Wei Ling San
    Polyporus Umbellatus
    Rhizoma Alismatis
    Rhizoma Atractylodis Macrocephalae
    Poria
    Ramulus Cinnamomi
    Rhizoma Atractylodis
    Cortex Magnoliae Officinalis
    Pericarpium Citri Reticulatae
    Radix Glycyrrhizae
    Rhizoma Zingiberis Recens
    Fructus Ziziphi Jujubae

Cattle Gallstone Pill to Clear the Heart
Niu Huang Qing Xin Wan
    Calculus Bovis
    Cinnabaris
    Rhizoma Coptidis
    Radix Scutellariae
    Fructus Gardeniae
    Radix Curcumae

Cephalanoplos Decoction
Xiao Ji Yin Zi
    Radix Rehmanniae
    Herba Cephalanoploris
    Talcum
    Caulis Akebiae
    Pollen Typhae
    Nodus Nelumbinis Rhizomatis
    Herba Lophatheri
    Radix Angelicae Sinensis
    Fructus Gardeniae
    Radix Glycyrrhizae Praeparata

Change Yellow [Discharge] Decoction
Yi Huang Tang
    Rhizoma Dioscoreae
    Semen Euryales
    Cortex Phellodendri
    Semen Plantaginis
    Semen Ginkgo

Chlorite-Schist Pill for Chronic Phlegm Syndromes
Mang Shi Gun Tan Wan
    Radix et Rhizoma Rhei
    Radix Scutellariae
    Chlorite-schist
    Lignum Aquilariae Resinatum

Cimicifuga and Kudzu Decoction
Sheng Ma Ge Gen Tang
    Rhizoma Cimicifugae
    Radix Puerariae
    Radix Paeoniae
    Radix Glycyrrhizae

Cinnabar Pill to Calm the Spirit
Zhu Sha An Shen Wan
    Cinnabaris
    Rhizoma Coptidis
    Radix Glycyrrhizae Praeparata
    Radix Rehmanniae
    Radix Angelicae Sinensis

Cinnamon Twig Decoction
Gui Zhi Tang
    Ramulus Cinnamomi
    Radix Paeoniae
    Rhizoma Zingiberis Recens
    Fructus Ziziphi Jujubae
    Radix Glycyrrhizae

Cinnamon Twig Decoction plus Ginseng
Gui Zhi Jia Ren Shen Tang
    Ramulus Cinnamomi
    Radix Glycyrrhizae Praeparata
    Rhizoma Atractylodis Macrocephalae
    Radix Ginseng
    Rhizoma Zingiberis

Cinnamon Twig Decoction plus Kudzu
Gui Zhi Jia Ge Gen Tang
    Ramulus Cinnamomi
    Radix Paeoniae

Radix Puerariae
Radix Glycyrrhizae
Rhizoma Zingiberis Recens
Fructus Ziziphi Jujubae

Cinnamon Twig Decoction plus Magnolia Bark and Apricot Kernel
Gui Zhi Jia Hou Po Xing Zi Tang
Ramulus Cinnamomi
Radix Paeoniae
Cortex Magnoliae Officinalis
Semen Armeniacae Amarum
Radix Glycyrrhizae
Rhizoma Zingiberis Recens
Fructus Ziziphi Jujubae

Cinnamon Twig Decoction plus Prepared Aconite
Gui Zhi Fu Zi Tang
Ramulus Cinnamomi
Radix Paeoniae
Radix Aconiti Praeparata
Radix Glycyrrhizae
Rhizoma Zingiberis Recens
Fructus Ziziphi Jujubae

Citrus aurantius Eliminating Stagnation Pill
Zhi Shi Dao Zhi Wan
Radix et Rhizoma Rhei
Fructus Aurantii Immaturus
Massa Fermentata Medicinalis
Poria
Radix Scutellariae
Rhizoma Coptidis
Rhizoma Atractylodis Macrocephalae

Clear Epidemics and Overcome Toxin Decoction
Qing Wen Bai Du Yin
Gypsum Fibrosum
Cornu Rhinoceri Asiatici
Rhizoma Coptidis
Fructus Gardeniae
Radix Platycodi
Radix Scutellariae
Rhizoma Anemarrhenae
Radix Paeoniae Rubra
Radix Scrophulariae
Fructus Forsythiae
Radix Glycyrrhizae
Cortex Moutan Radicis
Herba Lophatheri (*fresh*)

Clear Summer Heat and Augment the Qi Decoction
Qing Shu Yi Qi Tang
Radix Panacis Quinquefolii
Herba Dendrobii
Radix Ophiopogonis
Rhizoma Coptidis
Herba Lophatheri
Petiolus Nelumbinis
Rhizoma Anemarrhenae

Radix Glycyrrhizae
Rice (*Geng Mi*)
Watermelon peel

Clear the Nutritive Level Decoction
Qing Ying Tang
Cornu Rhinoceri Asiatici
Radix Rehmanniae
Radix Scrophulariae
Herba Lophatheri
Radix Ophiopogonis
Radix Salviae Miltiorrhizae
Rhizoma Coptidis
Flos Lonicerae
Fructus Forsythiae

Clearing Heat-Resolving Phlegm Pill
Qing Qi Hua Tan Wan
Fructus Trichosanthis
Pericarpium Citri Reticulatae
Radix Scutellariae
Semen Armeniacae Amarum
Fructus Aurantii Immaturus
Poria
Arisaema cum Bile
Rhizoma Pinelliae

Clearing the Stomach Powder
Qing Wei San
Radix Rehmanniae
Radix Angelicae Sinensis
Cortex Moutan Radicis
Rhizoma Coptidis
Rhizoma Cimicifugae

Clove and Persimmon Calyx Decoction
Ding Xiang Shi Di Tang
Flos Caryophylli
Calyx Kaki
Radix Ginseng
Rhizoma Zingiberis Recens

Coix Decoction
Yi Yi Ren Tang
Semen Coicis
Rhizoma Atractylodis
Herba Ephedrae
Ramulus Cinnamomi
Rhizoma seu Radix Notopterygii
Radix Angelicae Pubescentis
Radix Ledebouriellae
Radix Aconiti
Radix Angelicae Sinensis
Rhizoma Ligustici Chuanxiong
Radix Glycyrrhizae
Rhizoma Zingiberis Recens

Coptis Decoction to Relieve Toxicity
Huang Lian Jie Du Tang
Rhizoma Coptidis

Radix Scutellariae
Cortex Phellodendri
Fructus Gardeniae

Cyperus and Perilla Leaf Powder
Xiang Su San
Rhizoma Cyperi
Folium Perillae
Radix Glycyrrhizae Praeparata
Pericarpium Citri Reticulatae

Descurainia and Jujube Decoction to Drain the Lungs
Ting Li Da Zao Xie Fei Tang
Semen Lepidii seu Descurainiae
Fructus Ziziphi Jujubae

Decoction for Relieving Feverish Rash
Hua Ban Tang
Gypsum Fibrosum
Rhizoma Anemarrhenae
Radix Glycyrrhizae
Radix Scrophulariae
Cornu Rhinoceri Asiatici
White rice (*Bai Geng Mi*)

Arrest Seizures Pill
Ding Xian Wan
Rhizoma Gastrodiae
Bulbus Fritillariae Cirrhosae
Rhizoma Pinelliae
Poria
Poria cum Ligno Hospite
Arisaema cum Bile
Rhizoma Acori Graminei
Scorpio
Radix Glycyrrhizae
Bombyx Batryticatus
Succinum
Medulla Junci
Pericarpium Citri Reticulatae
Radix Polygalae
Radix Salviae Miltiorrhizae
Radix Ophiopogonis
Cinnabaris

Dioscoreae Hypoglauca Decoction to Separate the Clear
Bei Xie Fen Qing Yin
Fructus Alpiniae Oxyphyllae
Rhizoma Dioscoreae Hypoglauca
Rhizoma Acori Graminei
Radix Linderae

Drain the Epigastrium Decoction
Xie Xin Tang
Radix et Rhizoma Rhei
Rhizoma Coptidis
Radix Scutellariae

Drive Out Blood Stasis in the Lower Abdomen Decoction
Shao Fu Zhu Yu Tang
Radix Angelicae Sinensis

Rhizoma Ligustici Chuanxiong
Cortex Cinnamomi
Fructus Foeniculi
Rhizoma Zingiberis Praeparata
Pollen Typhae
Faeces Trogopterorum
Radix Paeoniae Rubra
Resina Myrrhae
Rhizoma Corydalis

Eight-Herb Powder for Rectification
Ba Zheng San
Semen Plantaginis
Herba Dianthi
Herba Polygoni Avicularis
Talcum
Fructus Gardeniae
Radix Glycyrrhizae Praeparata
Caulis Akebiae
Radix et Rhizoma Rhei

Eight-Precious Decoction
Ba Zhen Tang
Radix Angelicae Sinensis
Rhizoma Ligustici Chuanxiong
Radix Paeoniae Alba
Radix Rehmanniae Praeparata
Radix Ginseng
Rhizoma Atractylodis Macrocephalae
Poria
Radix Glycyrrhizae Praeparata

Eliminate Wind Powder
Xiao Feng San
Radix Angelicae Sinensis
Radix Rehmanniae
Radix Ledebouriellae
Periostracum Cicadae
Rhizoma Anemarrhenae
Radix Sophorae Flavescentis
Semen Sesami Indici
Herba Schizonepetae
Rhizoma Atractylodis
Fructus Arctii
Gypsum Fibrosum
Radix Glycyrrhizae
Caulis Akebiae

Eliminating Phlegm Decoction
Dao Tan Tang
Rhizoma Pinelliae
Rhizoma Arisaematis
Fructus Aurantii Immaturus
Poria
Exocarpium Citri Grandis
Radix Glycyrrhizae
Rhizoma Zingiberis

Eliminating Redness Powder
Dao Chi San
Radix Rehmanniae

Caulis Akebiae
Radix Glycyrrhizae (*tails*)
Herba Lophatheri

End Discharge Decoction
Wan Dai Tang
Rhizoma Atractylodis Macrocephalae
Rhizoma Dioscoreae
Radix Ginseng
Radix Paeoniae Alba
Semen Plantaginis
Rhizoma Atractylodis
Radix Glycyrrhizae
Pericarpium Citri Reticulatae
Herba Schizonepetae (*charred*)
Radix Bupleuri

Ephedra Decoction
Ma Huang Tang
Herba Ephedrae
Ramulus Cinnamomi
Semen Armeniacae Amarum
Radix Glycyrrhizae

Ephedra, Asarum and Prepared Aconite Decoction
Ma Huang Fu Zi Xi Xin Tang
Herba Ephedrae
Radix Aconiti Praeparata
Herba Asari

Ephedra-Prunus-Gypsum-Glycyrrhiza Decoction
Ma Xing Shi Gan Tang
Herba Ephedrae
Semen Armeniacae Amarum
Radix Glycyrrhizae
Gypsum Fibrosum

Evodia Decoction
Wu Zhu Yu Tang
Fructus Evodiae
Radix Ginseng
Fructus Ziziphi Jujubae
Rhizoma Zingiberis Recens

Expelling Whiteness Powder
Xie Bai San
Cortex Lycii Radicis
Cortex Mori Radicis
Radix Glycyrrhizae

Fetus Longevity Pill
Shou Tai Wan
Radix Dipsaci
Ramulus Loranthi
Colla Corii Asini
Semen Cuscutae

Five-Ingredient Decoction to Eliminate Toxin
Wu Wei Xiao Du Yin
Flos Lonicerae

Flos Chrysanthemi Indici
Herba Taraxaci
Herba Violae
Radix Semiaquilegiae

Five-Ingredient Powder with Poria
Wu Ling San
Polyporus Umbellatus
Rhizoma Alismatis
Rhizoma Atractylodis Macrocephalae
Poria
Ramulus Cinnamomi

Five-Juice Decoction
Wu Zhi Yin
Pear juice
Water chestnut juice
Juice of fresh Rhizoma Phragmitis
Juice of Radix Ophiopogonis
Lotus root juice

Five-Peel Powder
Wu Pi San
Peel of Rhizoma Zingiberis Recens
Cortex Mori Radicis
Pericarpium Citri Reticulatae
Pericarpium Arecae
Poria peel

Four Gentlemen Decoction
Si Jun Zi Tang
Radix Ginseng
Rhizoma Atractylodis Macrocephalae
Poria
Radix Glycyrrhizae

Four-Marvel Powder
Si Miao San
Cortex Phellodendri
Semen Coicis
Rhizoma Atractylodis
Radix Achyranthis Bidentatae

Four-Miracle Pill
Si Shen Wan
Semen Myristicae
Fructus Psoraleae
Fructus Schisandrae
Fructus Evodiae

Four-Preparation Cyperi Pill
Si Zhi Xiang Fu Wan
Rhizoma Cyperi
Rhizoma Ligustici Chuanxiong
Herba Lycopi
Pericarpium Citri Reticulatae
Radix Paeoniae Alba
Rhizoma Atractylodis Macrocephalae
Radix Rehmanniae Praeparata

Cortex Phellodendri
Radix Glycyrrhizae Praeparata

Four Rebellious Decoction
Si Ni Tang
Radix Aconiti Praeparata
Rhizoma Zingiberis
Radix Glycyrrhizae Praeparata

Four Rebellious Decoction with Ginseng
Si Ni Jia Ren Shen Tang
Radix Aconiti Praeparata
Rhizoma Zingiberis
Radix Glycyrrhizae
Radix Ginseng

Four Substance Decoction
Si Wu Tang
Radix Angelicae Sinensis
Rhizoma Ligustici Chuanxiong
Radix Paeoniae Alba
Radix Rehmanniae Praeparata

Four-Valiant Decoction for Well-Being
Si Miao Yong An Tang
Flos Lonicerae
Radix Scrophulariae
Radix Angelicae Sinensis
Radix Glycyrrhizae

Free and Relaxed Powder
Xiao Yao San
Radix Bupleuri
Radix Angelicae Sinensis
Radix Paeoniae Alba
Rhizoma Atractylodis Macrocephalae
Poria
Radix Glycyrrhizae

Free and Relaxed Powder with Moutan and Gardenia
Dan Zhi Xiao Yao San
Cortex Moutan Radicis
Fructus Gardeniae
Radix Bupleuri
Radix Angelicae Sinensis
Radix Paeoniae Alba
Rhizoma Atractylodis Macrocephalae
Poria
Radix Glycyrrhizae
Herba Menthae
Rhizoma Zingiberis Recens

Fritillaria-Trichosanthes Powder
Bei Mu Gua Lou San
Bulbus Fritillariae
Fructus Trichosanthis
Radix Trichosanthis
Poria Exocarpium Citri Grandis
Radix Platycodi

Galangal and Cyperus Pill
Liang Fu Wan
Rhizoma Alpiniae Officinalis
Rhizoma Cyperi

Gardenia and Prepared Soybean Decoction
Zhi Zi Dou Chi Tang
Fructus Gardeniae
Semen Sojae Praeparata

Gardenia-Ligusticum Pill
Yue Ju Wan
Rhizoma Atractylodis
Rhizoma Cyperi
Rhizoma Ligustici Chuanxiong
Massa Fermentata Medicinalis
Fructus Gardeniae

Gastrodia-Uncaria Decoction
Tian Ma Gou Teng Yin
Rhizoma Gastrodiae
Ramulus Uncariae cum Uncis
Concha Haliotidis
Fructus Gardeniae
Radix Scutellariae
Radix Achyranthis Bidentatae
Cortex Eucommiae
Herba Leonuri
Ramulus Loranthi
Caulis Polygoni Multiflori
Poria cum Ligno Hospite (*Cinnabaris coated*)

Generating the Pulse Powder
Sheng Mai San
Radix Ginseng
Radix Ophiopogonis
Fructus Schisandrae

Generation and Transformation Decoction
Sheng Hua Tang
Radix Angelicae Sinensis
Rhizoma Ligustici Chuanxiong
Semen Persicae
Rhizoma Zingiberis
Radix Glycyrrhizae

Gentian Draining the Liver Decoction
Long Dan Xie Gan Tang
Radix Gentianae
Radix Scutellariae
Fructus Gardeniae
Rhizoma Alismatis
Caulis Akebiae
Semen Plantaginis
Radix Angelicae Sinensis
Radix Rehmanniae
Radix Bupleuri
Radix Glycyrrhizae

Ginseng and Gecko Powder
Ren Shen Ge Jie San
Gecko
Semen Armeniacae Amarum
Radix Glycyrrhizae
Radix Ginseng
Poria
Bulbus Fritillariae
Cortex Mori Radicis
Rhizoma Anemarrhenae

Ginseng and Walnut Decoction
Ren Shen Hu Tao Tang
Radix Ginseng
Semen Juglandis

Ginseng Decoction to Nourish the Nutritive Qi
Ren Shen Yang Rong Tang
Radix Paeoniae Alba
Radix Angelicae Sinensis
Pericarpium Citri Reticulatae
Radix Astragali seu Hedysari
Cortex Cinnamomi
Radix Ginseng
Rhizoma Atractylodis Macrocephalae
Radix Glycyrrhizae Praeparata
Radix Rehmanniae Praeparata
Fructus Schisandrae
Poria
Radix Polygalae

Ginseng Powder to Overcome Pathogenic Influences
Ren Shen Bai Du San
Radix Bupleuri
Radix Peucedani
Rhizoma Ligustici Chuanxiong
Fructus Aurantii
Rhizoma seu Radix Notopterygii
Radix Angelicae Pubescentis
Poria
Radix Platycodi
Radix Ginseng
Radix Glycyrrhizae

Glehnia-Ophiopogon Decoction
Sha Shen Mai Dong Tang
Radix Adenophorae
Rhizoma Polygonati Odorati
Radix Glycyrrhizae
Folium Mori
Semen Dolichoris
Radix Trichosanthis
Radix Ophiopogonis

Glycyrrhiza Decoction
Zhi Gan Cao Tang
Radix Glycyrrhizae Praeparata
Radix Ginseng
Ramulus Cinnamomi
Rhizoma Zingiberis Recens

Colla Corii Asini
Radix Rehmanniae
Radix Ophiopogonis
Semen Sesami
Fructus Ziziphi Jujubae

Great Tonify the Source Decoction
Da Bu Yuan Jian
Fructus Corni
Radix Glycyrrhizae Praeparata
Rhizoma Dioscoreae
Cortex Eucommiae
Radix Angelicae Sinensis
Fructus Lycii
Radix Ginseng
Radix Rehmanniae Praeparata

Great Tonify the Yin Pill
Da Bu Yin Wan
Cortex Phellodendri
Rhizoma Anemarrhenae
Radix Rehmanniae Praeparata
Plastrum Testudinis

Great Tranquillity Pill
Da An Wan
Fructus Crataegi
Massa Fermentata Medicinalis
Rhizoma Pinelliae
Poria
Pericarpium Citri Reticulatae
Fructus Forsythiae
Semen Raphani
Rhizoma Atractylodis Macrocephalae

Greatest Treasure Special Pill
Zhi Bao Dan
Cornu Rhinoceri Asiatici
Cinnabaris
Realgar
Carapax Eretmochaelydis
Succinum
Moschus
Borneolum Syntheticum
Gold leaf (*Jin Bo*)
Silver leaf (*Yin Bo*)
Calculus Bovis
Benzoinum

Half-Decoction of Ephedra and Cinnamon Twig
Ma Huang Gui Zhi Ge Ban Tang
Equal amounts of **Ephedra Decoction** and **Cinnamon Twig Decoction**

Heavenly Emperor Tonifying the Heart Pill
Tian Wan Bu Xin Dan
Radix Rehmanniae
Radix Ginseng
Radix Salviae Miltiorrhizae
Radix Scrophulariae

Poria
Fructus Schisandrae
Radix Polygalae
Radix Platycodi
Radix Angelicae Sinensis
Radix Asparagi
Radix Ophiopogonis
Semen Biotae
Semen Ziziphi Spinosae

Hemp Seed Pill
Ma Zi Ren Wan
Fructus Cannabis
Radix Paeoniae
Fructus Aurantii Immaturus
Radix et Rhizoma Rhei
Cortex Magnoliae Officinalis
Semen Armeniacae Amarum

Hidden Tiger Pill
Hu Qian Wan
Radix Rehmanniae Praeparata
Radix Paeoniae Alba
Plastrum Testudinis
Rhizoma Anemarrhenae
Cortex Phellodendri
Herba Cynomorii
Tiger bone (*Hu Gu*)
Rhizoma Zingiberis
Pericarpium Citri Reticulatae

Honeysuckle and Forsythia Powder
Yin Qiao San
Fructus Forsythiae
Flos Lonicerae
Radix Platycodi
Herba Menthae
Herba Lophatheri
Radix Glycyrrhizae
Herba Schizonepetae
Semen Sojae Praeparata
Fructus Arctii

Immature Bitter Orange Pill to Reduce Focal Distension
Zhi Shi Xiao Pi Wan
Radix et Rhizoma Rhei
Fructus Aurantii Immaturus
Massa Fermentata Medicinalis
Poria
Radix Scutellariae
Rhizoma Coptidis
Rhizoma Atractylodis Macrocephalae

Important Formula for Painful Diarrhoea
Tong Xie Yao Fang
Rhizoma Atractylodis Macrocephalae
Radix Paeoniae Alba
Pericarpium Citri Reticulatae
Radix Ledebouriellae

Increase the Fluids and Order the Qi Decoction
Zeng Ye Cheng Qi Tang
Radix Scrophulariae
Radix Ophiopogonis
Radix Rehmanniae
Radix et Rhizoma Rhei
Natrii Sulfas

Indigo Naturalis-Concha Meretricis Powder
Dai Ge San
Indigo Naturalis
Concha Meretricis seu Cyclinae

Invigorate the Kidney Pill
Ji Sheng Shen Qi Wan
Radix Rehmanniae Praeparata
Rhizoma Dioscoreae
Fructus Corni
Rhizoma Alismatis
Poria
Cortex Moutan Radicis
Cortex Cinnamomi
Radix Aconiti Praeparata
Radix Achyranthis Bidentatae
Semen Plantaginis

Jade Wind-Screen Powder
Yu Ping Feng San
Radix Ledebouriellae
Radix Astragali seu Hedysari
Rhizoma Atractylodis Macrocephalae

Jade Woman Decoction
Yu Nu Jian
Gypsum Fibrosum
Radix Rehmanniae Praeparata
Radix Ophiopogonis
Rhizoma Anemarrhenae
Radix Achyranthis Bidentatae

Kidney Qi Pill
Shen Qi Wan
Radix Rehmanniae Praeparata
Rhizoma Dioscoreae
Fructus Corni
Rhizoma Alismatis
Poria
Cortex Moutan Radicis
Ramulus Cinnamomi
Radix Aconiti Praeparata

Kudzu, Coptis and Scutellaria Decoction
Ge Gen Qin Lian Tang
Radix Puerariae
Radix Glycyrrhizae
Radix Scutellariae
Rhizoma Coptidis

Lead to Symmetry Powder
Qian Zheng San
Rhizoma Typhonii
Bombyx Batryticatus
Scorpio

Left Metal Pill
Zuo Jin Wan
Rhizoma Coptidis
Fructus Evodiae

Ligusticum-Green Tea Regulating Powder
Chuan Xiong Cha Tiao San
Rhizoma Ligustici Chuanxiong
Herba Schizonepetae
Radix Angelicae Dahuricae
Rhizoma seu Radix Notopterygii
Radix Glycyrrhizae
Herba Asari
Radix Ledebouriellae
Herba Menthae

Licorice, Wheat and Jujube Decoction
Gan Mai Da Zao Tang
Radix Glycyrrhizae
Wheat
Fructus Ziziphi Jujubae

Lift the Source decoction
Ju Yuan Jian
Radix Ginseng
Radix Astragali seu Hedysari
Radix Glycyrrhizae Praeparata
Rhizoma Cimicifugae
Rhizoma Atractylodis Macrocephalae

Lily Bulb Decoction to Preserve the Metal
Bai He Gu Jin Tang
Radix Rehmanniae
Radix Rehmanniae Praeparata
Radix Ophiopogonis
Bulbus Lilii
Radix Paeoniae Alba
Radix Angelicae Sinensis
Bulbus Fritillariae
Radix Glycyrrhizae Praeparata
Radix Scrophulariae
Radix Platycodi

Linking Decoction
Yi Guan Jian
Radix Glehniae
Radix Ophiopogonis
Radix Angelicae Sinensis
Radix Rehmanniae
Fructus Lycii
Fructus Meliae Toosendan

Lophatheri-Tamarix-Arctii Decoction
Zhu Ye Liu Bang Tang
Cacumen Tamaricis

Herba Schizonepetae
Radix Puerariae
Periostracum Cicadae
Herba Menthae
Fructus Arctii
Rhizoma Anemarrhenae
Radix Scrophulariae
Radix Glycyrrhizae
Radix Ophiopogonis
Herba Lophatheri

Lophatherus and Gypsum Decoction
Zhu Ye Shi Gao Tang
Herba Lophatheri
Gypsum Fibrosum
Rhizoma Pinelliae
Radix Ophiopogonis
Radix Ginseng
Radix Glycyrrhizae
Rice (Geng Mi)

Lycium Fruit, Chrysanthemum and Rehmannia Pill
Qi Ju Di Huang Wan
Radix Rehmanniae Praeparata
Fructus Corni
Rhizoma Dioscoreae
Rhizoma Alismatis
Poria
Cortex Moutan Radicis
Fructus Lycii
Flos Chrysanthemi

Magnetite and Cinnabar Pill
Ci Zhu Wan
Magnetitum
Cinnabaris
Massa Fermentata Medicinalis

Magnolia Bark Decoction for Warming the Middle
Hou Po Weng Zhong Tang
Cortex Magnoliae Officinalis
Pericarpium Citri Reticulatae
Radix Glycyrrhizae Praeparata
Poria
Semen Alpiniae Katsumadai
Radix Aucklandiae
Rhizoma Zingiberis

Major Arrest Wind Pearl
Da Ding Feng Zhu
Radix Paeoniae Alba
Colla Corii Asini
Plastrum Testudinis
Radix Rehmanniae
Fructus Cannabis
Fructus Schisandrae
Concha Ostreae
Radix Ophiopogonis
Radix Glycyrrhizae Praeparata

Egg yolk
Carapax Trionycis

Major Blue-Green Dragon Decoction
Da Qing Long Tang
Herba Ephedrae
Ramulus Cinnamomi
Radix Glycyrrhizae Praeparata
Semen Armeniacae Amarum
Gypsum Fibrosum
Rhizoma Zingiberis Recens
Fructus Ziziphi Jujubae

Major Order the Qi Decoction
Da Cheng Qi Tang
Radix et Rhizoma Rhei
Cortex Magnoliae Officinalis
Fructus Aurantii Immaturus
Natrii Sulfas

Major Sinking into the Chest Decoction
Da Xian Xiong Tang
Radix et Rhizoma Rhei
Natrii Sulfas
Radix Euphorbiae Kansui

Major Strengthening the Middle Decoction
Da Jian Zhong Tang
Pericarpium Zanthoxyli
Rhizoma Zingiberis
Radix Ginseng

Mantis Egg-Case Powder
Sang Piao Xiao San
Ootheca Mantidis
Radix Polygalae
Rhizoma Acori Graminei
Os Draconis
Radix Ginseng
Poria cum Ligno Hospite
Radix Angelicae Sinensis
Plastrum Testudinis

Melia Toosendan Powder
Jin Ling Zi San
Fructus Meliae Toosendan
Rhizoma Corydalis

Metal Lock Pill to Stabilize the Essence
Jin Suo Gu Jing Wan
Semen Astragali Complanati
Semen Euryales
Stamen Nelumbinis
Os Draconis
Concha Ostreae

Minor Invigorate the Collaterals Special Pill
Xiao Huo Luo Dan
Radix Aconiti
Radix Aconiti Kusnezoffii

Lumbricus
Rhizoma Arisaematis
Resina Olibani
Resina Myrrhae

Minor Order the Qi Decoction
Xiao Cheng Qi Tang
Radix et Rhizoma Rhei
Cortex Magnoliae Officinalis
Fructus Aurantii Immaturus

Minor Strengthening the Middle Decoction
Xiao Jian Zhong Tang
Radix Paeoniae
Ramulus Cinnamomi
Radix Glycyrrhizae Praeparata
Rhizoma Zingiberis Recens
Fructus Ziziphi Jujubae
Saccharum Granorum

Modified Polygonatum Odoratum Decoction
Jia Jian Wei Rui Tang
Rhizoma Polygonati Odorati
Bulbus Allii Fistulosi
Radix Platycodi
Radix Cynanchi Atrati
Semen Sojae Praeparata
Herba Menthae
Radix Glycyrrhizae Praeparata
Fructus Ziziphi Jujubae

Moisten the Intestines Pill
Run Chang Wan
Radix et Rhizoma Rhei
Radix Angelicae Sinensis (*thin ends*)
Rhizoma seu Radix Notopterygii
Semen Persicae
Fructus Cannabis

Mulberry Leaf and Apricot Kernel Decoction
Sang Xing Tang
Folium Mori
Semen Armeniacae Amarum
Radix Adenophorae
Bulbus Fritillariae Thunbergii
Semen Sojae Praeparata
Fructus Gardeniae
Pear peel

Mulberry Leaf and Chrysanthemum Decoction
Sang Ju Yin
Folium Mori
Flos Chrysanthemi
Semen Armeniacae Amarum
Fructus Forsythiae
Herba Menthae
Radix Platycodi
Radix Glycyrrhizae
Rhizoma Phragmitis

Nine-Herb Decoction with Notopterygium

Jiu Wei Qiang Huo Tang
Rhizoma seu Radix Notopterygii
Radix Ledebouriellae
Rhizoma Atractylodis
Herba Asari
Rhizoma Ligustici Chuanxiong
Radix Angelicae Dahuricae
Radix Rehmanniae
Radix Scutellariae
Radix Glycyrrhizae

Notopterygium Dispelling Dampness Decoction

Qiang Huo Sheng Shi Tang
Rhizoma seu Radix Notopterygii
Radix Angelicae Pubescentis
Rhizoma Ligustici
Radix Ledebouriellae
Radix Glycyrrhizae Praeparata
Rhizoma Ligustici Chuanxiong
Fructus Viticis

Nourish the Yin and Clear the Lungs Decoction

Yang Yin Qing Fei Tang
Radix Rehmanniae
Radix Ophiopogonis
Radix Glycyrrhizae
Radix Scrophulariae
Bulbus Fritillariae
Cortex Moutan Radicis
Herba Menthae
Radix Paeoniae Alba

Oyster Shell Powder

Mu Li San
Radix Astragali seu Hedysari
Radix Ephedrae
Concha Ostreae

Pacifying the Liver and Subduing Wind Decoction

Zhen Gan Xi Feng Tang
Radix Achyranthis Bidentatae
Haematitum
Os Draconis
Concha Ostreae
Plastrum Testudinis
Radix Paeoniae
Radix Scrophulariae
Radix Asparagi
Fructus Meliae Toosendan
Fructus Hordei Germinatus
Herba Artemisiae Scopariae
Radix Glycyrrhizae

Panax-Aconitum Decoction

Shen Fu Tang
Radix Ginseng
Radix Aconiti Praeparata

Panax-Aconitum Decoction with Long Gu and Mu Li

Shen Fu Long Mu Tang
Radix Ginseng
Radix Aconiti Praeparata
Os Draconis
Concha Ostreae (*calcined*)

Panax-Poria-Atractylodis Powder

Shen Ling Bai Zhu San
Semen Nelumbinis
Semen Coicis
Fructus Amomi
Radix Platycodi
Semen Dolichoris Album
Poria
Radix Ginseng
Radix Glycyrrhizae
Rhizoma Atractylodis Macrocephalae
Rhizoma Dioscoreae

Peach Pit Decoction to Order the Qi

Tao Ren Cheng Qi Tang
Semen Persicae
Radix et Rhizoma Rhei
Ramulus Cinnamomi
Radix Glycyrrhizae
Natrii Sulfas

Peony Decoction

Shao Yao Tang
Radix Paeoniae
Radix Angelicae Sinensis
Rhizoma Coptidis
Semen Arecae
Radix Aucklandiae
Radix Glycyrrhizae
Radix et Rhizoma Rhei
Radix Scutellariae
Cortex Cinnamomi

Perilla Seed Lowering Qi Decoction

Su Zi Jiang Qi Tang
Fructus Perillae
Rhizoma Pinelliae
Radix Angelicae Sinensis
Radix Glycyrrhizae
Radix Peucedani
Cortex Magnoliae Officinalis
Cortex Cinnamomi

Pill Requiring a Change of Clothes

Geng Yi Wan
Cinnabaris
Aloe

Pinellia and Magnolia Bark Decoction

Ban Xia Hou Po Tang
Rhizoma Pinelliae
Cortex Magnoliae Officinalis

Poria
Rhizoma Zingiberis Recens
Folium Perillae

Pinelliae-Atractylodis-Gastrodia Decoction
Ban Xia Bai Zhu Tian Ma Tang
Rhizoma Pinelliae
Rhizoma Gastrodiae
Poria
Exocarpium Citri Grandis
Rhizoma Atractylodis Macrocephalae
Radix Glycyrrhizae

Polyporus Decoction
Zhu Ling Tang
Polyporus Umbellatus
Poria
Rhizoma Alismatis
Colla Corii Asini
Talcum

Poria-Glycyrrhiza-Schisandra-Zingiber-Asarum Decoction
Ling Gan Wu Wei Jiang Xin Tang
Poria
Radix Glycyrrhizae
Rhizoma Zingiberis
Herba Asari
Fructus Schisandrae

Poria-Ramulus Cinnamomi-Atractylodis-Glycyrrhiza Decoction
Ling Gui Zhu Gan Tang
Poria
Ramulus Cinnamomi
Rhizoma Atractylodis Macrocephalae
Radix Glycyrrhizae Praeparata

Powder to Take at Cock's Crow
Ji Ming San
Semen Arecae
Pericarpium Citri Reticulatae
Fructus Chaenomelis
Fructus Evodiae
Folium Perillae
Radix Platycodi
Rhizoma Zingiberis Recens

Prepared Aconite Pill to Regulate the Middle
Fu Zi Li Zhong Wan
Radix Ginseng
Rhizoma Atractylodis Macrocephalae
Rhizoma Zingiberis
Radix Glycyrrhizae
Radix Aconiti Praeparata

Prescription to Treat Diabetes
Xiao Ke Fang
Rhizoma Coptidis
Radix Trichosanthis
Juice of Radix Rehmanniae

Juice of Lotus Root
Radix Asparagi
Radix Ophiopogonis
Radix Scutellariae

Preserving and Harmonizing Pill
Bao He Wan
Fructus Crataegi
Massa Fermentata Medicinalis
Rhizoma Pinelliae
Poria
Pericarpium Citri Reticulatae
Fructus Forsythiae
Semen Raphani

Protect the Yin Decoction
Bao Yin Jian
Radix Rehmanniae
Radix Rehmanniae Praeparata
Radix Paeoniae Alba
Rhizoma Dioscoreae
Radix Dipsaci
Radix Scutellariae
Cortex Phellodendri
Radix Glycyrrhizae

Purple Snow Special Pill
Zi Xue Dan
Gypsum Fibrosum
Calcitum (*Han Shui Shi*)
Talcum
Magnetitum
Cornu Rhinoceri Asiatici
Cornu Antelopis
Radix Aristolochiae
Lignum Aquilariae Resinatum
Radix Scrophulariae
Rhizoma Cimicifugae
Radix Glycyrrhizae
Flos Caryophylli
Natrii Sulfas
Nitrum
Moschus
Cinnabaris
Gold (Huang Jin)

Rectify the Qi Powder Worth More Than Gold
Bu Huan Jin Zheng Qi San
Cortex Magnoliae Officinalis
Herba Agastachis
Radix Glycyrrhizae
Rhizoma Pinelliae
Rhizoma Atractylodis
Pericarpium Citri Reticulatae
Rhizoma Zingiberis Recens
Fructus Ziziphi Jujubae

Reed Decoction
Wei Jing Tang
Rhizoma Phragmitis

Semen Coicis
Semen Benincasae
Semen Persicae

Regulate the Stomach and Order the Qi Decoction
Tiao Wei Cheng Qi Tang
Radix et Rhizoma Rhei
Radix Glycyrrhizae Praeparata
Natrii Sulfas

Regulating the Middle Pill
Li Zhong Wan
Radix Ginseng
Rhizoma Zingiberis
Radix Glycyrrhizae
Rhizoma Atractylodis Macrocephalae

Rehmannia Decoction
Di Huang Yin Zi
Radix Rehmanniae Praeparata
Radix Morindae Officinalis
Fructus Corni
Herba Dendrobii
Herba Cistanchis
Radix Aconiti Praeparata
Fructus Schisandrae
Cortex Cinnamomi
Poria
Radix Ophiopogonis
Rhizoma Acori Graminei
Radix Polygalae

Renewal Powder
Zai Zao San
Radix Astragali seu Hedysari
Radix Ginseng
Ramulus Cinnamomi
Radix Glycyrrhizae
Radix Aconiti Praeparata
Herba Asari
Rhizoma seu Radix Notopterygii
Radix Ledebouriellae
Rhizoma Ligustici Chuanxiong
Rhizoma Zingiberis Recens (roasted)

Restore Collapsed Yang Decoction
Hui Yang Jiu Ji Tang
Radix Aconiti Praeparata
Rhizoma Zingiberis
Cortex Cinnamomi
Radix Ginseng
Rhizoma Atractylodis Macrocephalae
Poria
Pericarpium Citri Reticulatae
Radix Glycyrrhizae
Fructus Schisandrae
Rhizoma Pinelliae

Restoring the Left Decoction
Zuo Gui Yin
Radix Rehmanniae Praeparata

Rhizoma Dioscoreae
Fructus Lycii
Radix Glycyrrhizae Praeparata
Poria
Fructus Corni

Restoring the Left Pill
Zuo Gui Wan
Radix Rehmanniae Praeparata
Rhizoma Dioscoreae
Fructus Lycii
Fructus Corni
Radix Achyranthis Bidentatae
Semen Cuscutae
Colla Cornus Cervi
Plastrum Testudinis

Restoring the Right Pill
You Gui Wan
Radix Rehmanniae Praeparata
Rhizoma Dioscoreae
Fructus Corni
Fructus Lycii
Semen Cuscutae
Cortex Eucommiae
Radix Angelicae Sinensis
Cortex Cinnamomi
Radix Aconiti Praeparata

Revised Major Order the Qi Decoction
Fu Fang Cheng Qi Tang
Cortex Magnoliae Officinalis
Semen Raphani
Fructus Aurantii Immaturus
Semen Persicae
Radix Paeoniae Rubra
Radix et Rhizoma Rhei
Natrii Sulfas

Revive Health by Invigorating the Blood Decoction
Fu Yuan Huo Xue Tang
Radix Bupleuri
Radix Trichosanthis
Radix Angelicae Sinensis
Flos Carthami
Radix Glycyrrhizae
Squama Manitis
Radix et Rhizoma Rhei
Semen Persicae

Rhinoceros Horn and Rehmannia Decoction
Xi Jiao Di Huang Tang
Cornu Rhinoceri
Radix Rehmanniae
Radix Paeoniae

Rhubarb and Moutan Decoction
Da Huang Mu Dan Tang
Radix et Rhizoma Rhei
Cortex Moutan Radicis

Semen Persicae
Semen Benincasae
Natrii Sulfas

Rhubarb and Prepared Aconite Decoction
Da Huang Fu Zi Tang
Radix et Rhizoma Rhei
Radix Aconiti Praeparata
Herba Asari

Sargentodoxa Decoction
Hong Teng Jian
Caulis Sargentodoxae
Herba Violae
Resina Olibani
Resina Myrrhae
Radix et Rhizoma Rhei
Fructus Forsythiae
Rhizoma Corydalis
Cortex Moutan Radicis
Flos Lonicerae
Radix Glycyrrhizae

Schizonepeta and Ledebouriella Powder to Overcome Pathogenic Influences
Jing Fang Bai Du San
Rhizoma seu Radix Notopterygii
Radix Angelicae Pubescentis
Radix Bupleuri
Radix Peucedani
Fructus Aurantii
Poria .
Herba Schizonepetae
Radix Ledebouriellae
Radix Platycodi
Rhizoma Ligustici Chuanxiong
Radix Glycyrrhizae

Six-Flavour Rehmannia Pill
Liu Wei Di Huang Wan
Radix Rehmanniae Praeparata
Fructus Corni
Rhizoma Dioscoreae
Rhizoma Alismatis
Poria
Cortex Moutan Radicis

Six-Flavour Rehmannia Pill with Anemarrhena and Phellodendron
Zhi Bai Di Huang Wan
Radix Rehmanniae Praeparata
Fructus Corni
Rhizoma Dioscoreae
Rhizoma Alismatis
Poria
Cortex Moutan Radicis
Rhizoma Anemarrhenae
Cortex Phellodendri

Six Gentlemen Decoction
Liu Jun Zi Tang
Radix Ginseng
Rhizoma Atractylodis Macrocephalae
Poria
Radix Glycyrrhizae
Pericarpium Citri Reticulatae
Rhizoma Pinelliae

Six Gentlemen Decoction with Aucklandia and Amomum
Xiang Sha Liu Jun Zi Tang
Radix Ginseng
Rhizoma Atractylodis Macrocephalae
Poria
Radix Glycyrrhizae
Pericarpium Citri Reticulatae
Rhizoma Pinelliae
Rhizoma Cyperi
Fructus Amomi

Six-to-One Powder
Liu Yi San
Talcum
Radix Glycyrrhizae

Small Bupleurum Decoction
Xiao Chai Hu Tang
Radix Bupleuri
Radix Scutellariae
Radix Ginseng
Rhizoma Pinelliae
Radix Glycyrrhizae Praeparata
Rhizoma Zingiberis Recens
Fructus Ziziphi Jujubae

Small Green Dragon Decoction
Xiao Qing Long Tang
Herba Ephedrae
Radix Paeoniae
Herba Asari
Rhizoma Zingiberis
Radix Glycyrrhizae
Ramulus Cinnamomi
Rhizoma Pinelliae
Fructus Schisandrae

Small Sinking Chest Decoction
Xiao Xian Xiong Tang
Rhizoma Coptidis
Rhizoma Pinelliae
Fructus Trichosanthis

Spring Onion and Prepared Soybean Decoction
Cong Chi Tang
Bulbus Allii Fistulosi
Semen Sojae Praeparata

Spring Onion and Prepared Soybean Decoction with Platycodon
Cong Chi Jie Geng Tang
 Bulbus Allii Fistulosi
 Semen Sojae Praeparata
 Radix Platycodi
 Fructus Gardeniae
 Herba Menthae
 Herba Lophatheri
 Radix Glycyrrhizae

Spring Onion Decoction with Seven Ingredients
Cong Bai Qi Wei Yin
 Bulbus Allii Fistulosi
 Radix Puerariae
 Semen Sojae Praeparata
 Rhizoma Zingiberis Recens
 Radix Ophiopogonis
 Radix Rehmanniae

Sour Jujube Decoction
Suan Zao Ren Tang
 Semen Ziziphi Spinosae
 Radix Glycyrrhizae
 Rhizoma Anemarrhenae
 Poria
 Rhizoma Ligustici Chuanxiong

Stabilize Gushing Decoction
Gu Chong Tang
 Rhizoma Atractylodis Macrocephalae
 Radix Astragali seu Hedysari
 Os Draconis
 Concha Ostreae
 Fructus Corni
 Radix Paeoniae Alba
 Os Sepiellae seu Sepiae
 Radix Rubiae
 Cortex Trachycarpi (*charred*)
 Fructus Schisandrae

Stabilize the Menses Pill
Gu Jing Wan
 Cortex Ailanthi
 Plastrum Testudinis
 Radix Scutellariae
 Cortex Phellodendri
 Radix Paeoniae Alba
 Rhizoma Cyperi

Sophora Japonica Flower Powder
Huai Hua San
 Flos Sophorae
 Cacumen Biotae
 Herba Schizonepetae
 Fructus Aurantii

Special Pill to Promote Lactation
Tong Ru Dan
 Radix Codonopsis Pilosulae

 Radix Astragali seu Hedysari
 Radix Angelicae Sinensis
 Radix Ophiopogonis
 Medulla Tetrapanacis
 Radix Platycodi
 Leg of pork (*Zhu Ti*)

Stephania and Astragalus Decoction
Fang Ji Huang Qi Tang
 Radix Stephaniae Tetrandrae
 Radix Astragali seu Hedysari
 Radix Glycyrrhizae
 Rhizoma Atractylodis Macrocephalae

Strengthen the Spleen Pill
Jian Pi Wan
 Rhizoma Atractylodis Macrocephalae
 Radix Aucklandiae
 Rhizoma Coptidis
 Radix Glycyrrhizae
 Poria
 Radix Ginseng
 Massa Fermentata Medicinalis
 Pericarpium Citri Reticulatae
 Fructus Amomi
 Fructus Hordei Germinatus
 Fructus Crataegi
 Rhizoma Dioscoreae
 Semen Myristicae

Strengthening the Spleen Powder
Shi Pi San
 Cortex Magnoliae Officinalis
 Rhizoma Atractylodis Macrocephalae
 Fructus Chaenomelis
 Radix Aucklandiae
 Fructus Tsaoko
 Semen Arecae
 Radix Aconiti Praeparata
 Poria
 Rhizoma Zingiberis
 Radix Glycyrrhizae

Styrax Pill
Su He Xiang Wan
 Rhizoma Atractylodis Macrocephalae
 Radix Aristolochiae
 Cornu Rhinoceri Asiatici
 Rhizoma Cyperi
 Cinnabaris
 Fructus Chebulae
 Lignum Santalum
 Benzoinum
 Lignum Aquilariae Resinatum
 Moschus
 Flos Caryophylli
 Fructus Piperis Longi
 Borneolum Syntheticum
 Styrax Liquidus
 Resina Olibani

Sublime Formula for Sustaining Life
Xian Fang Huo Ming Yin
Radix Angelicae Dahuricae
Bulbus Fritillariae
Radix Ledebouriellae
Radix Paeoniae Rubra
Radix Angelicae Sinensis (*extension*)
Radix Glycyrrhizae
Spina Gleditsiae
Squama Manitis
Radix Trichosanthis
Resina Olibani
Resina Myrrhae
Flos Lonicerae
Pericarpium Citri Reticulatae

Sudden Smile Powder
Shi Xiao San
Faeces Trogopterorum
Pollen Typhae

Sweet Dew Special Pill to Eliminate Toxin
Gan Lu Xiao Du Dan
Talcum
Herba Artemisiae Scopariae
Radix Scutellariae
Rhizoma Acori Graminei
Bulbus Fritillariae Cirrhosae
Caulis Akebiae
Herba Agastachis
Rhizoma Belamcandae
Fructus Forsythiae
Herba Menthae
Semen Amomi Cardamomi

Tangerine Peel and Bamboo Shaving Decoction
Ju Pi Zhu Ru Tang
Pericarpium Citri Reticulatae
Caulis Bambusae in Taeniam
Fructus Ziziphi Jujubae
Rhizoma Zingiberis Recens
Radix Glycyrrhizae
Radix Ginseng

Ten-Jujube Decoction
Shi Zao Tang
Flos Genkwa
Radix Euphorbiae Kansui
Radix Euphorbiae Pekinensis

Ten Partially-charred Substance Powder
Shi Hui San
Herba seu Radix Cirsii Japonici
Herba Cephalanoploris
Folium Nelumbinis
Cacumen Biotae
Rhizoma Imperatae
Radix Rubiae
Fructus Gardeniae
Radix et Rhizoma Rhei

Cortex Moutan Radicis
Cortex Trachycarpi

Three-Nut Decoction
San Ren Tang
Semen Armeniacae Amarum
Talcum
Medulla Tetrapancis
Semen Amomi Cardamomi
Herba Lophatheri
Cortex Magnoliae Officinalis
Semen Coicis
Rhizoma Pinelliae

Three-Seed Nourishing Parents Decoction
San Zi Yang Qin Tang
Semen Sinapis Albae
Fructus Perillae
Semen Raphani

Three-Substance Pill for Emergencies
San Wu Bei Ji Wan
Radix et Rhizoma Rhei
Rhizoma Zingiberis
Fructus Crotonis

Tonify the Yang to Restore Five-Tenths Decoction
Bu Yang Huan Wu Tang
Radix Astragali seu Hedysari
Radix Angelicae Sinensis
Radix Paeoniae Rubra
Lumbricus
Rhizoma Ligustici Chuanxiong
Flos Carthami
Semen Persicae

Tonifying the Lung Decoction with Ass-Hide Gelatin
Bu Fei E Jiao Tang
Colla Corii Asini
Fructus Arctii
Radix Glycyrrhizae Praeparata
Fructus Aristolochiae
Semen Armeniacae Amarum
Glutinous rice (*Nuo Mi*)

Tonifying the Middle and Benefiting Qi Decoction
Bu Zhong Yi Qi Tang
Radix Astragali seu Hedysari
Radix Glycyrrhizae Praeparata
Radix Ginseng
Radix Angelicae Sinensis
Pericarpium Citri Reticulatae
Rhizoma Cimicifugae
Radix Bupleuri
Rhizoma Atractylodis Macrocephalae

Tonifying the Spleen Decoction
Gui Pi Tang
Rhizoma Atractylodis Macrocephalae
Poria cum Ligno Hospite

Radix Astragali seu Hedysari
Arillus Longan
Semen Ziziphi Spinosae
Radix Ginseng
Radix Aucklandiae
Radix Glycyrrhizae Praeparata
Radix Angelicae Sinensis
Radix Polygalae

Top-Quality Lindera Powder
Tian Tai Wu Yao San
Radix Linderae
Radix Aucklandiae
Fructus Foeniculi
Pericarpium Citri Reticulatae Viride
Rhizoma Alpiniae Officinalis
Semen Arecae
Fructus Meliae Toosendan
Fructus Crotonis

Trichosanthes-Allium-Pinellia Decoction
Gua Lou Xie Bai Ban Xia Tang
Fructus Trichosanthis
Bulbus Allii Macrostemi
Rhizoma Pinelliae
Wine

True Man's Decoction to Nourish the Organs
Zhen Ren Yang Zang Tang
Radix Ginseng
Radix Angelicae Sinensis
Rhizoma Atractylodis Macrocephalae
Semen Myristicae
Cortex Cinnamomi
Radix Glycyrrhizae Praeparata
Radix Paeoniae Alba
Radix Aucklandiae
Fructus Chebulae
Pericarpium Papaveris

True Warrior Decoction
Zhen Wu Tang
Poria
Radix Paeoniae
Rhizoma Atractylodis Macrocephalae
Rhizoma Zingiberis Recens
Radix Aconiti Praeparata

Turtle Shell Pill
Bie Jia Jian Wan
Carapax Trionycis
Rhizoma Belamcandae
Radix Scutellariae
Armadillidium vulgare (*Shu Fu*)
Rhizoma Zingiberis
Radix et Rhizoma Rhei
Ramulus Cinnamomi
Folium Pyrrosiae
Cortex Magnoliae Officinalis
Herba Dianthi

Flos Campsis Grandiflorae (*Zi Wei*)
Colla Corii Asini
Radix Bupleuri
Dung Beetle (*Qiang Lang*)
Radix Paeoniae
Cortex Moutan Radicis
Eupolyphaga seu Steleophaga
Honeycomb (*Feng Cao*)
Nitrum
Semen Persicae
Radix Ginseng
Rhizoma Pinelliae
Semen Lepidii seu Descurainiae

Two-Old Decoction
Er Chen Tang
Rhizoma Pinelliae
Exocarpium Citri Grandis
Poria
Radix Glycyrrhizae Praeparata

Universal Benefit Decoction to Eliminate Toxin
Pu Ji Xiao Du Yin
Radix Scutellariae
Rhizoma Coptidis
Pericarpium Citri Reticulatae
Radix Glycyrrhizae
Radix Scrophulariae
Radix Bupleuri
Radix Platycodi
Fructus Forsythiae
Radix Isatidis
Lasiosphaera seu Calvatia
Fructus Arctii
Herba Menthae
Bombyx Batryticatus
Rhizoma Cimicifugae

Warm the Liver Decoction
Nuan Gan Jian
Radix Angelicae Sinensis
Fructus Lycii
Fructus Foeniculi
Cortex Cinnamomi
Radix Linderae
Lignum Aquilariae Resinatum
Poria

Warm the Menses Decoction
Wen Jing Tang
Fructus Evodiae
Radix Angelicae Sinensis
Radix Paeoniae
Rhizoma Ligustici Chuanxiong
Radix Ginseng
Ramulus Cinnamomi
Colla Corii Asini
Cortex Moutan Radicis
Rhizoma Zingiberis Recens
Radix Glycyrrhizae

Rhizoma Pinelliae
Radix Ophiopogonis

Warm the Spleen Decoction
Wen Pi Tang
Radix et Rhizoma Rhei
Radix Aconiti Praeparata
Rhizoma Zingiberis
Radix Ginseng
Radix Glycyrrhizae

Warming the Gall Bladder Decoction
Wen Dan Tang
Rhizoma Pinelliae
Caulis Bambusae in Taeniam
Fructus Aurantii Immaturus
Pericarpium Citri Reticulatae
Radix Glycyrrhizae
Poria

Water and Earth Immortals Special Pill
Shui Lu Er Xian Dan
Semen Euryales
Fructus Rosae Laevigatae

White Tiger Decoction
Bai Hu Tang
Gypsum Fibrosum
Rhizoma Anemarrhenae
Radix Glycyrrhizae Praeparata
Rice (*Geng Mi*)

White Tiger Decoction for Ordering the Qi
Bai Hu Cheng Qi Tang
Gypsum Fibrosum
Radix et Rhizoma Rhei (*raw*)
Radix Glycyrrhizae
Rhizoma Anemarrhenae
Natrii Sulfas Exsiccatus
Old rice (*Chen Cang Mi*)

White Tiger Decoction with Atractylodis
Bai Hu Jia Cang Zhu Tang
Rhizoma Anemarrhenae
Radix Glycyrrhizae Praeparata
Gypsum Fibrosum
Rhizoma Atractylodis
Rice (*Geng Mi*)

White Tiger plus Ginseng Decoction
Bai Hu Jia Ren Shen Tang
Rhizoma Anemarrhenae
Gypsum Fibrosum
Radix Glycyrrhizae Praeparata
Rice (*Geng Mi*)
Radix Ginseng

White Tiger Decoction with Antelopis and Gastrodia
Ling Ma Bai Hu Tang
Cornu Antelopis

Rhizoma Gastrodiae
Gypsum Fibrosum
Rhizoma Anemarrhenae
Radix Glycyrrhizae
Rice (*Geng Mi*)

White Tiger Ramulus Cinnamomi Decoction
Bai Hu Jia Gui Zhi Tang
Rhizoma Anemarrhenae
Radix Glycyrrhizae Praeparata
Gypsum Fibrosum
Rice (*Geng Mi*)
Ramulus Cinnamomi

Yellow Dragon Decoction
Huang Long Tang
Radix et Rhizoma Rhei
Natrii Sulfas
Fructus Aurantii Immaturus
Cortex Magnoliae Officinalis
Radix Glycyrrhizae
Radix Ginseng
Radix Angelicae Sinensis

Yellow Earth Decoction
Huang Tu Tang
Radix Glycyrrhizae
Radix Rehmanniae
Rhizoma Atractylodis Macrocephalae
Radix Aconiti Praeparata
Colla Corii Asini
Radix Scutellariae
Terra Flava Usta

Yong Quan Powder to Promote Lactation
Xia Ru Yong Quan San
Radix Angelicae Sinensis
Radix Paeoniae Alba
Radix Rehmanniae
Rhizoma Ligustici Chuanxiong
Radix Bupleuri
Pericarpium Citri Reticulatae Viride
Radix Trichosanthis
Squama Manitis
Radix Angelicae Dahuricae
Semen Vaccariae
Radix Platycodi
Caulis Akebiae
Medulla Tetrapanacis
Radix Rhapontici seu Echinopsis
Radix Glycyrrhizae

Index

Printed and bound by CPI Group (UK) Ltd, Croydon, CR0 4YY

03/10/2024

01040366-0017